WITHDRAWN

HISTOPATHOLOGY OF DISEASE

HISTOPATHOLOGY OF DISEASE

JAY H. LEFKOWITCH, M.D.

Professor of Clinical Pathology
Department of Pathology
Columbia University College of Physicians and Surgeons
New York, New York

Illustrated by the Author

Foreword by
Peter J. Scheuer, M.D., DSc (Med), FRC Path

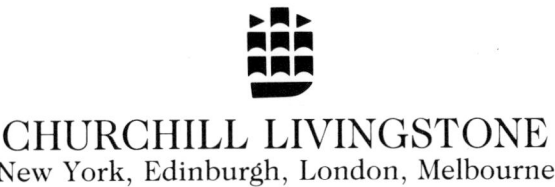

CHURCHILL LIVINGSTONE
New York, Edinburgh, London, Melbourne

Library of Congress Cataloging in Publication Data

Lefkowitch, Jay H.
  Histopathology of disease / Jay H. Lefkowitch ; illustrated by the author ; foreword by Peter J. Scheuer.
    p.   cm.
  Includes index.
  ISBN 0-443-08566-8
  1. Histology, Pathological—Atlases.   I. Title.
  [DNLM: 1. Histology.   2. Pathology.   QZ 4 L493h]
RB33.L44   1989
611'.018—dc19
DNLM/DLC   88-20417
for Library of Congress   CIP

© Churchill Livingstone Inc. 1989

All rights reserved. No part of this publication may be reproduced, stored in a retrieval system, or transmitted in any form or by any means, electronic, mechanical, photocopying, recording, or otherwise, without prior permission of the publisher (Churchill Livingstone Inc., 1560 Broadway, New York, NY 10036).

Distributed in the United Kingdom by Churchill Livingstone, Robert Stevenson House, 1–3 Baxter's Place, Leith Walk, Edinburgh EH1 3AF, and by associated companies, branches, and representatives throughout the world.

Accurate indications, adverse reactions, and dosage schedules for drugs are provided in this book, but it is possible that they may change. The reader is urged to review the package information data of the manufacturers of the medications mentioned.

The Publishers have made every effort to trace the copyright holders for borrowed material. If they have inadvertently overlooked any, they will be pleased to make the necessary arrangements at the first opportunity.

Acquisitions Editor: *Robert A. Hurley*
Copy Editor: *Kamely Dahir*
Book Designer: *Gloria Brown*

Printed and bound in Hong Kong

First published in 1989

To Donald West King, M.D.
for his support and vision.

FOREWORD

Today's medical student needs a sound knowledge of pathology as much as his or her predecessor. The rapid and accelerating developments of modern medicine have accentuated rather than reduced this need. Without a clear understanding of the structural changes that underlie clinical symptoms and signs, much of the student's experience becomes empirical and superficial. Disease processes cannot be understood without consideration of their structural and cellular basis and their correlation with physiological and biochemical data.

This essential understanding of structural change can be acquired in different ways. Practical work at the microscope helps to train the eye to observe accurately, and it is retained in many modern curricula. A book such as Dr. Jay Lefkowitch's lavishly illustrated text ensures that the observations made are correctly correlated and integrated into a comprehensible mental picture of disease. The student and trainee pathologist need guidance to obtain the full benefit of viewing tissue sections, and a good annotated atlas is one way in which this guidance can be provided.

Good photomicrography requires several skills. Telling examples of lesions must be selected and shown in tissue sections of high quality. These must then be photographed competently. Choice of microscope field and magnification is important and requires both knowledge of pathology and aesthetic judgement. Dr. Lefkowitch has fulfilled these criteria in the production of a fine book that is greatly enhanced by a historic perspective and carefully prepared diagrams that help the reader to understand the clinical relevance of the structural changes illustrated.

An important function of a good text is to attract, motivate, and stimulate the reader. It is rare indeed to find a pathologist who is not fascinated by pathology, with its extensive span of all organs, tissues, and systems; its endless variety and complexity; and its relevance to patient care. *Histopathology of Disease* will surely help to transmit the pathologist's enthusiasm to others.

Peter J. Scheuer, M.D., D.Sc. (Med), FRC Path
Professor of Histopathology
Royal Free Hospital School of Medicine
University of London, England

PREFACE

I first contemplated writing this book several years ago after many of our medical students requested a reference source for assistance in pathology microscopic laboratories. Such a project posed a number of problems—deciding which histopathologic images in basic and systemic pathology comprise fundamental knowledge, providing clear and representative illustrations with concise descriptions, and making the book an attractive "friend" for use at the microscope and, hopefully, for future review. Thousands of photomicrographs later, I sadly realized that a microscopic slide, like life, is imperfect, and that no single microscopic field can convey the entire histopathologic picture of a disease process. Nevertheless, the book progressed to its current form, imperfections and all.

Those of us who teach pathology hope to endow our students and residents with enthusiasm and excitement for the field, and for the spirit of inquisitiveness that should rightly inform all who practice medicine. Microscopy continues to be a linchpin for clinical medicine and laboratory research a century after the ascendancy of Rudolph Virchow. Yet, the medical curriculum has become alarmingly dense and students face growing time constraints in acquiring their microscopic skills in the midst of explosive growth in other medical disciplines. I am hopeful that this book will ease the way over some of these hurdles.

The text is organized into major sections on pathobiology and organ system pathology, with additional chapters on cytopathology and infectious agents. I have included a somewhat selective pictorial history of pathology and medicine as a reminder of the remarkable achievements that have preceded us. Magnifications for the photomicrographs have been omitted for the sake of clarity. The stains used throughout are, except where noted, hematoxylin and eosin or hematoxylin, phloxine, and saffron. The "overview" diagrams for each organ system should be useful as introduction and for later review.

This book is for medical students, residents in postgraduate training programs in pathology, and others whose work or interest entails an understanding of fundamental histopathology. Schleiden wrote that "to see is a difficult art." I hope the reader will find this practical guide helpful in meeting that challenge.

Jay H. Lefkowitch, M.D.

ACKNOWLEDGMENTS

Production of any major work involves concessions from colleagues, family, and friends, and I am grateful for the consideration shown to me from everyone during the months of preparation of this book. I must especially thank Professor Peter J. Scheuer for his unfailing generosity and encouragement; Dr. Margaret Grimes, who put up with me in her office taking photomicrographs all these many months; and Mr. Ulises Martin, our expert departmental photographer, who taught me most of what I know about taking pictures. Mrs. Mildred Shemesh provided continuous sustenance through listening and advice, and Lourdes Waters assisted me in manuscript preparation. Mr. Alfred Lamme was instrumental in getting my photographic slides to me on time. Our excellent resident staff was of enormous help in alerting me to important specimens and was most accommodating. This was also true of many other colleagues in the divisions of medical and surgical pathology. In developing the chapter on the history of pathology and medicine, I was reminded that Dr. John J. Fenoglio, Jr. first interested me in this area while I was a medical student at Columbia. Aurelia Chattock, of our cytology division, was very kind in providing me access to the cytopathology specimens depicted in Chapter 3. Unquestionably, I could not have taken the photomicrographs without help from Liwayway Mallavo, Jean Beidl, and Susan Cassaro, who had the onerous job of pulling slides. Carole Miller, Barbara Fegeley, and Lee Stecher gave me their years of practical experience with our diagnostic files in assisting me to find the pathologic lesions I needed. The administrative staff of the National Library of Medicine was most cooperative in finding the prints for Chapter 1.

My family, of course, has been very special in giving ongoing support. In particular, I must thank my sisters who, by this time, are experts in the study of my workaholism. Mr. Robert Hurley and the production staff at Churchill Livingstone have, from the first glimmer of this textbook, provided it a warm and enthusiastic environment in which it could flourish.

I must thank the following individuals who directly provided me with kodachromes and photographs used in this book:

Dr. Vivette D'Agati and Dr. Conrad Pirani, Department of Pathology, Columbia University College of Physicians and Surgeons, New York, New York (Figs. 8.3, 8.5, 8.6, 8.7, 8.9, 8.10, 8.11, 8.12, 8.13, 8.14, 8.15, 8.16, and 8.19)

Dr. Florabel Mullick, Department of Drug and Environmental Pathology, The Armed Forces Institute of Pathology, Washington, DC (Fig. 5.19).

Dr. Zachary Goodman and Dr. Kamal Ishak, Department of Hepatic Pathology, The Armed Forces Institute of Pathology, Washington, DC (Fig. 4.12).

Dr. Arthur Hays, Department of Pathology, Columbia University College of Physicians and Surgeons, New York, New York (Fig. 16.28).

Dr. Maria Paoletti, Department of Pathology, The University of Chicago Pritzker School of Medicine, Chicago, Illinois (Fig. 7.25).

Dr. A. Sùbietas, Department of Pathology, City Hospital Center at Elmhurst, Elmhurst, New York (Figs. 4.16 and 4.17).

Dr. David Silvers, Department of Dermatopathology, Columbia University College of Physicians and Surgeons, New York, New York, for access to his teaching file.

Dr. Jerome Cantor, Department of Pathology, St. Luke's–Roosevelt Hospital Center, New York, New York (autoradiography for Fig. 10.60).

UPI/Bettmann Newsphotos (Fig. 1.17).

Dr. Cesar Milstein (Fig. 1.18).

Ms. Sylvia Ford, Division of Clinical Hematology, Presbyterian Hospital, New York, New York, for access to the hematology teaching collection.

The National Library of Medicine, Washington, DC (Figs. 1.1 through 1.16).

The sources for organ weights used in this text were the following:

Ludwig J: Current Methods of Autopsy Practice. 2nd. Ed. WB Saunders, Philadelphia, 1979

Robbins SL, Cotran RS, Kumar V: Pathologic Basis of Disease. 3rd Ed. WB Saunders, Philadelphia, 1984

CONTENTS

1	History of Pathology	1
2	Principles of Pathobiology	7
3	Cell Ultrastructure and Cytopathology	23
4	Infectious Agents	29
5	Cardiovascular Pathology	39
6	Pulmonary Pathology	49
7	Hematopathology	65
8	Renal and Lower Urinary Tract Pathology	87
9	Gastrointestinal Pathology	103
10	Liver Pathology	121
11	Gallbladder and Pancreas Pathology	145
12	Reproductive Organ Pathology	151
13	Endocrine Pathology	173
14	Bone and Soft Tissue Pathology	185
15	Dermatopathology	199
16	Neuropathology	211
	Index	223

CHAPTER 1

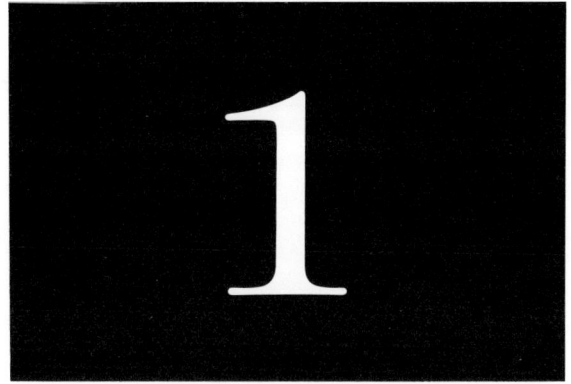

HISTORY OF PATHOLOGY

The history of the medical sciences is a noble one, brimming with landmark developments and colorful personal triumphs of individuals responsible for them. Within the broad scope of medical history, pathology (the study of disease, both its causes and effects) has left a major legacy, threading its way through discoveries in medicine, often inseparable from them. The following pictorial history traces the beginnings of pathology, from antiquity and the "humoral pathology," to the "cellular pathology" of Virchow and developments in our own century. It is an "overview" and, as such, is rather selective and cannot be considered all-inclusive. One hopes that the reader's appetite will be whetted for additional study.

ANTIQUITY

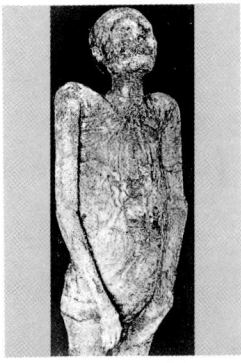

Figure 1.1
Egyptian mummy (3000–1000 BC)

Plate II, Figure 1 of Mummy from Mémoires présentés à L'Institut Égyptien et publiés sous les auspices de S.A. Abbas II by G.E. Smith, 1906. The field of paleopathology utilizes the relics of antiquity, such as mummies, to determine pathologic conditions that existed in earlier times. The Edwin Smith papyrus of 1600 BC chronicles numerous pathologic lesions, including fractures, wound infections, and tumors.

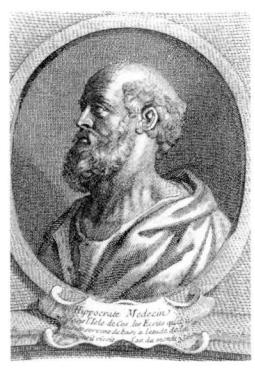

Figure 1.2
Hippocrates (460–375 BC)

The school of Greek thought in this period (humoral pathology) was based on attribution of diseases to disorders of body fluids and humors (blood from the heart, phlegm from the brain, bile from the liver, black bile from the spleen, etc.).

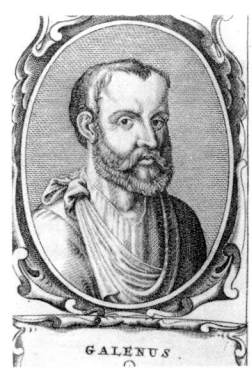

Figure 1.3
Galen (130–200 AD)

Drawing on Alexandrian and Hippocratic principles of humoral pathology, Galen's physiological and humoral theories were based on the principles of the natural spirit *(pneuma)* and its mode of "presentation" and "adhesion" to various internal anatomic sites. His observations were based on limited knowledge of animal dissections and external examinations of human lesions. Galen's influence lasted for some 1500 years, into the Middle Ages.

THE RISE OF THE RENAISSANCE AND MORBID ANATOMY

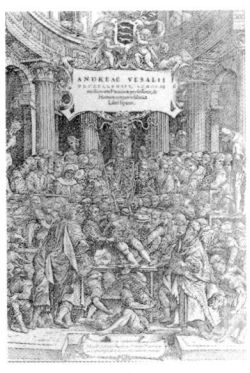

Figure 1.4
Andreas Vesalius title page (c.1543)

The dissections of Vesalius and Leonardo da Vinci (1452–1519) invested their illustrations with truth and challenged the doctrines of Galen. In this period, Antonio Benivenii (1440–1502), the "father of pathological anatomy," performed 20 postmortem examinations to specifically determine the cause of death and explain symptoms.

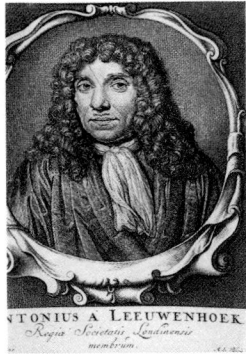

Figure 1.5
Anton Von Leeuwenhoek (1632–1723)

The Dutch lens grinder built several hundred simple microscopes that were variants of magnifying lenses. He is credited with the first descriptions and/or illustrations of spermatozoa, striations in the muscle fibers composing voluntary muscle, and, in 1683, bacteria.

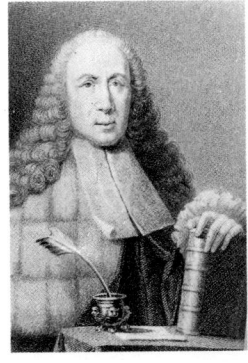

Figure 1.6
Giovanni Battista Morgagni (1682–1771)

The anatomy professor from Padua authored the seminal volume *De sedibus, et causis morborum per anatomem indagatis (The Seats and Causes of Disease)* in 1761, in which the relations between postmortem data and disease symptoms and manifestations during life were described in extreme detail. Masterly expositions on the circulation (aneurysms, endocarditis, cardiac rupture) and lobar pneumonia are among his contributions.

History of Pathology

PATHOLOGY OF TISSUES AND CELLS

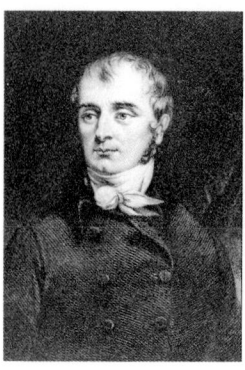

Figure 1.7
Marie-François-Xavier Bichat (1771–1802)

Along with Morgagni and Virchow, Bichat is considered one of the founders of modern pathology. Despite his brief life (cut short by tuberculosis), he provided the landmark concept that organs are composed of *tissues*. He was the first to posit the major classification of pathology into conditions common to all organ systems (general pathology) and those specific to individual organs (organ system pathology).

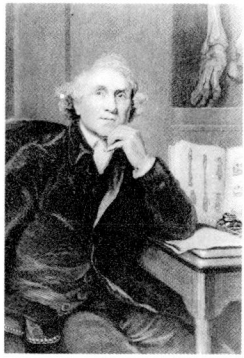

Figure 1.8
John Hunter (1728–1793)

English anatomist and surgeon who pursued a zealous penchant for collecting anatomic specimens and developed a large teaching museum (later endowed to the Royal College of Surgeons). The expansive museum was highly influential in the teaching of morbid anatomy in his time.

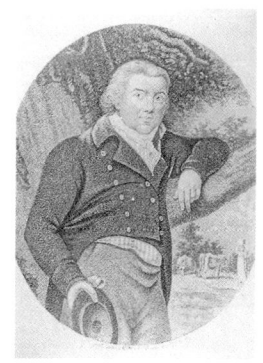

Figure 1.9
Edward Jenner (1749–1823)

A country doctor and pupil of John Hunter, Jenner's contribution to immunology was the use of cow-pox vaccination to prevent smallpox.

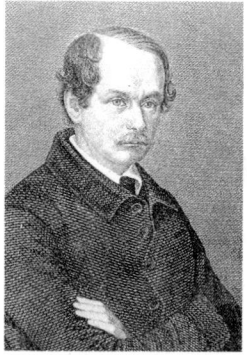

Figure 1.10
Mathias Jakob Schleiden (1804–1881)

Credited (along with Schwann) with establishing the "cell theory," Schleiden as botanist described nuclei and nucleoli in plants in his *"Contributions to Phytogenesis."*

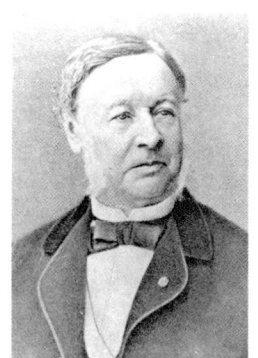

Figure 1.11
Theodor Schwann (1810–1882)

The zoologist's principle that complex tissues were composed of cells was, even more so than Schleiden's work, critical to the "cell theory." He described cellular modifications during development as well as secretory substances which subserved specific functions in tissues.

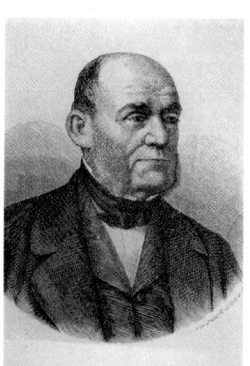

Figure 1.12
Carl Rokitansky (1804–1878)

The Viennese pathologist refined an en bloc technique for postmortem dissection and, largely through gross observations of 30,000 autopsies he personally performed (and 60,000 to which he had access), brought descriptive gross pathology to its height.

CELLULAR AND EXPERIMENTAL PATHOLOGY

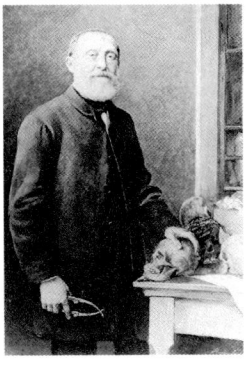

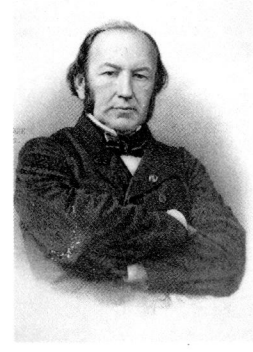

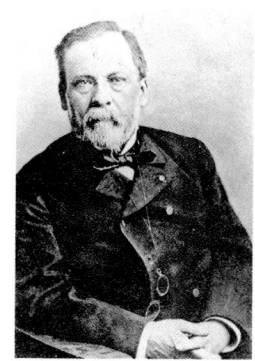

Figure 1.13
Rudolph Virchow (1821–1902)

Considered the greatest of all pathologists, Virchow's work consisted of autopsies combined with microscopic studies by which he developed the renowned *Cellularpathologie*. This concept, that basic changes in disease are related to abnormalities in cells, is still the root of modern pathophysiology.

Figure 1.14
Claude Bernard (1813–1878)

The French physiologist founded the field of experimental medicine. His greatest work was the discovery of glycogen in liver tissue and its metabolism.

Figure 1.15
Louis Pasteur (1822–1895)

Training in chemistry informed the French scientist's studies of fermentation and, later, infectious diseases. A pioneer in the field of bacteriology, Pasteur recorded the specificity of microbial infections for certain diseases and developed immunizations for anthrax, chicken cholera, and rabies.

NEW TECHNIQUES

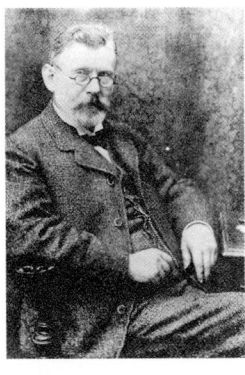

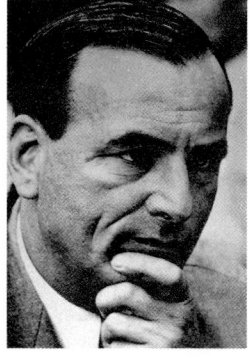

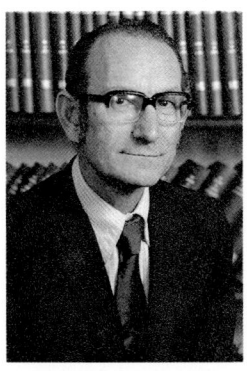

Figure 1.16
Paul Ehrlich (1854–1915)

Nobel Prize winner in 1908 for his work on chemotherapy (then referring to synthetic agents used in treatment of microbial diseases), particularly the arsenical Salvarsan, which revolutionized therapy for syphilis. His "side-chain theory" described binding of chemical substances to receptors on cells and set the groundwork for studies of toxins and antitoxins.

Figure 1.17
Ernst Ruska (1907–1988)

1986 Nobel Prize winner in Physics for his invention of the electron microscope in 1931, by which electrons are focussed through a magnetic coil to provide images of the internal structures of cells.

Figure 1.18
Cesar Milstein (1927–   )

British molecular biologist awarded the 1984 Nobel Prize in Physiology or Medicine for his work on monoclonal antibodies and hybridomas. The development of high-specificity antibodies has dramatically augmented the field of immunopathology and tissue localization of antigens, and has afforded promising inroads in cancer chemotherapy.

History of Pathology

CHAPTER 2

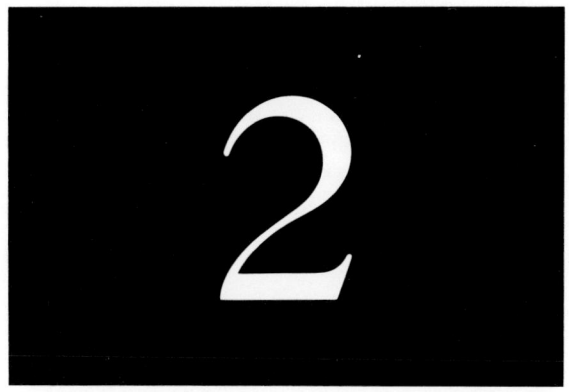

PRINCIPLES OF PATHOBIOLOGY

The tissue responses to cellular injury consist of inflammation, repair, and neoplasia. The inflammatory cells involved in these processes and histologic changes of acute inflammation, granulation tissue repair, chronic inflammation, granulomas, abscesses and scar, and thrombosis are shown in the following pages. The major morphologic forms of neoplasia (tumors), both benign and malignant, are also illustrated.

INFLAMMATORY CELLS

Figure 2.1
Neutrophilic leukocytes

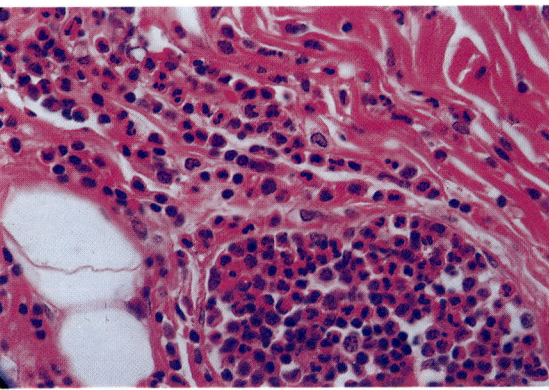

Cytologic features include multilobated nucleus and cytoplasmic lysosomal granules.

Figure 2.2
Eosinophils

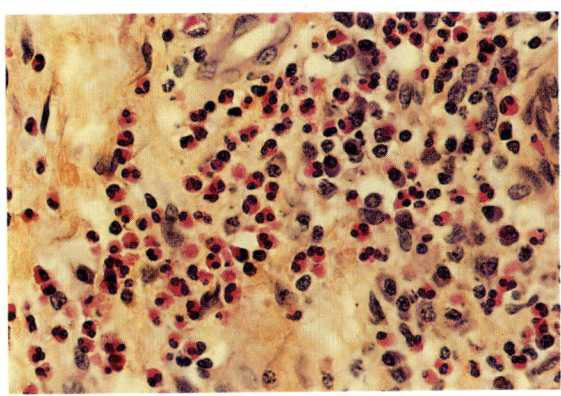

Cytologic features include bilobed nucleus and eosinophilic cytoplasmic granules.

Figure 2.3
Mast cells

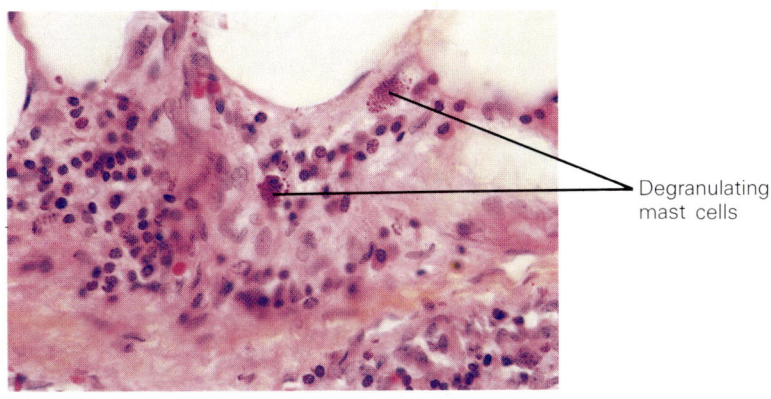

Degranulating mast cells

Cytologic features include ovoid nuclei and ample cytoplasm with granules.

Figure 2.4
Lymphocytes

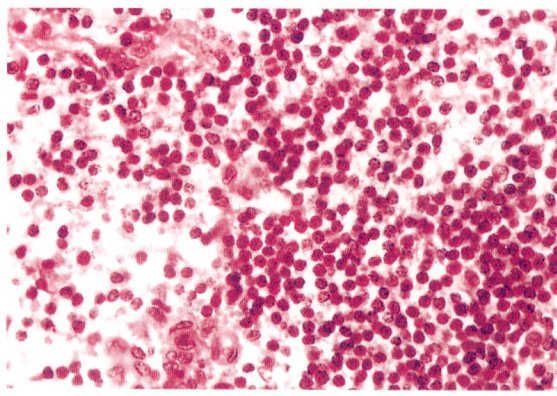

Cytologic features include small, round, dark nuclei and scant cytoplasm.

Figure 2.5
Plasma cells

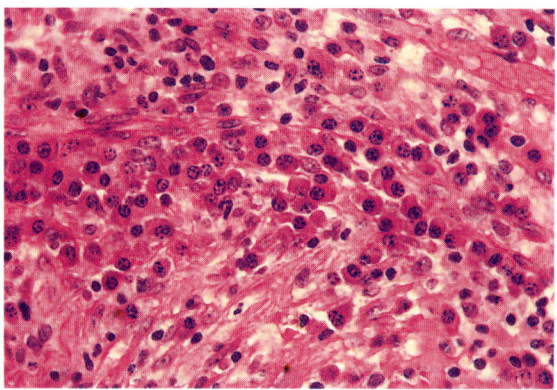

Cytologic features include a cartwheel or clockface nucleus and ample pink cytoplasm with perinuclear clear zone (Golgi apparatus).

Figure 2.6
Macrophages (histiocytes)

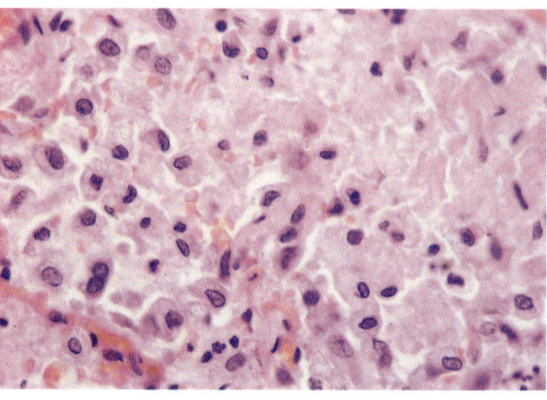

Cytologic features include an ovoid, vesicular nucleus and ample pink cytoplasm.

Figure 2.7
Giant cell

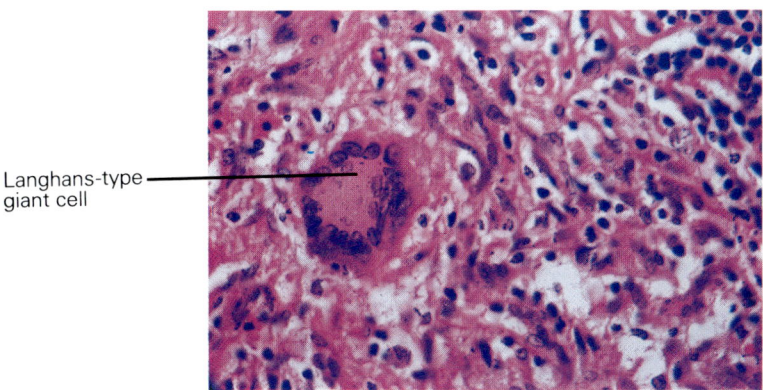

Giant cells result from fusion of macrophages. The Langhans' giant cell has its multiple nuclei arranged in a peripheral rim and is seen in tuberculosis. Foreign body giant cells have haphazard, often centrally arranged nuclei.

Figure 2.8
Pavementing and emigration of neutrophils

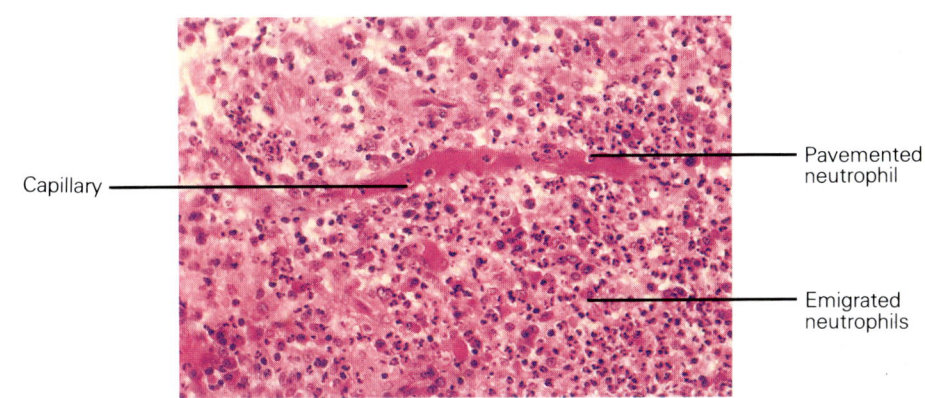

In acute inflammation, adherence of neutrophils to the capillary endothelium (pavementing) is followed by their emigration into the extravascular space.

Figure 2.9
Cellular necrosis

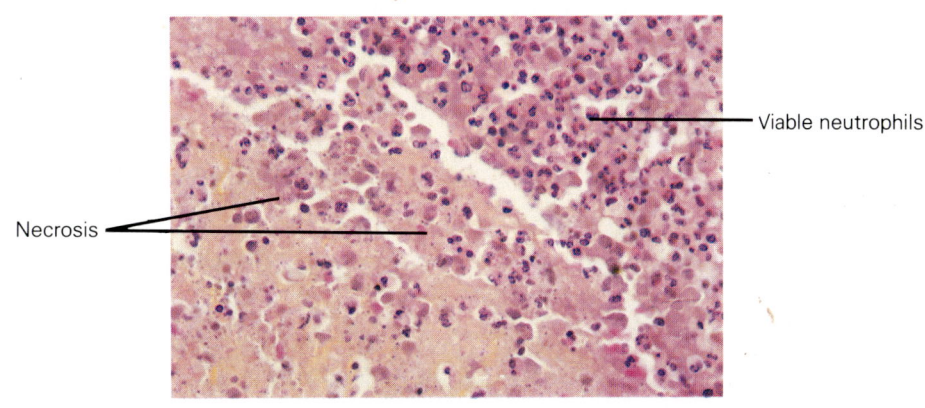

All forms of cellular necrosis result in breakdown of the cell (its nucleus and its cytoplasm) to fragmented acidophilic debris with interspersed basophilic nuclear dust.

Figure 2.10
Nuclear pyknosis and karyorrhexis

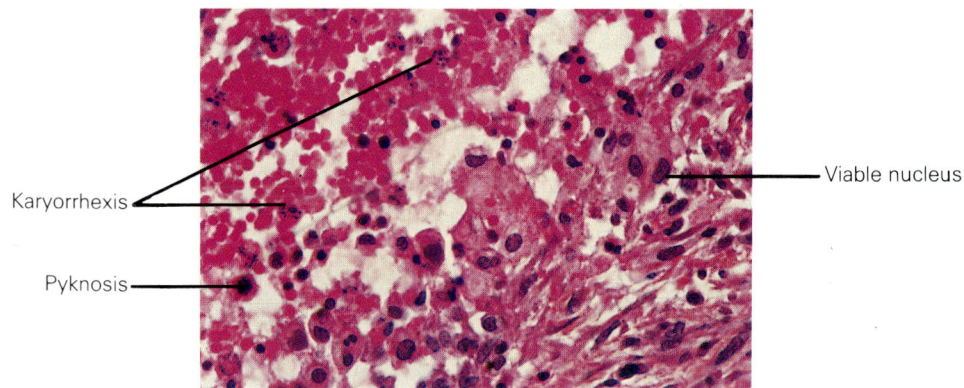

The nuclear changes after cell death include shrinkage with condensation of chromatin (pyknosis), nuclear fragmentation (karyorrhexis), and lysis (karyolysis).

Figure 2.11
Granulation tissue

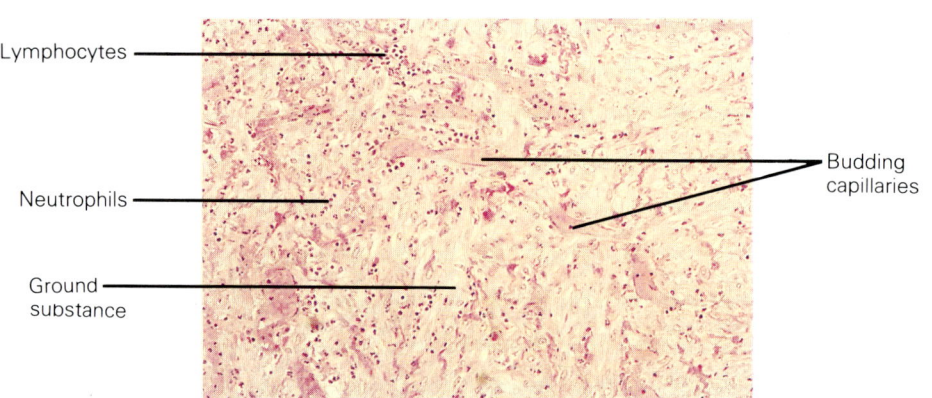

Wounds with extensive loss of tissue substance heal by deposition of granulation tissue, which consists of budding capillaries, mixed inflammatory cells, and new matrix ground substance.

COMPLICATIONS OF INFLAMMATION

Figure 2.12
Granuloma (noncaseating)

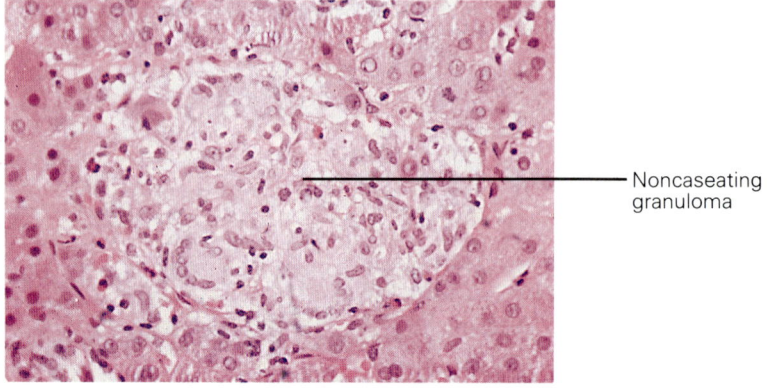

Granulomas are collections of mature, apposed macrophages. The noncaseating variety shown above (in the liver) is seen in numerous disorders, particularly in sarcoidosis.

Figure 2.13
Granuloma (caseating)

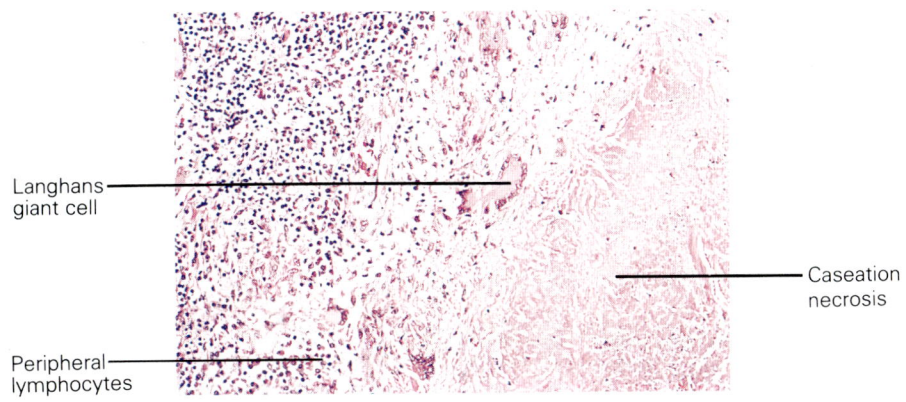

Necrosis at the center of granulomas (cheeselike or caseation necrosis) is a feature of tuberculous granulomas.

Figure 2.14
Abscess

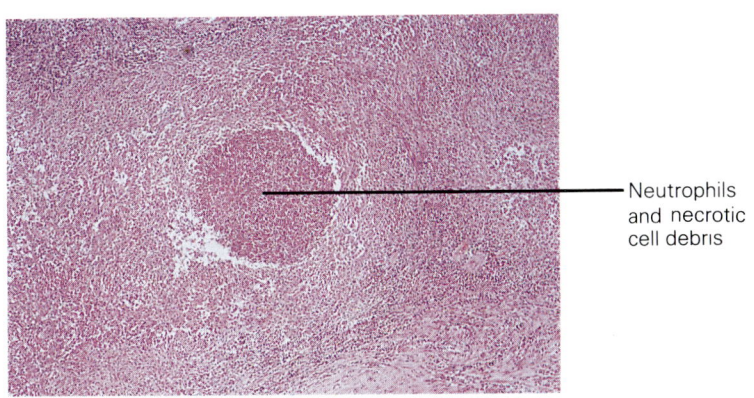

Abscesses are localized collections of purulent exudate and necrotic cells with or without a fibrous tissue capsule.

Figure 2.15
Scar tissue (myocardial infarction)

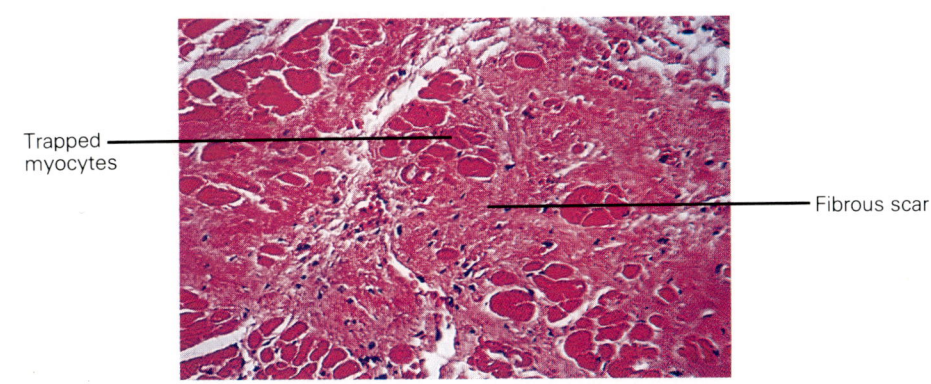

Death of postmitotic cardiac myocytes results in their replacement by fibrous scar tissue.

Figure 2.16
Vascular thrombosis

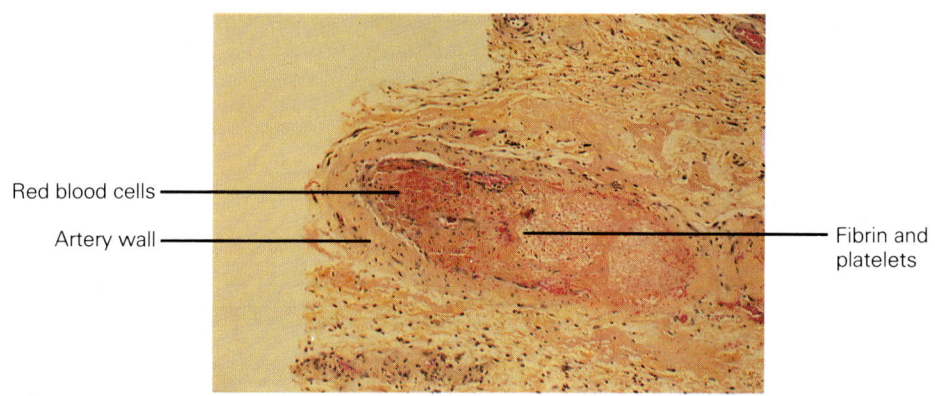

A thrombus consisting of red blood cells, fibrin, and platelets fills the lumen of an artery. The passage of a thrombus from an initiating to a distal site, sometimes associated with infarction of the distal tissue, is known as thromboembolism (see Figure 6.7).

Figure 2.17
Thrombus: lines of Zahn

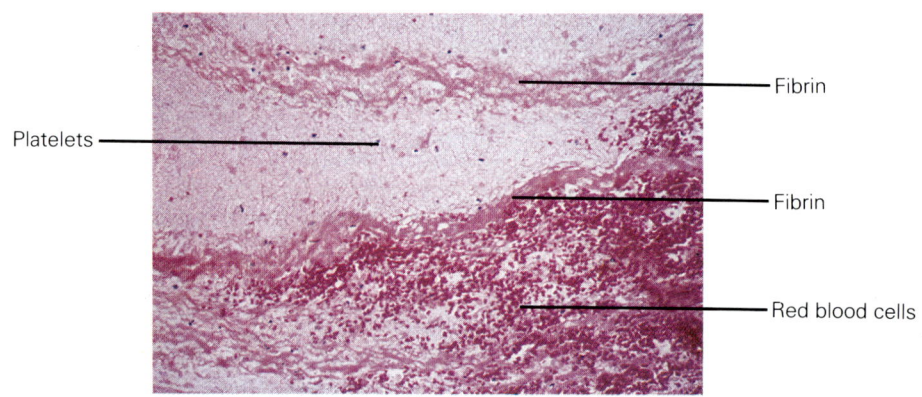

Thrombi form by progressive deposition of layers (lines of Zahn) of fibrin, platelets, and red blood cells.

Figure 2.18
Disseminated intravascular coagulation

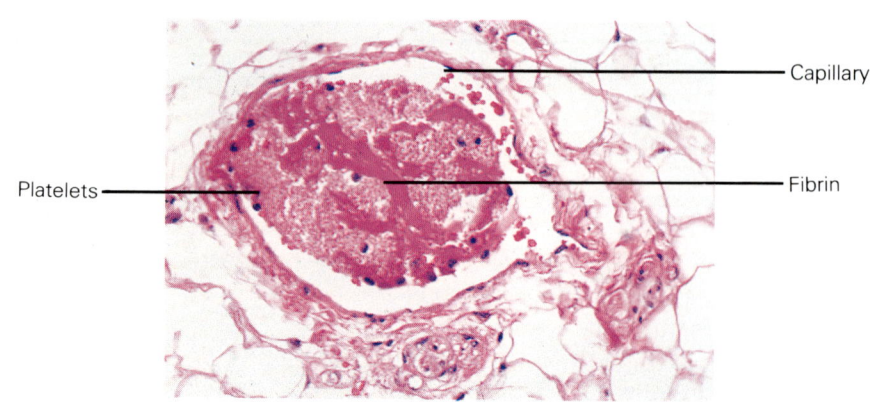

Activation of the intrinsic coagulation pathway by sepsis or other conditions results in small platelet-fibrin thrombi forming within the microvasculature.

14 *Histopathology of Disease*

Figure 2.19
Vascular and cellular responses in inflammation

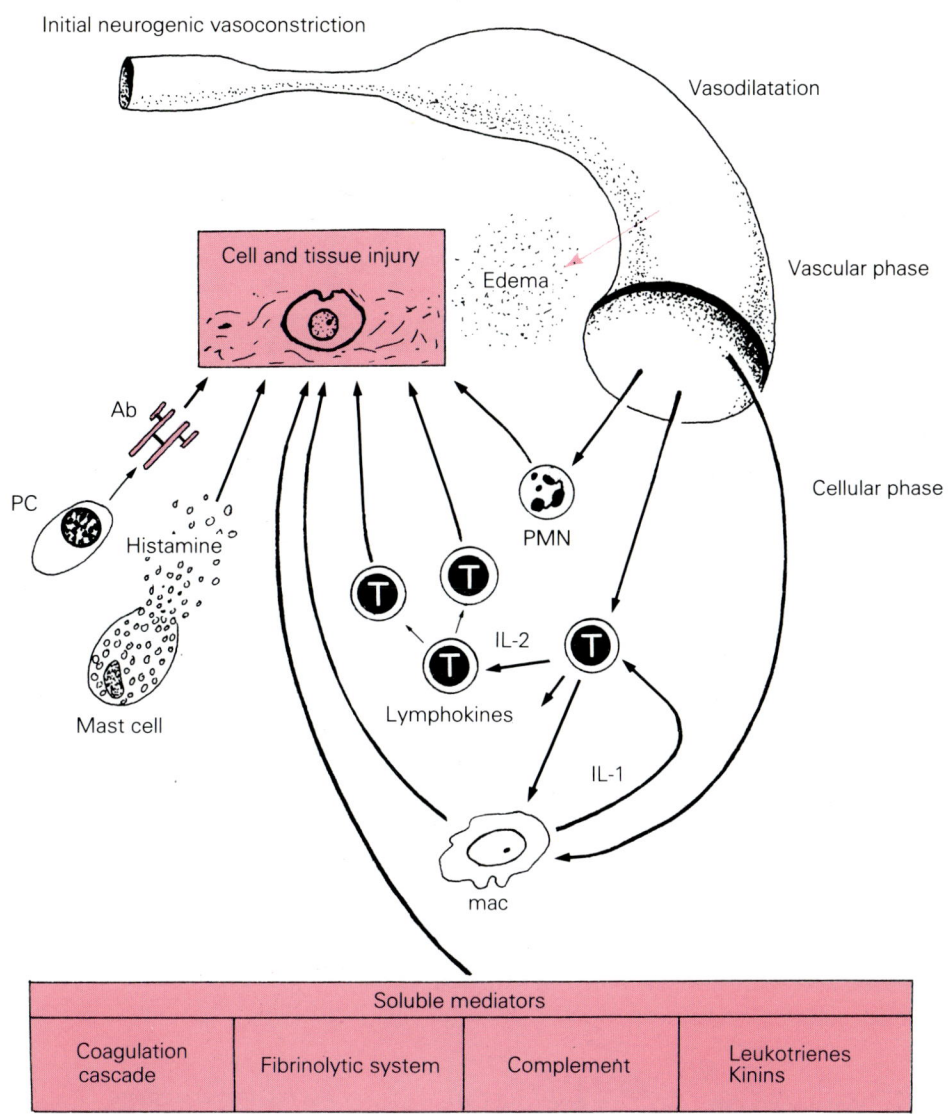

The vascular and cellular phases of inflammation are shown schematically above. In acute inflammation, polymorphonuclear leukocytes (PMN) and other mediators such as leukotrienes and kinins result in five cardinal signs: *rubor* (redness), *calor* (heat), *dolor* (pain), *tumor* (swelling), and *functio laesa* (loss of function). Other components of the inflammatory response (often more prominent in cell-mediated immune reactions and chronic inflammation) include secretion of interleukin-1 (IL-1) by macrophages (mac) serving to activate T-lymphocytes; T-cell secretion of interleukin-2 (IL-2), a clonal expander; and antibody (Ab) synthesis by plasma cells (PC).

Principles of Pathology 15

Figure 2.20
Features of reactive and neoplastic growth processes

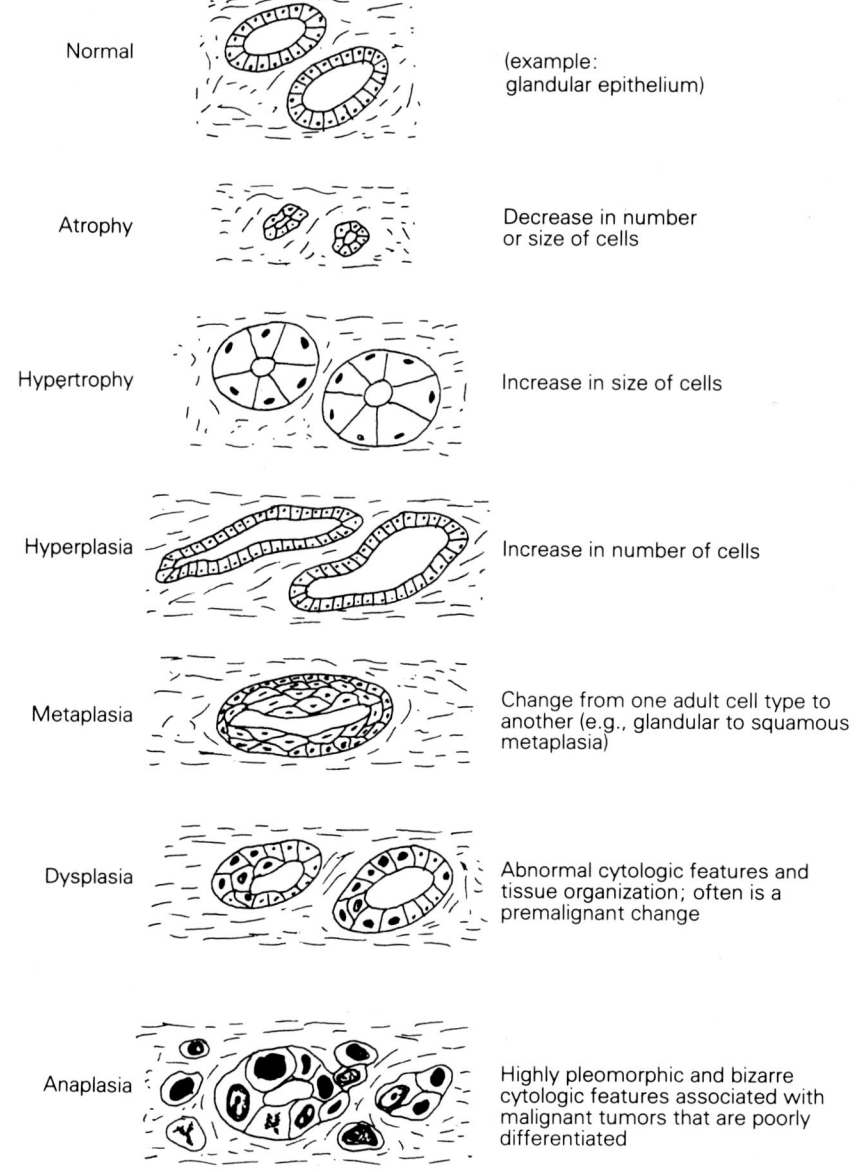

16 *Histopathology of Disease*

Figure 2.21
Classification of neoplasms

Type of tumor	Cell of origin	Benign	Malignant
Epithelial	Squamous cell	Papilloma	Squamous cell carcinoma
	Glandular cell	Adenoma	Adenocarcinoma
Mesenchymal	Lipocyte	Lipoma	Liposarcoma
	Smooth muscle cell	Leiomyoma	Leiomyosarcoma
	Fibroblast	Fibroma	Fibrosarcoma

Figure 2.22
Features of malignant neoplasms

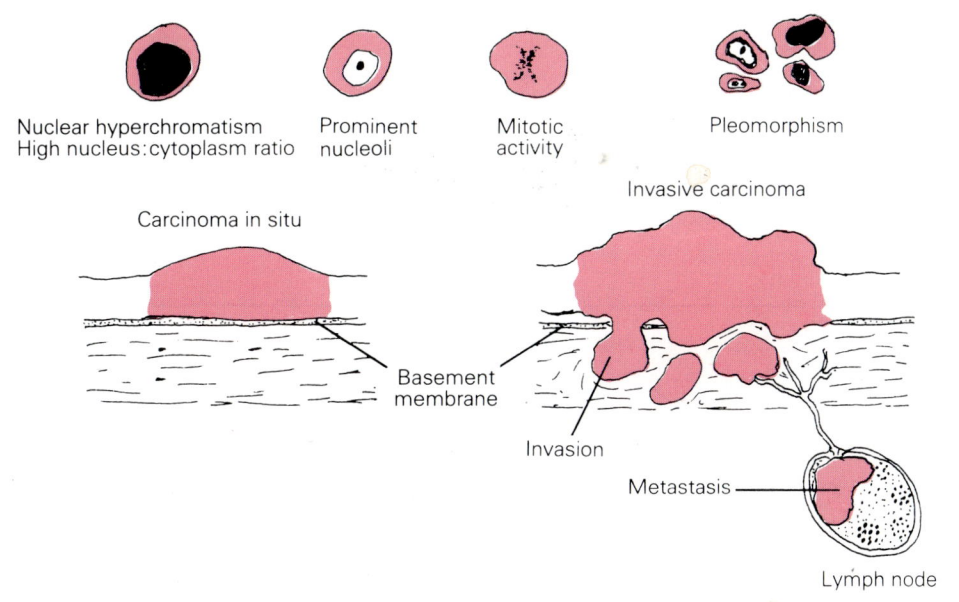

NEOPLASIA

Figure 2.23
Adenoma

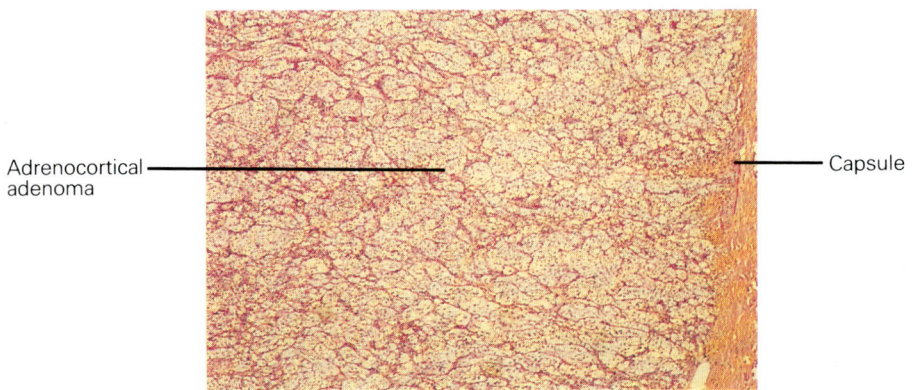

Adenomas (benign tumors of glandular epithelium) histologically resemble the tissue or origin, show little pleomorphism and few, if any, mitoses, and are either well-circumscribed or encapsulated.

Figure 2.24
Malignant cells

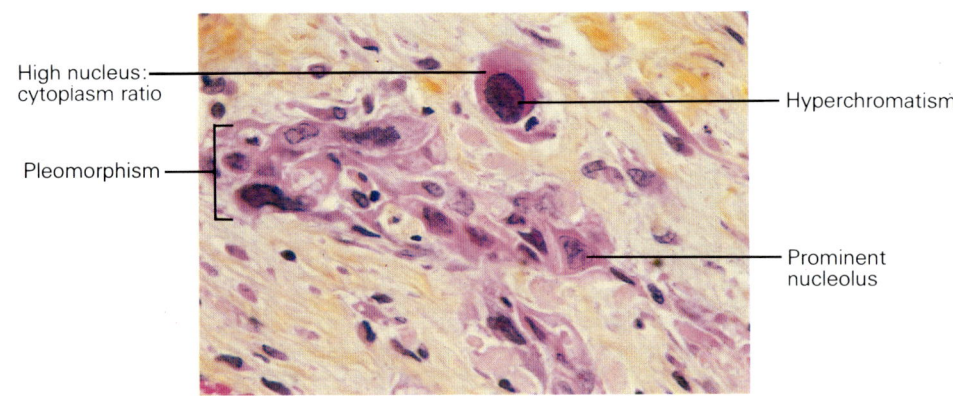

Malignant squamous cells are shown invading adjacent stroma (stained yellow). Note the cytologic features of malignancy.

Figure 2.25
Invasion (stromal)

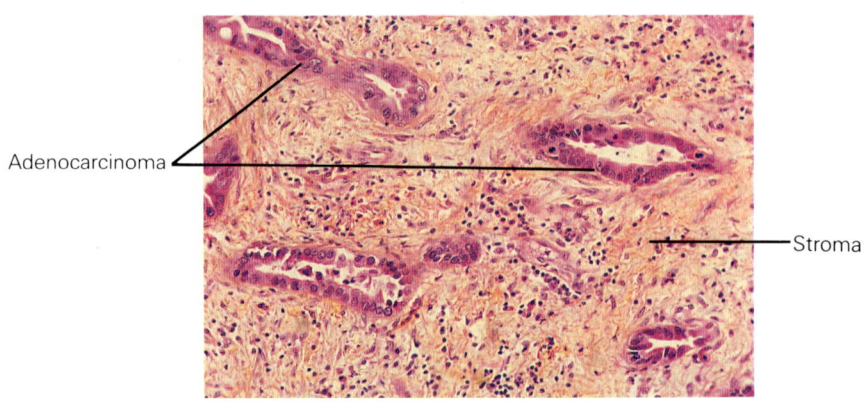

Malignant tumors have the capacity to invade adjacent tissues. The example above shows glands of adenocarcinoma invading nearby stroma.

Figure 2.26
Invasion (vascular)

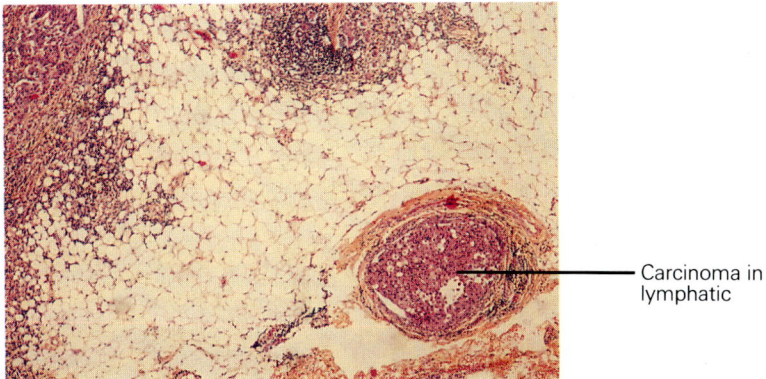

Malignant tumors can invade lymphatics and veins. This example shows breast carcinoma in a lymphatic.

Figure 2.27
Invasion (perineural)

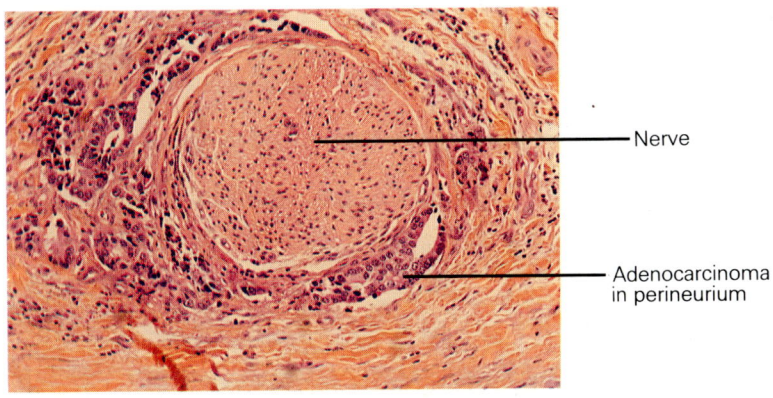

Certain malignant tumors, such as adenocarcinoma of the prostate and of bile ducts, display perineural invasion.

Figure 2.28
Metastasis (lymph node)

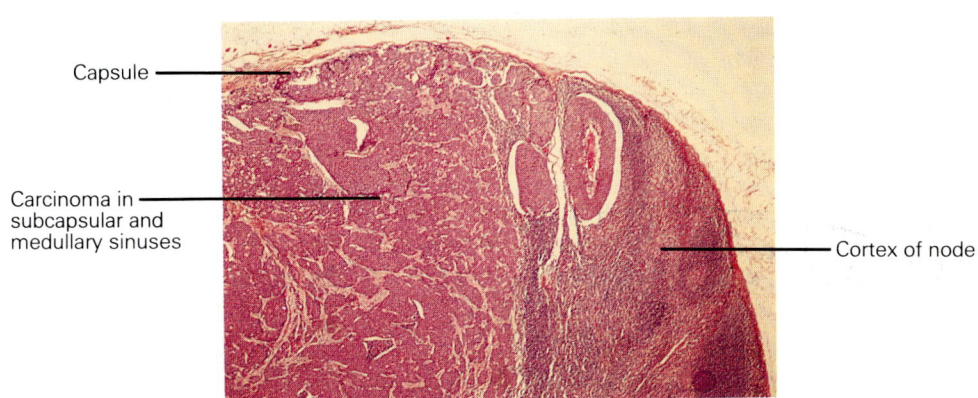

Distal spread of malignant tumors (metastasis) may be to regional lymph nodes or parenchymal organs such as lungs, liver, and bone. Carcinomas tend to metastasize to lymph nodes, while sarcomas invade veins and spread to the lungs.

Principles of Pathology

HISTOLOGIC TYPES OF MALIGNANT TUMORS

Figure 2.29
Adenocarcinoma

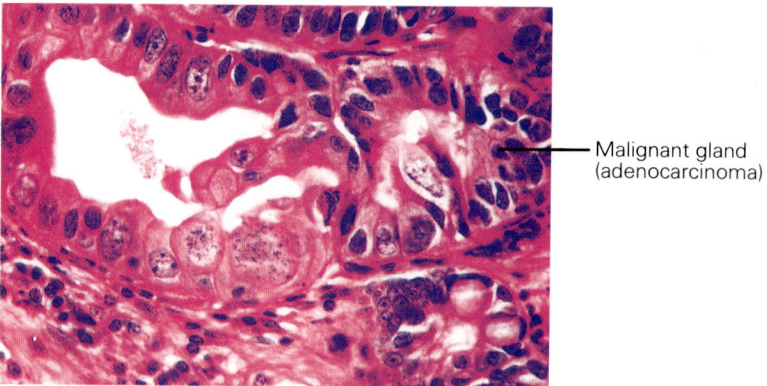

These epithelial malignancies are derived from glandular tissues and, when well differentiated, show growth as glands.

Figure 2.30
Papillary adenocarcinoma

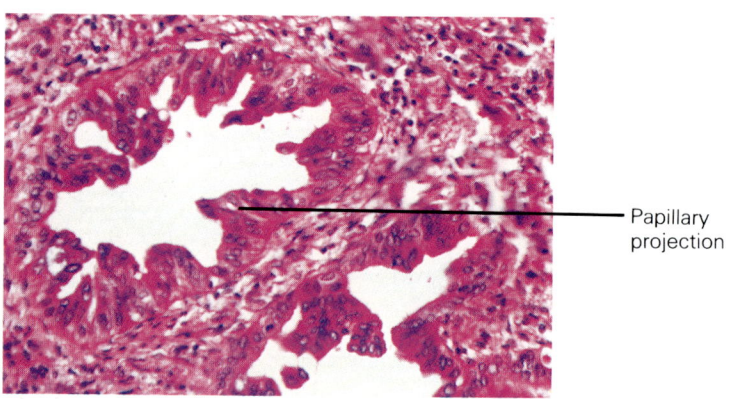

This histologic variant of adenocarcinoma shows growth of tumor cells in papillary projections.

Figure 2.31
Mucinous adenocarcinoma

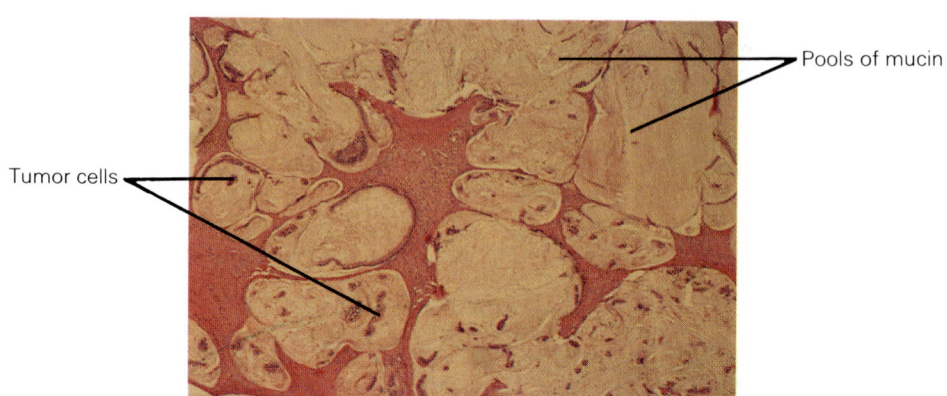

This variant of adenocarcinoma is characterized by tumor cell secretion of pools of mucin. Scattered carcinoma cells, often inconspicuous or cytologically bland, are floating in the mucin.

Figure 2.32
Squamous cell carcinoma

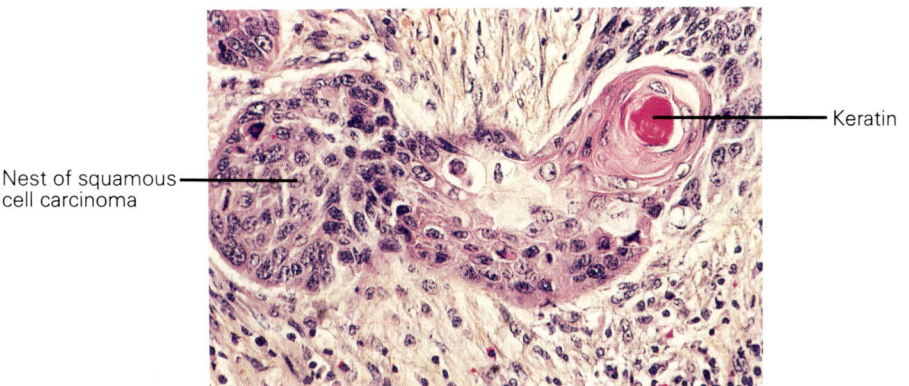

Malignancies arising in squamous epithelium grow as nests and islands. Better differentiated tumors may show keratin production (above) in the midst of whirls of squamous cells called keratin pearls.

Figure 2.33
Poorly differentiated carcinoma

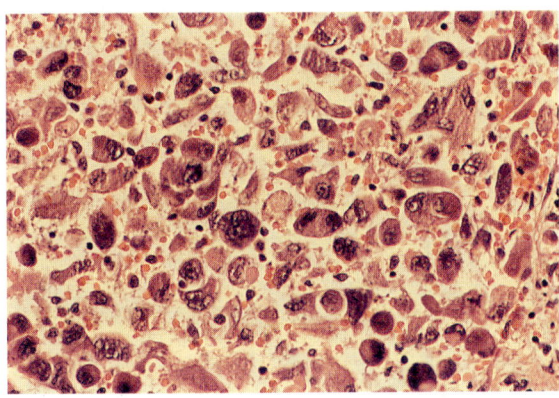

Tumor cells here are markedly pleomorphic and bizarre with few features by which to determine their histogenesis.

Figure 2.34
Sarcoma

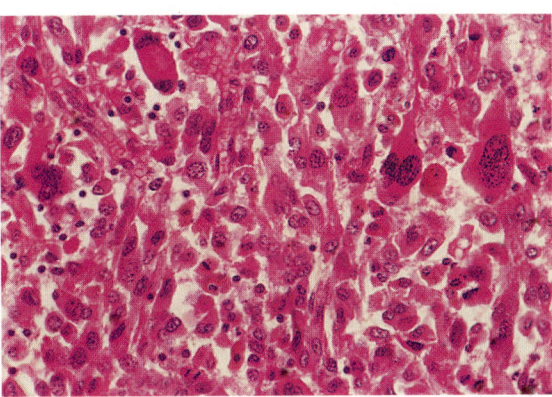

Sarcomas are malignant tumors of mesenchymal origin. That shown above is a rhabdomyosarcoma, derived from skeletal muscle. Sarcomas often show spindle cells histologically.

Figure 2.35
Carcinosarcoma

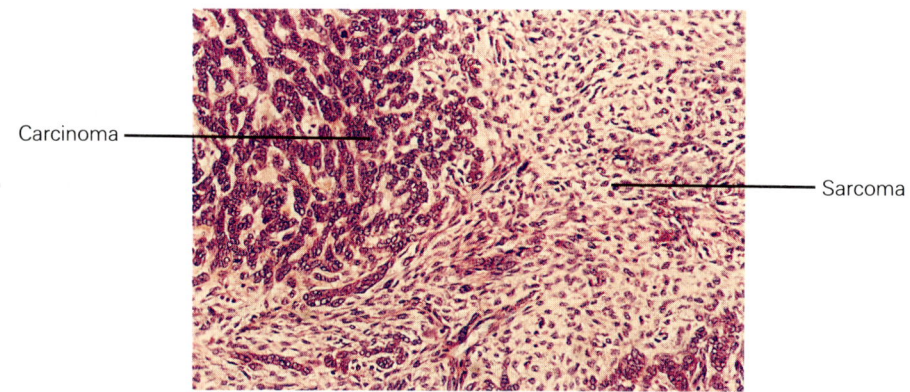

This rare malignant tumor consists of cells which differentiate along both carcinomatous (epithelial) and sarcomatous (mesenchymal) pathways.

Figure 2.36
Malignant lymphoma

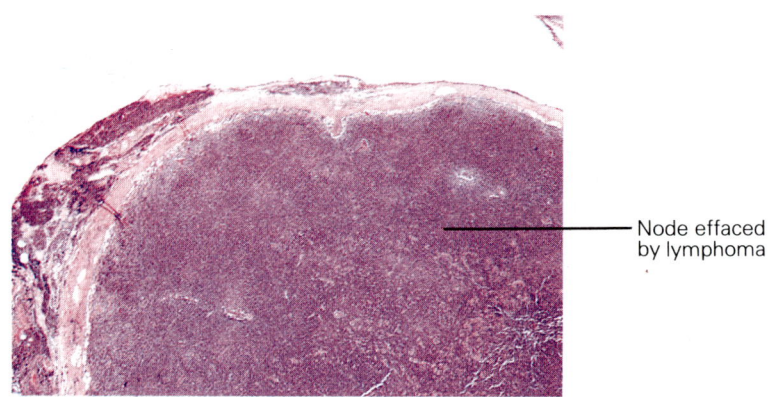

Lymphomas (shown above) are malignancies of lymphocytes and histiocytes. Leukemias are malignancies of hematopoietic cells.

Figure 2.37
Expression of tumor cell antigens

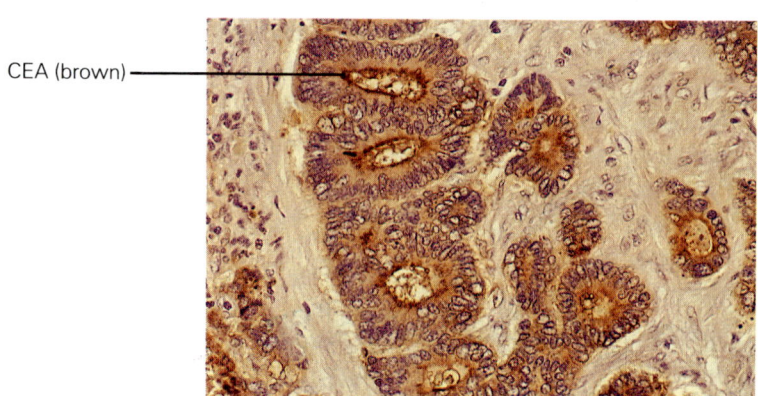

Certain oncofetal antigens such as carcinoembryonic antigen (CEA) and alphafetoprotein (AFP) may be expressed by malignant tumor cells. Above, CEA is stained brown by immunoperoxidase within cells of colon adenocarcinoma.

CHAPTER 3

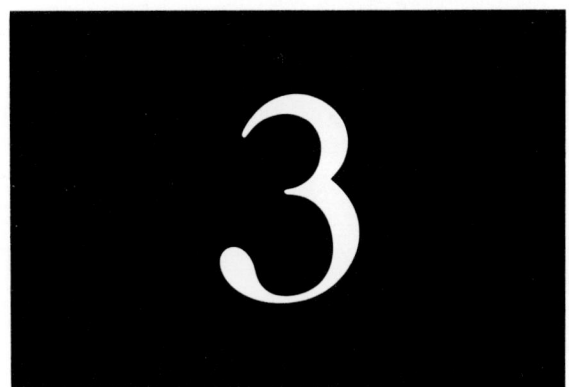

CELL ULTRASTRUCTURE AND CYTOPATHOLOGY

Electron microscopy and examination of tissue fluids or aspirates for cytopathology are useful diagnostic techniques that supplement routine histopathology. The normal cell organelles (shown below) may be altered in disease (e.g., degranulation of rough endoplasmic reticulum (RER), proliferation of smooth endoplasmic reticulum). This chapter includes a number of representative examples of cytopathology, as seen in everyday practice.

Figure 3.1
Transmission electron micrograph (liver tissue)

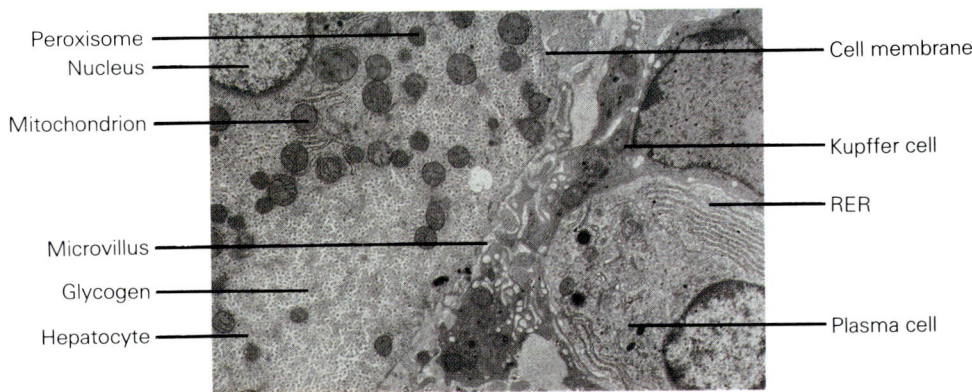

This field shows a hepatocyte and a Kupffer cell and plasma cell within the adjacent sinusoidal space. The basic organelles of cells are shown.

Figure 3.2
Slide of pleural fluid for cytology

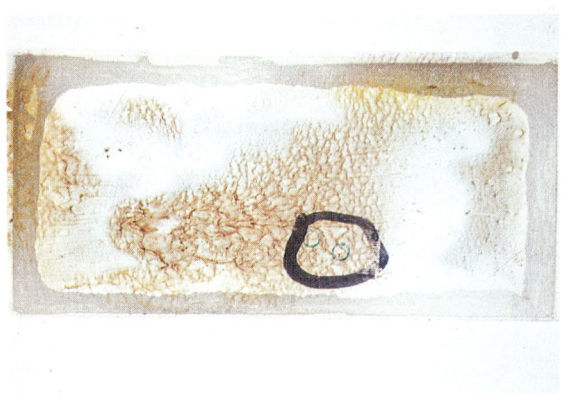

Examination of slides of pleural fluid and other samples for abnormal cells involves screening and marking of suspicious areas, as shown above.

Figure 3.3
Normal squamous cells (PAP smear)

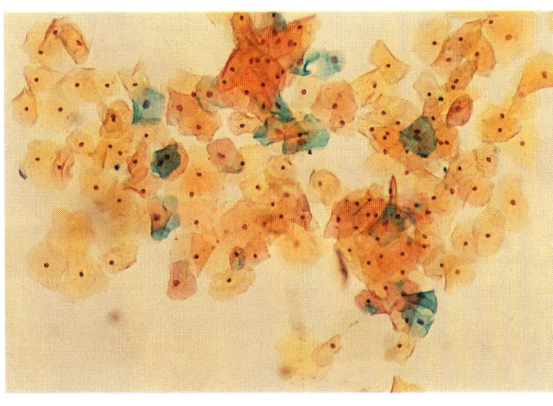

Superficial squamous cells of the cervix have small, inconspicuous nuclei.

Figure 3.4
Intermediate and parabasal cells (PAP smear)

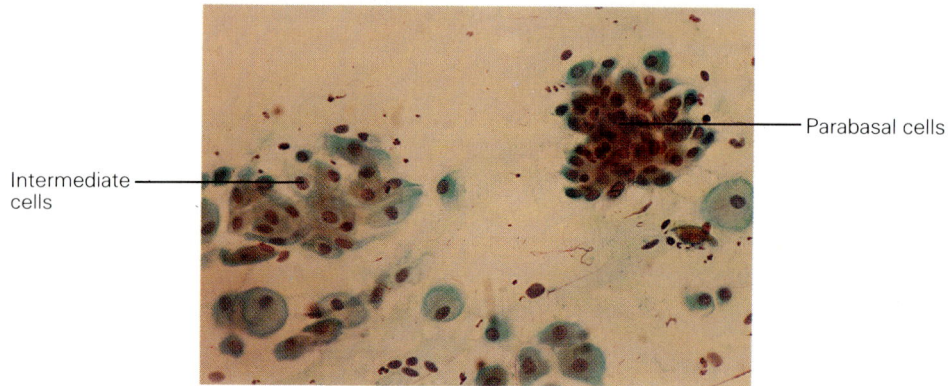

Cervical PAP smear.

Figure 3.5
Squamous cell carcinoma of cervix

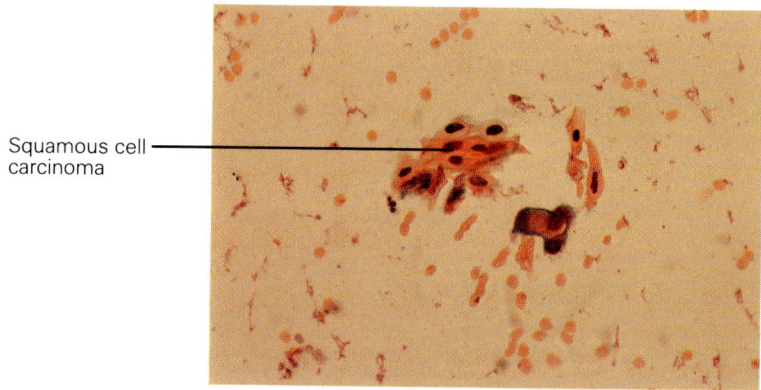

Compare the hyperchromatic nuclei of these malignant cells to the benign nuclei in normal cervical squamous cells (see Figure 3.3).

Figure 3.6
Adenocarcinoma of lung

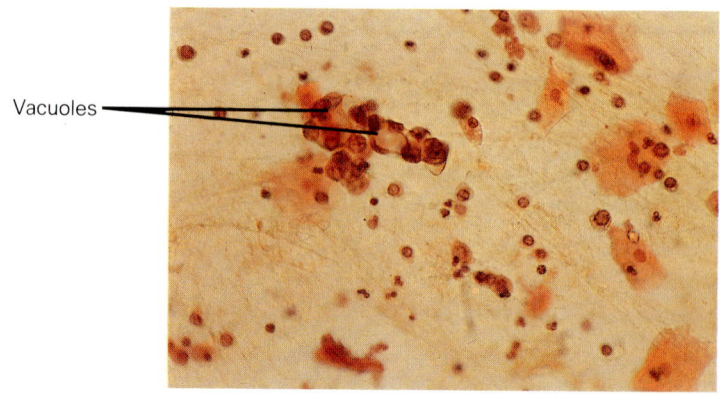

A cluster of adenocarcinoma cells with characteristic vacuoles is present. The vacuoles reflect the glandular (secretory) function of these cells.

Figure 3.7
Oat cell carcinoma of lung

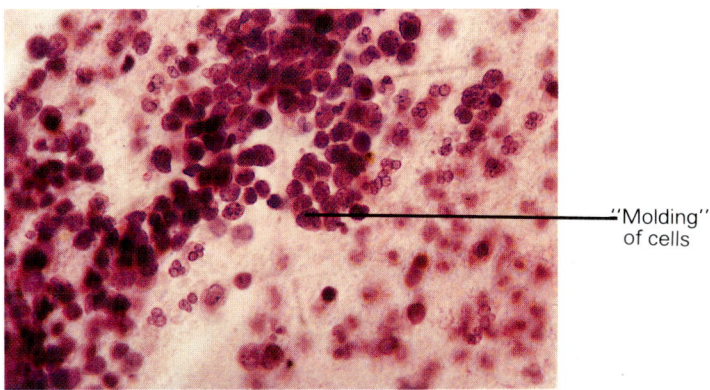

Sputum specimen showing clusters of oat cell carcinoma cells with finely stippled chromatin and typical "molding" of one cell into another.

Figure 3.8
Poorly differentiated lymphocytic lymphoma

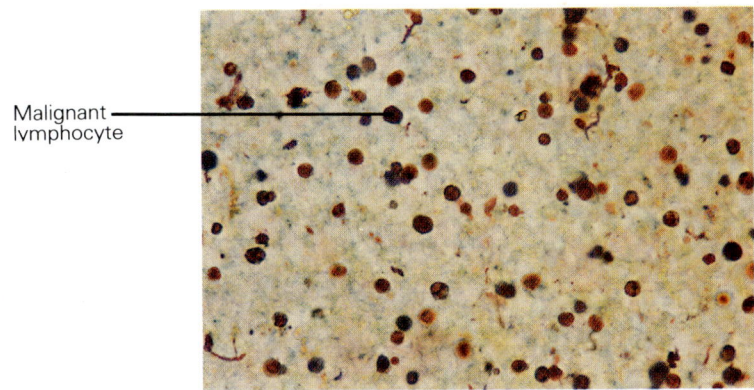

Pleural fluid specimen showing scattered lymphoma cells. Cellular debris and fragmentation in this field are effects of chemotherapy.

Figure 3.9
"Histiocytic" lymphoma

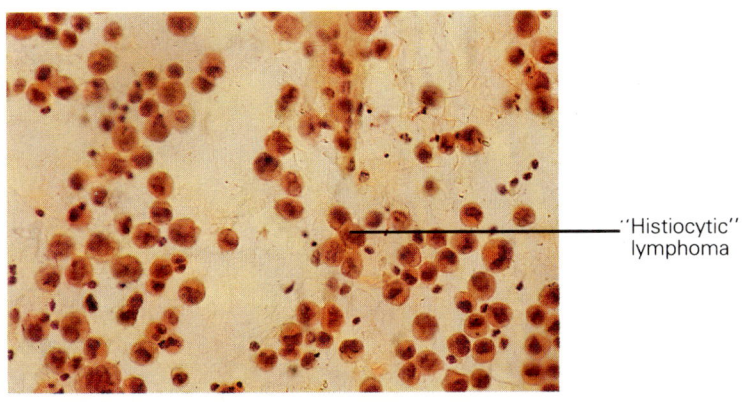

The lymphoma cells have vesicular nuclei. The cells were found in pleural fluid.

Figure 3.10
Candida in cervical PAP smear

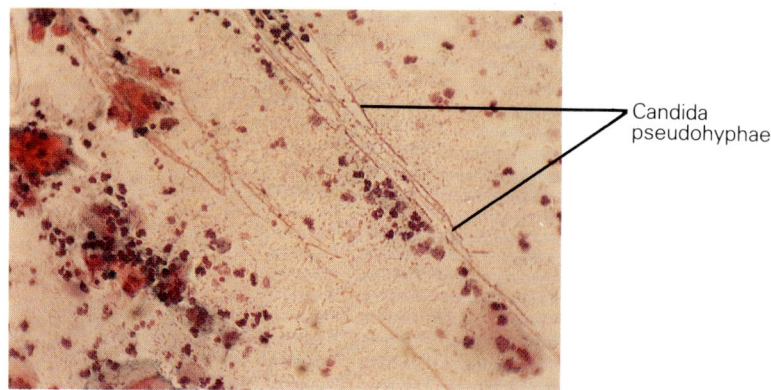

This fungal infection was diagnosed on PAP smear. Compare the fungal morphology to that in tissue (see Figure 4.6).

Figure 3.11
Trichomonas (cervical PAP smear)

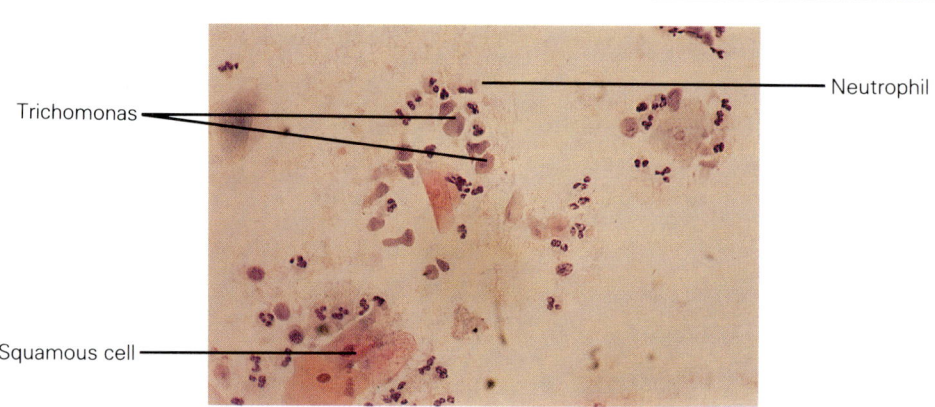

This flagellated, pear-shaped protozoan is a common gynecologic pathogen. Compare its size to adjacent neutrophils and squamous cells.

CHAPTER 4

INFECTIOUS AGENTS

This chapter provides an overview of the more commonly encountered bacterial, fungal, viral, and parasitic infections and their histologic appearances on routine and special stains.

BACTERIA

Figure 4.1
Gram-positive cocci

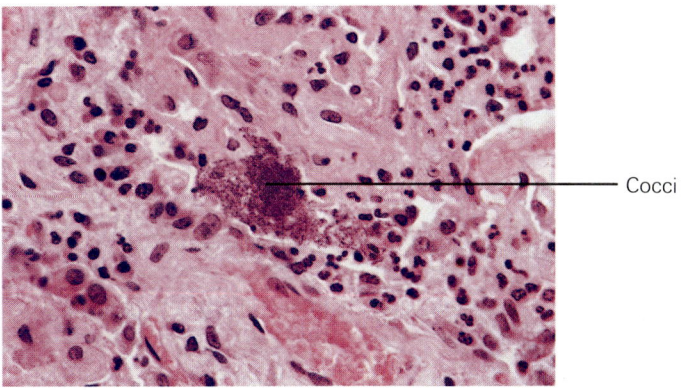

Hematoxylin and eosin stain.

Figure 4.2
Gram-negative rods

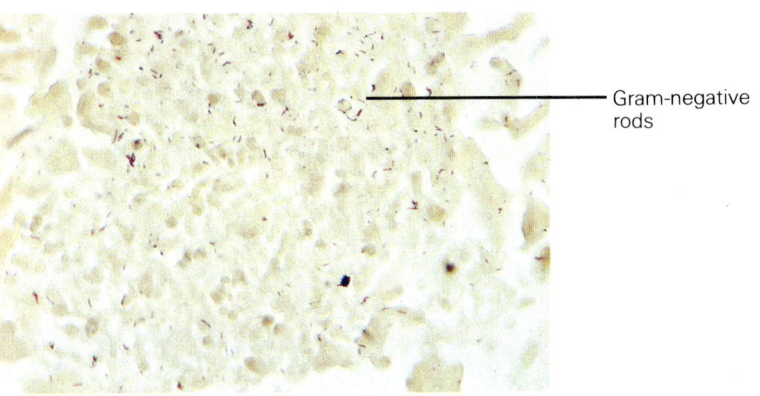

Brown-Brenn stain.

Figure 4.3
Mycobacterium tuberculosis

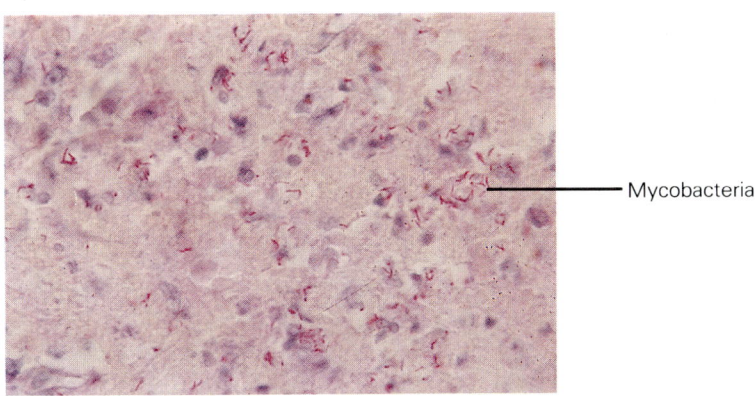

Ziehl-Neelsen stain.

Figure 4.4
Spirochetes

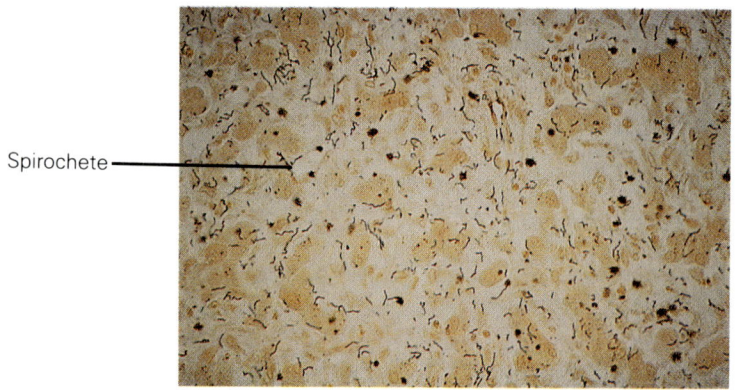

This field shows the liver in congenital syphilis, due to the spirochete *Treponema pallidum*. (Warthin-Starry stain.)

FUNGI

Figure 4.5
Cryptococcus

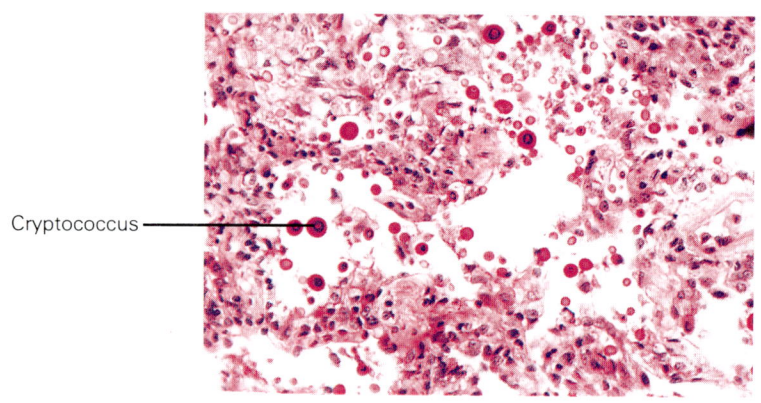

Cryptococci show a target-like appearance because of their thick outer capsule. (Hematoxylin and eosin stain.)

Figure 4.6
Candida

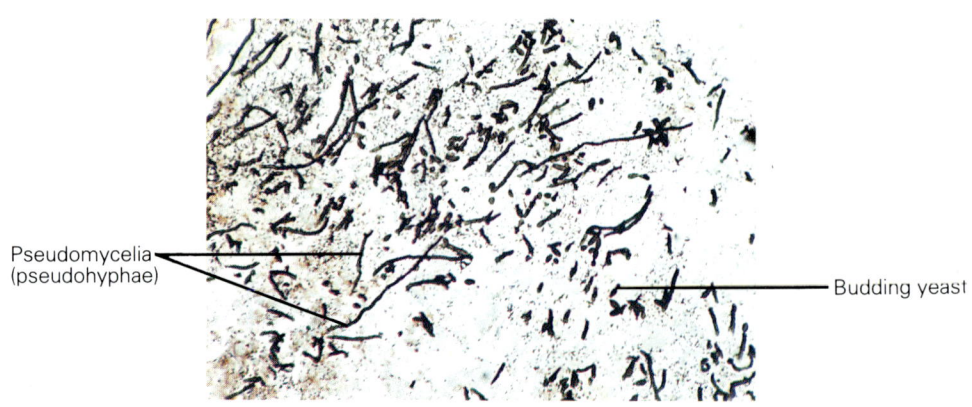

Candida in tissue grows in both budding yeast and elongated pseudomycelial form. (Gomori Methenamine Silver stain.)

Figure 4.7
Aspergillus

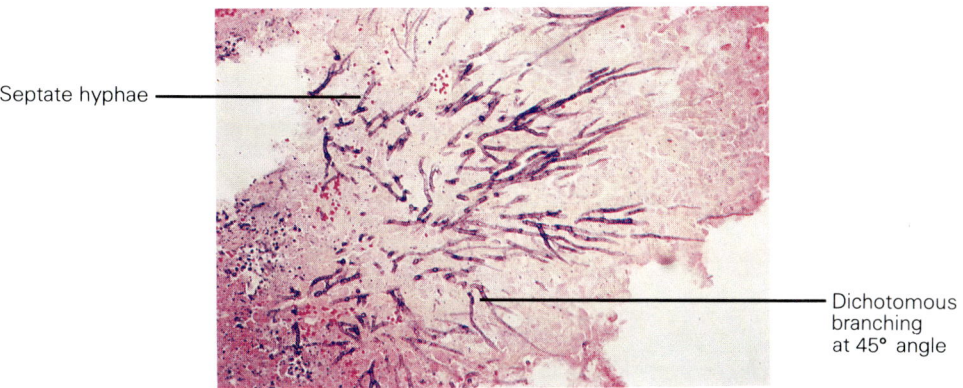

Aspergillus grows as dichotomously branching, septate hyphae. (PAS stain with diastase.)

Figure 4.8
Mucormycosis

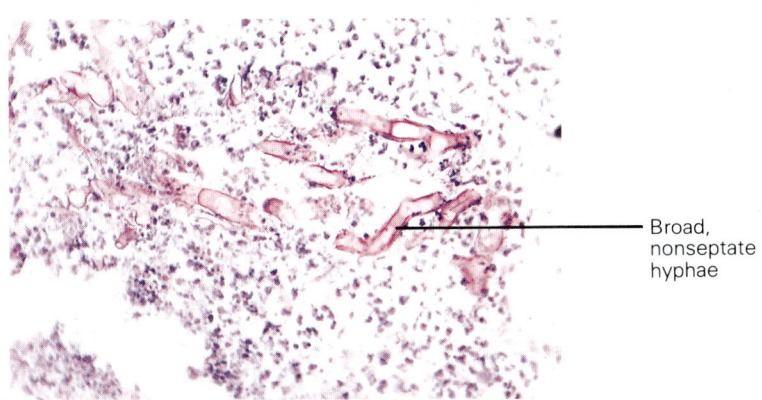

This fungus grows as broad, nonseptate hyphae. (Hematoxylin, phloxine, and saffron stain.)

Figure 4.9
Histoplasmosis

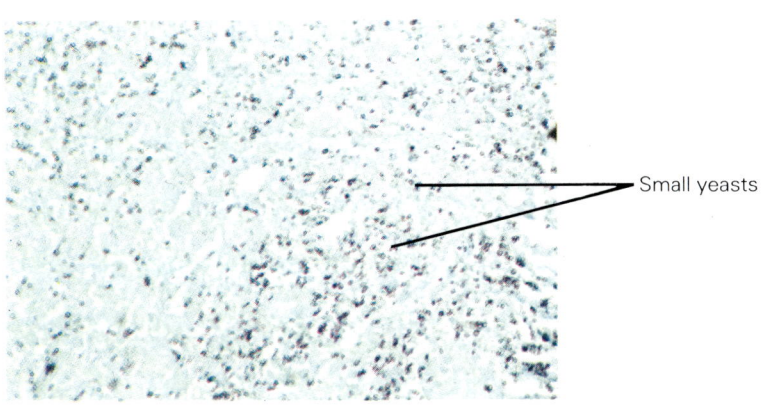

Growth is in small, round 2 to 4 μm diameter yeasts. (Gomori Methenamine Silver stain.)

Infectious Agents **33**

Figure 4.10
Coccidioidomycosis

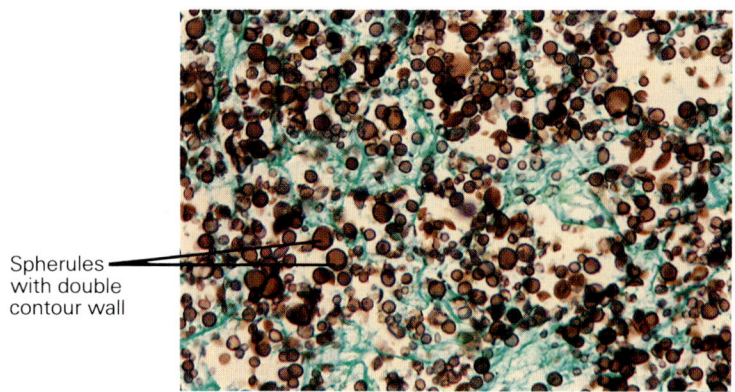

Spherules with double contour wall

Growth is in spherules with thick, doubly refractile walls. (Gomori Methenamine Silver stain.)

VIRUSES

Figure 4.11
Cytomegalovirus (CMV)

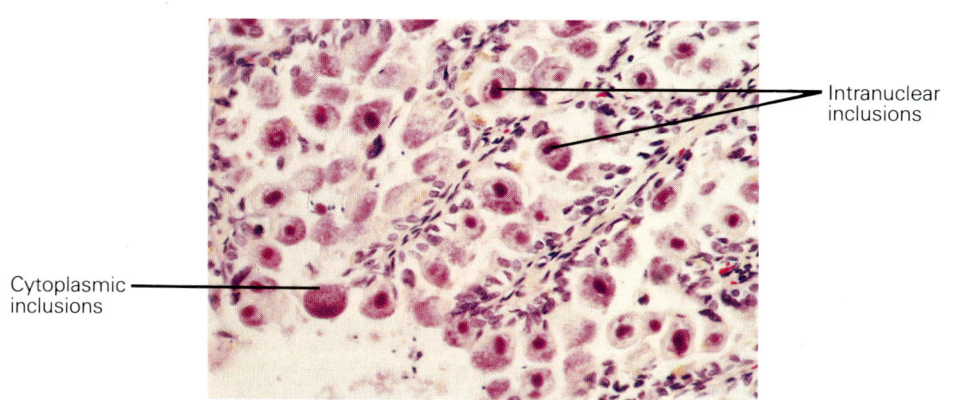

Intranuclear inclusions

Cytoplasmic inclusions

CMV is identified by large, basophilic intranuclear inclusions separated from the nuclear membrane by a halo. Smaller intracytoplasmic basophilic inclusions (virions) occur in the cytoplasm of infected cells. This section is of seminal vesicles.

Figure 4.12
Herpes virus

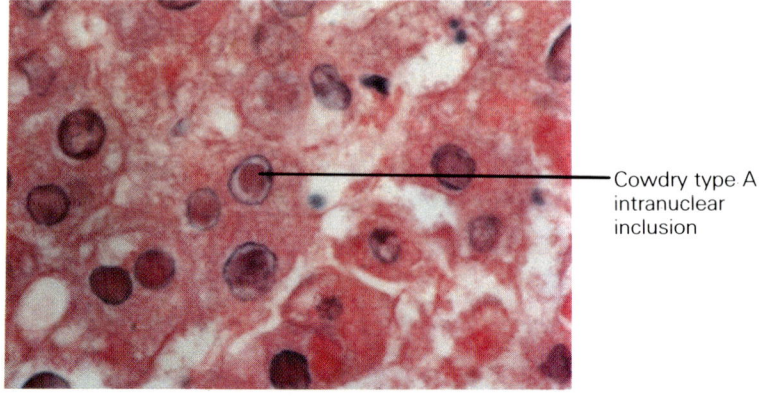

Cowdry type A intranuclear inclusion

Section of liver from immunosuppressed host with herpes virus infection. A round, acidophilic Cowdry type A intranuclear inclusion is seen within a hepatocyte.

PARASITES

Figure 4.13
Schistosomiasis

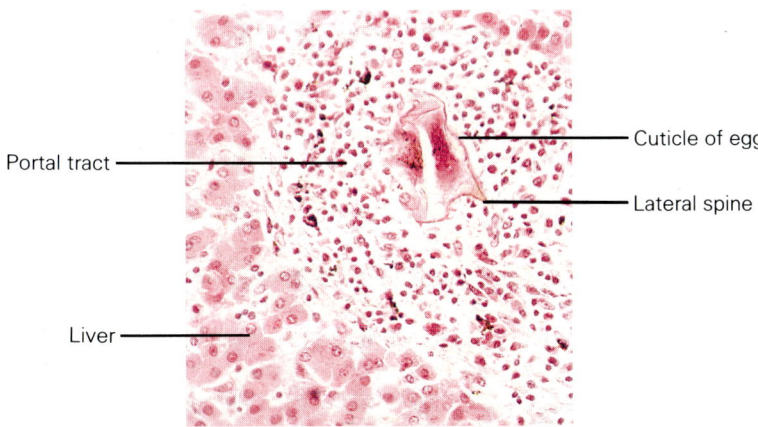

Schistosoma mansoni (shown above, with lateral spine on egg), *hematobium*, and *japonicum* cause granulomatous disease in the liver and urinary bladder.

Figure 4.14
Echinococcus (hydatid disease)

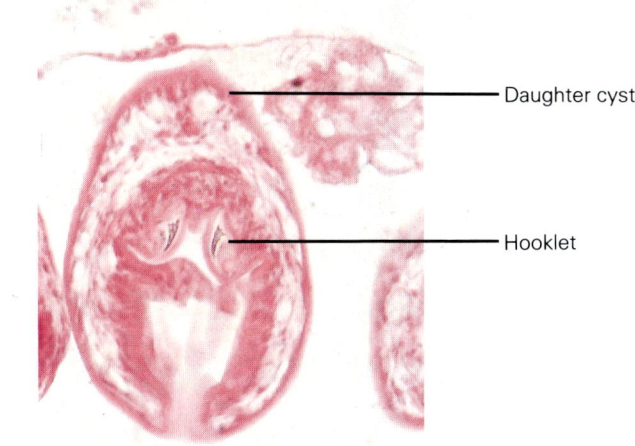

This parasite encysts in organs such as the liver and contains daughter cysts with refractile hooklets (scolices).

Figure 4.15
Amebiasis

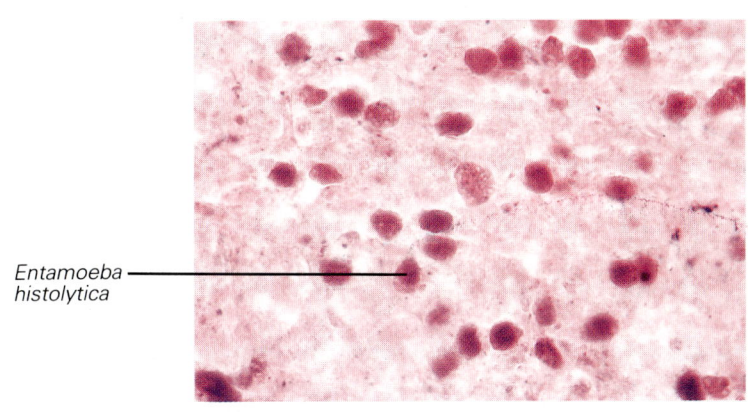

These protozoan parasites cause diarrhea as well as hepatic abscesses. They are unicellular organisms with large nuclei.

Figure 4.16
Pneumocystis carinii

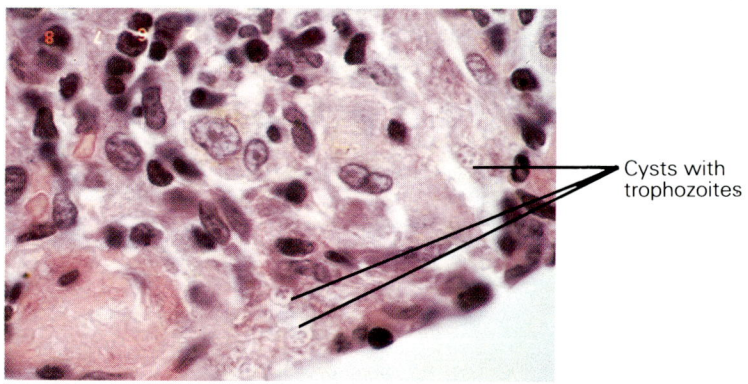

Section of lung from a patient with acquired immune deficiency syndrome (AIDS). A lymphocytic and histiocytic reaction has developed around several Pneumocystis cysts.

Figure 4.17
Pneumocystis (touch preparation)

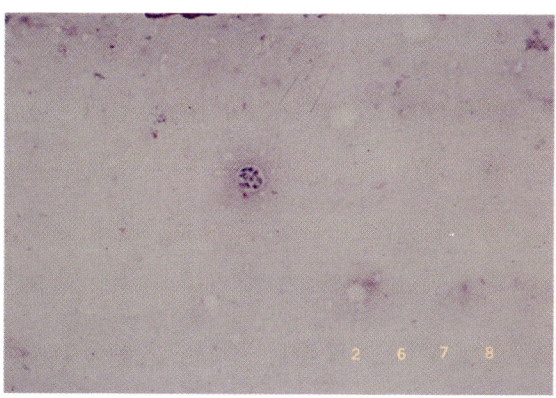

Giemsa stain of touch preparation from transbronchial biopsy. A cyst containing nine trophozoites is seen.

Figure 4.18
Pneumocystis in postmortem lung tissue

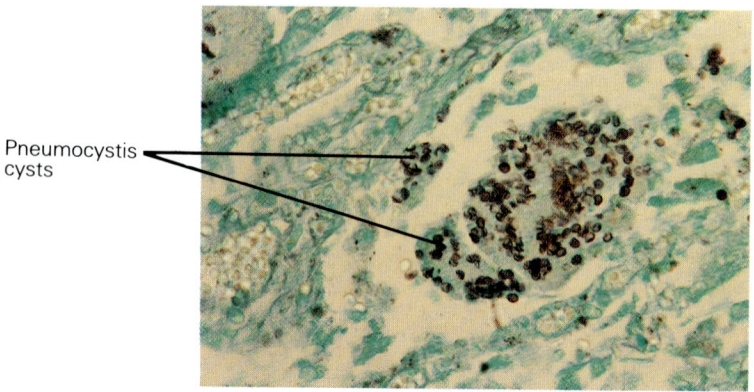

Gomori Methenamine Silver stain demonstrates darkly stained Pneumocystis cysts within an alveolar space. The cysts resemble indented or crushed ping-pong balls. Routine stains usually show a foamy alveolar exudate (see Figure 6.19).

Figure 4.19
Toxoplasmosis

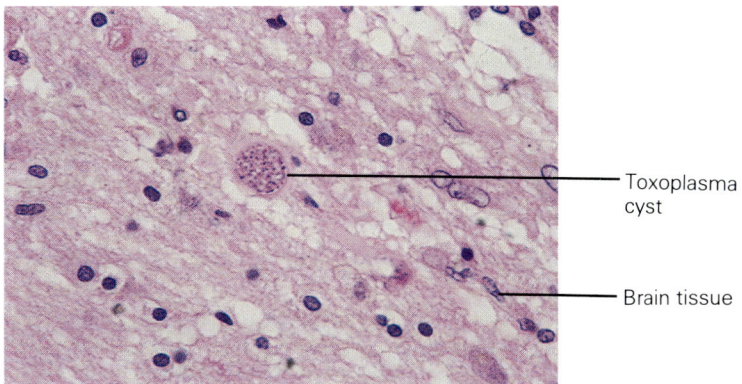

This protozoan encysts in the brain and is a common infective agent in patients with AIDS.

Figure 4.20
Cryptosporidia

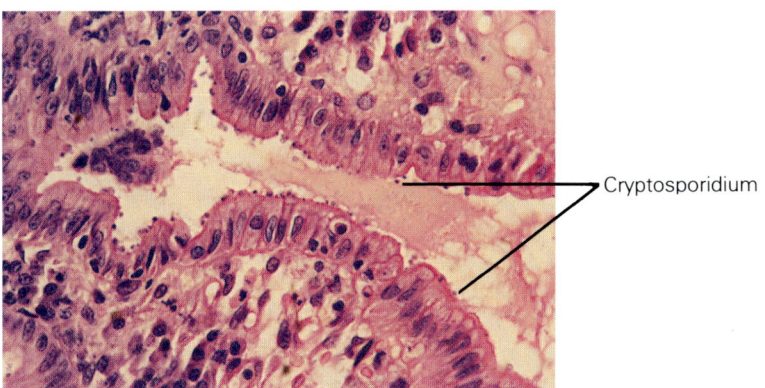

Cryptosporidia attach to the surfaces of epithelial cells within the intestine (seen as blue dots above) and are associated with diarrhea, often in AIDS patients.

Figure 4.21
Giardiasis

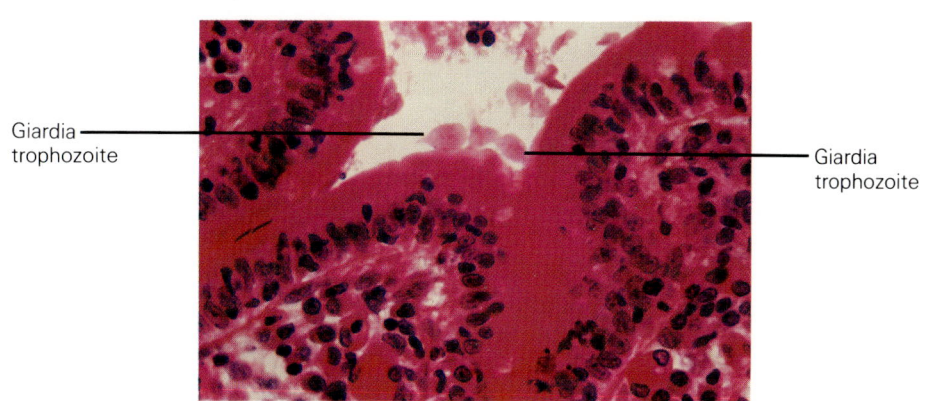

Several giardia are attached to the surface of intestinal villi. Their double nuclei endow them with "face-like" features.

CHAPTER 5

CARDIOVASCULAR PATHOLOGY

Figure 5.1
Normal heart

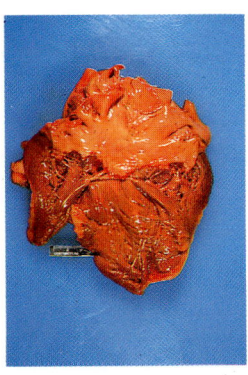

View of opened left atrium and left ventricle. Normal weight: male (300 to 350 g), female (250 to 300 g).

Figure 5.2
Normal heart

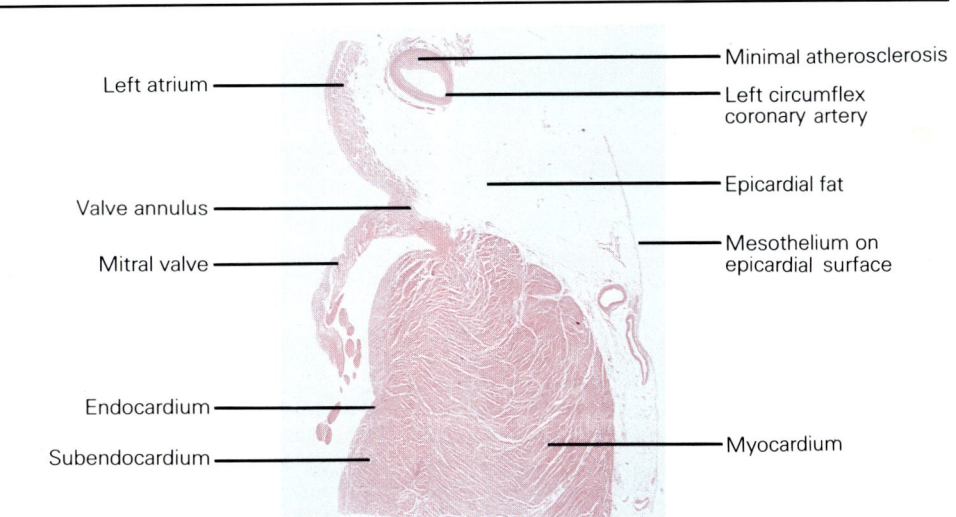

Section through lateral left ventricle.

Figure 5.3
Normal heart

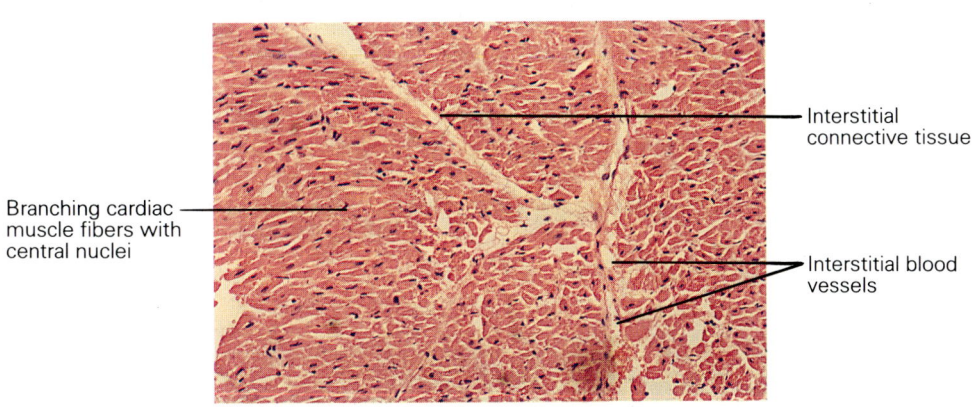

Section of myocardium.

Cardiovascular Pathology

Figure 5.4
Cardiovascular system: major pathologic lesions

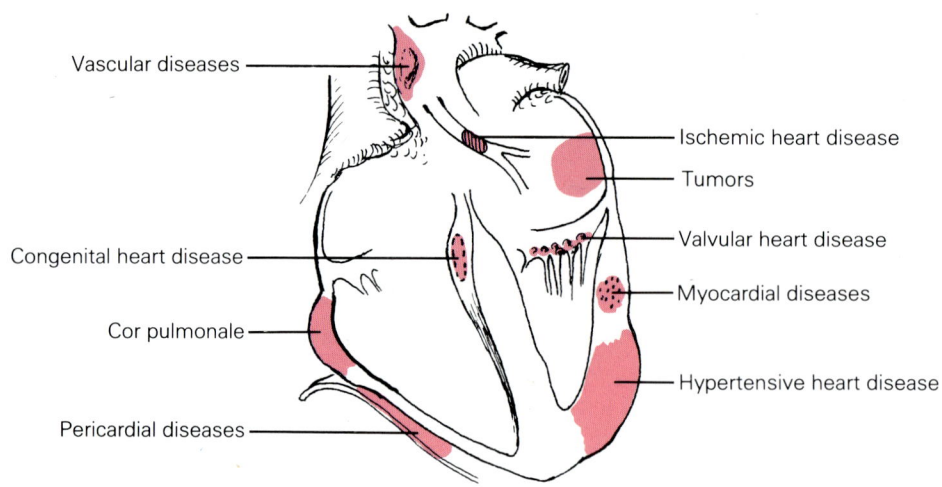

Ischemic heart disease: Myocardial infarction (MI) may develop as a consequence of atherosclerotic narrowing of coronary arteries. Pathogenesis is related to endothelial damage, hyperlipidemia, smooth muscle proliferation, fibrosis, and formation of atheromatous plaques.

Tumors: Benign atrial myxoma is the most common primary tumor.

Valvular heart disease: Includes rheumatic heart disease, mitral prolapse, aortic valvular stenosis, infective endocarditis, and marantic (nonbacterial, thrombotic) endocarditis.

Myocardial diseases: Includes myocarditis and cardiomyopathy.

Hypertensive heart disease: Left ventricular hypertrophy associated with systemic hypertension.

Vascular diseases: Arteriosclerosis (includes atherosclerosis, Mönckeberg's calcific sclerosis and arteriolosclerosis); arteritis (includes polyarteritis nodosa, giant cell or temporal arteritis, Takayasu's pulseless aortitis, and thromboangiitis obliterans or Buerger's disease); aneurysms; varicose veins; and thrombophlebitis.

Congenital heart disease: Ventricular septal defect (VSD) is the most common. In adults, atrial septal defect (ASD) is most common. Others include tetralogy of Fallot (VSD, aorta overriding VSD, pulmonic stenosis, and right ventricular hypertrophy), coarctation of aorta, and transposition of great vessels.

Cor pulmonale: Pulmonary heart disease consisting of right ventricular enlargement and pulmonary arterial hypertension. Seen in pulmonary embolism, chronic obstructive pulmonary disease, bronchiectasis, interstitial fibrosis, and sarcoidosis.

Pericardial diseases: Inflammation of the pericardium due to primary cardiac disease, system disease involving the heart, or local reaction to tumor. Constrictive pericarditis is a late sequela.

Figure 5.5
Endocarditis

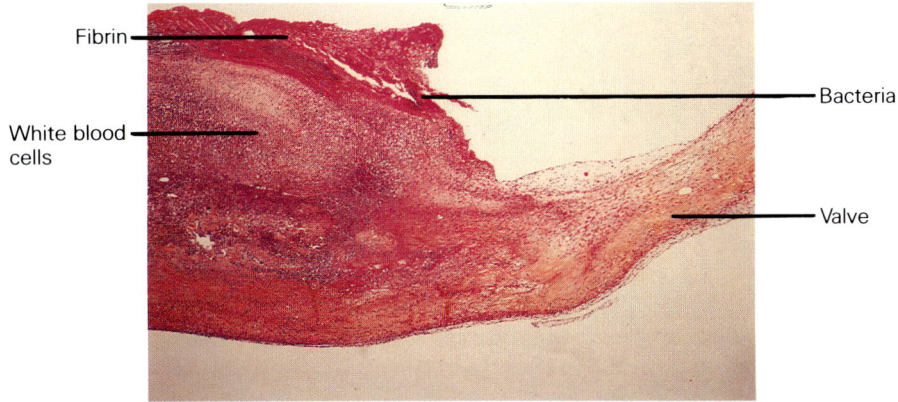

Valve vegetations consist of amorphous masses of fibrin, platelets, and red blood cells. Bacteria and inflammatory cells are seen within vegetations in infective endocarditis, in contrast to nonbacterial thrombotic (marantic) endocarditis. Vegetations may embolize to brain, spleen, coronary arteries, and kidneys with resultant infarcts.

Figure 5.6
Rheumatic heart disease

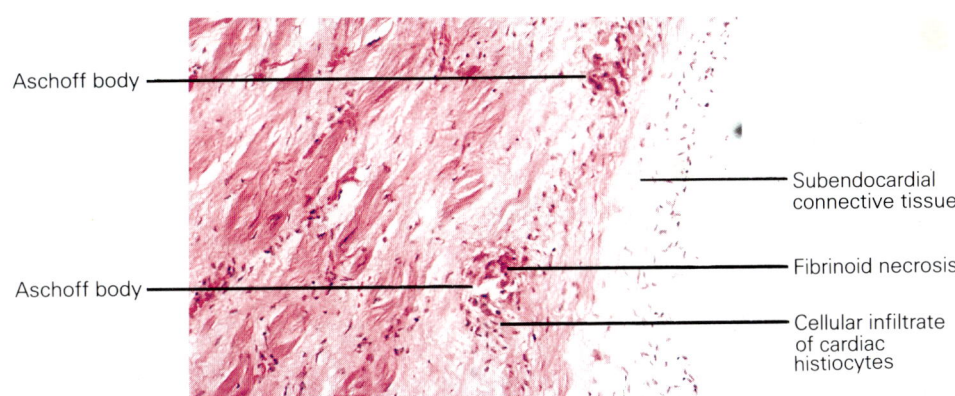

Aschoff bodies, the pathognomonic cellular lesions of rheumatic fever, are seen in the subendocardial region shown above. They consist of foci of smudged collagen, ground substance, and fibrin deposits ("fibrinoid necrosis") surrounded by cardiac macrophages also known as Anitchkow cells or Aschoff cells.

Figure 5.7
Atherosclerosis

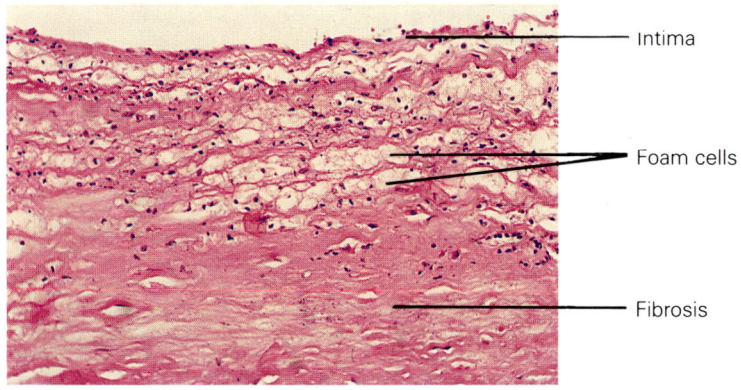

Atherosclerotic lesion of aorta consists of lipid-laden myointimal cells ("foam cells") with fibrosis of intima and media.

Cardiovascular Pathology 43

Figure 5.8
Atherosclerosis

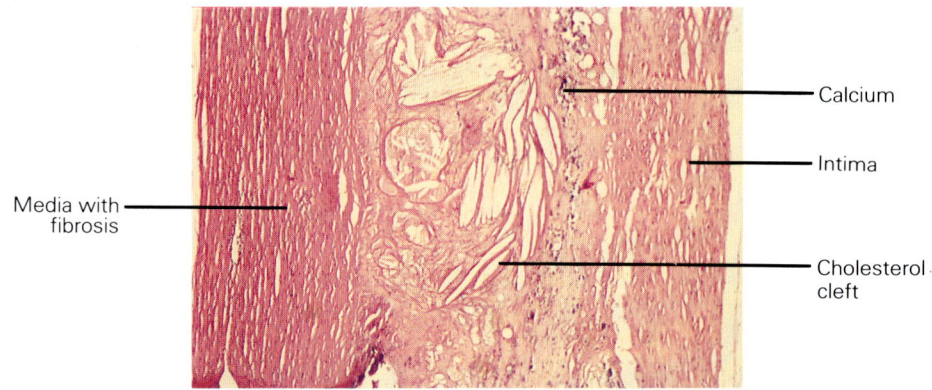

Section of aorta with atherosclerosis. Cholesterol and other lipids appear as cleft-like empty spaces following histologic processing.

Figure 5.9
Coronary atherosclerosis and thrombosis

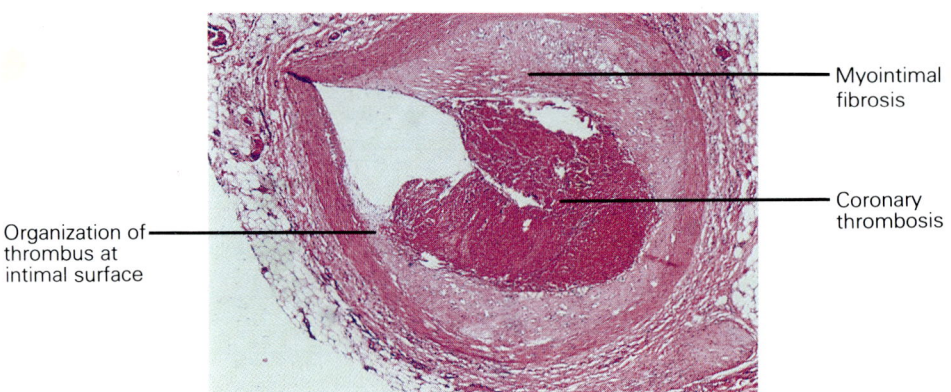

A recent thrombus is organizing within the atherosclerotic left anterior descending coronary artery. Note penetration of thrombus at left by endothelial cells and new ground substance ("organization").

Figure 5.10
Acute myocardial infarction (2 hours)

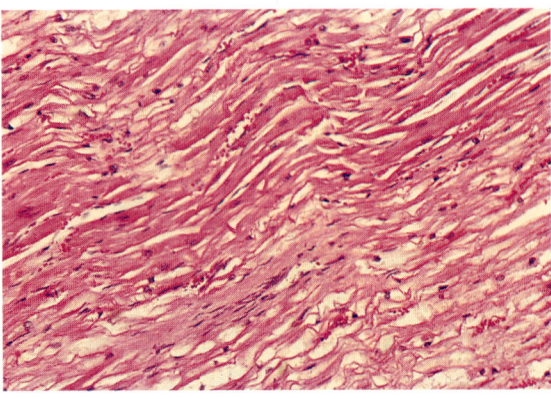

Wavy fibers, interstitial edema.

Figure 5.11
Acute myocardial infarction (1 to 2 days)

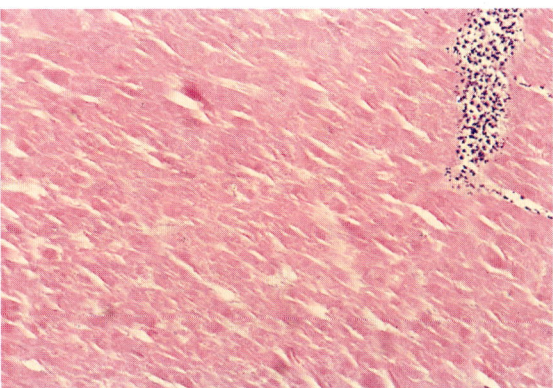

Coagulative necrosis of myocytes, scant neutrophils.

Figure 5.12
Acute myocardial infarction (2 to 3 days)

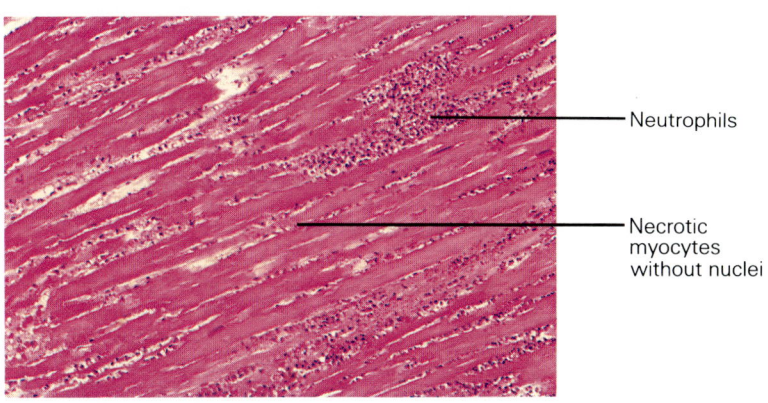

Heavy neutrophil infiltrate with coagulative necrosis.

Figure 5.13
Acute myocardial infarction (4 to 7 days)

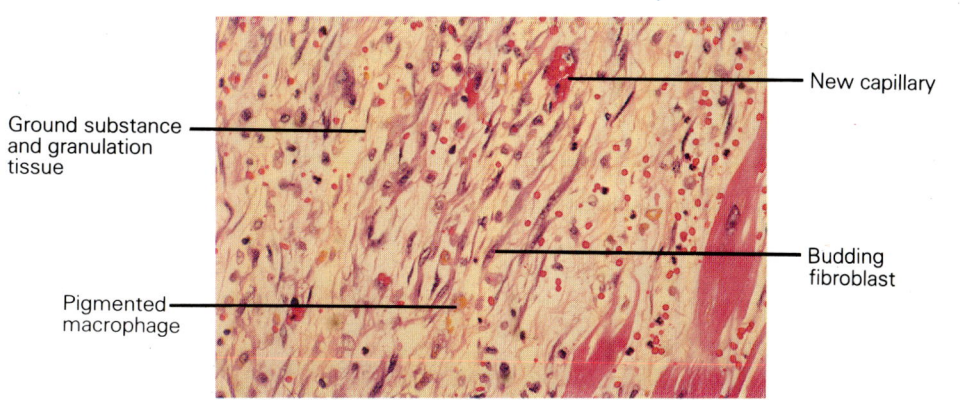

Ingrowth of fibrovascular granulation tissue.

Cardiovascular Pathology

Figure 5.14
Healed myocardial infarction (6 weeks)

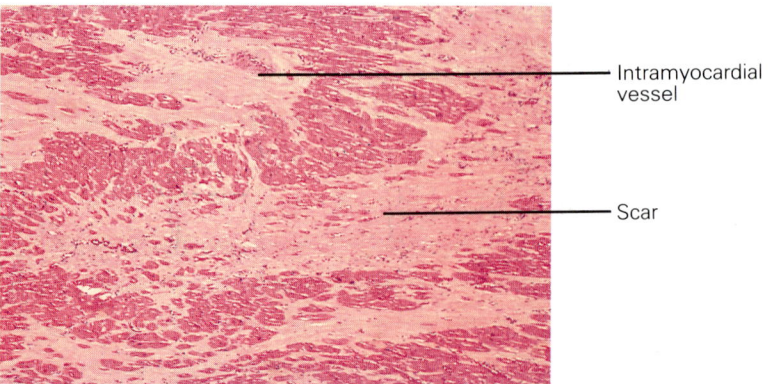

Healed myocardial infarction shows collagenous scar tissue replacing myocytes, usually with a perivascular distribution.

Figure 5.15
Left ventricular hypertrophy

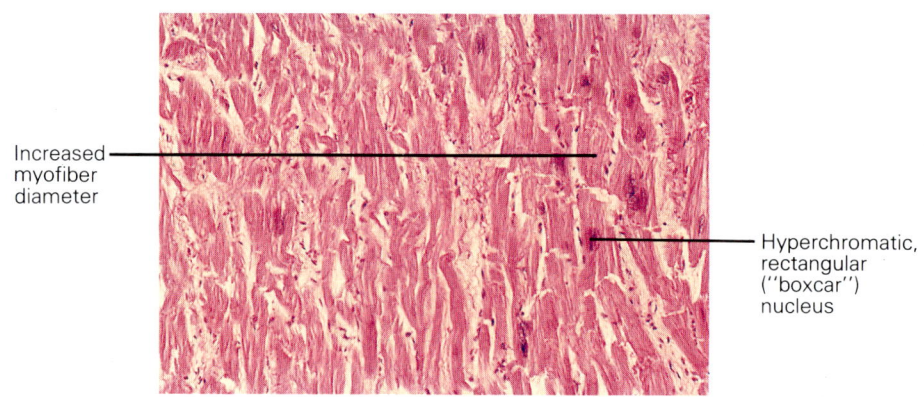

The microscopic changes of hypertrophy are associated with hypertensive heart disease and an increase in heart weight.

Figure 5.16
Myocarditis

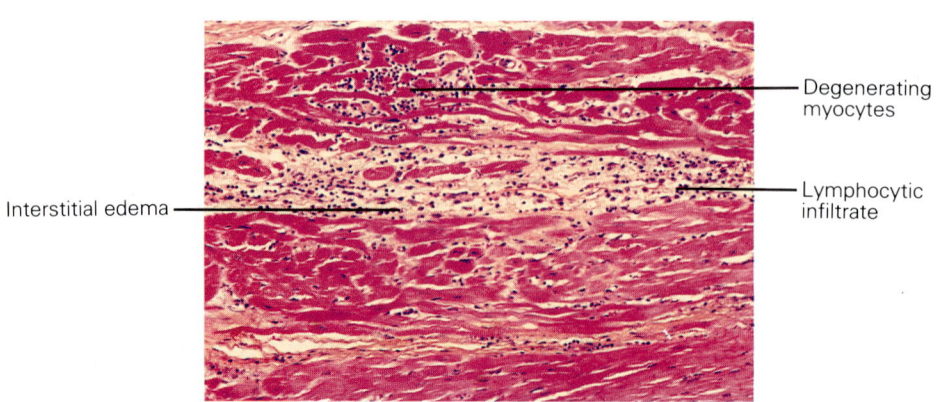

Myocarditis is defined as inflammation and necrosis or degeneration of myocardium.

Figure 5.17
Cardiomyopathy

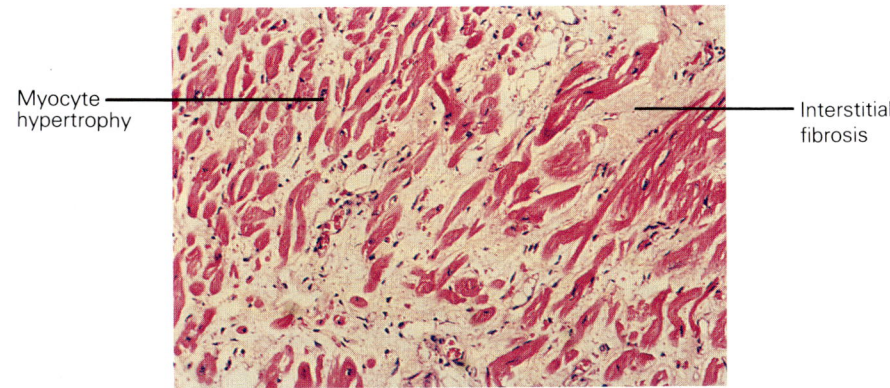

Histologic changes in cardiomyopathy are nonspecific. Classification is usually dependent on clinical data, gross appearances of the heart, and exclusion of coronary atherosclerosis, valvular disease, and hypertension.

Figure 5.18
Fibrinous pericarditis

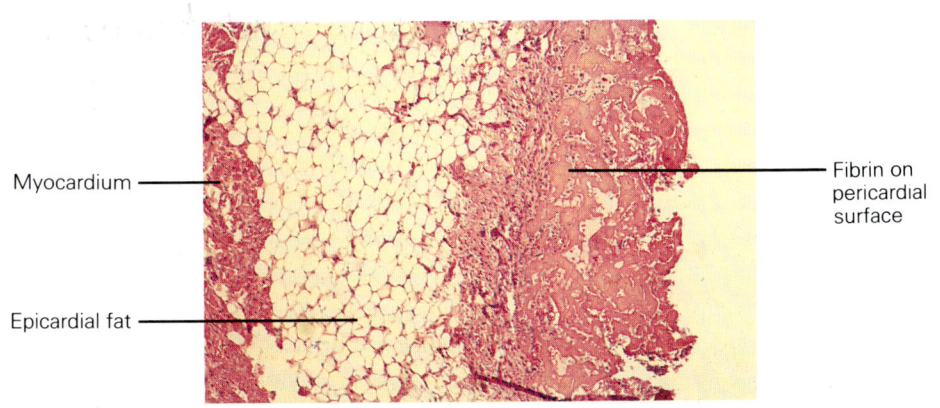

This is the most common form of pericarditis.

Figure 5.19
Hypersensitivity vasculitis

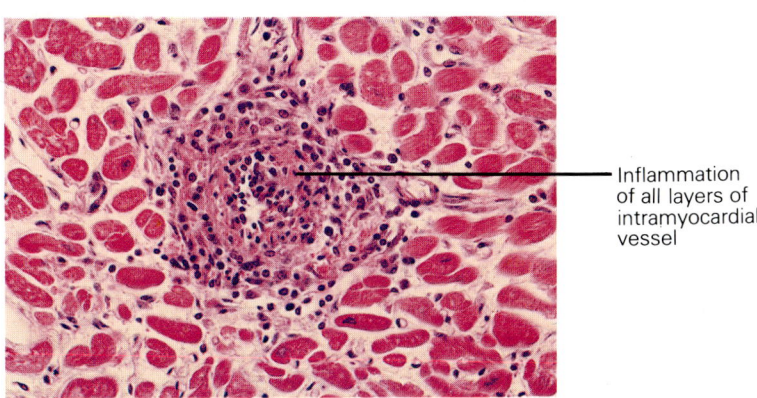

A hypersensitivity reaction to an antibiotic was responsible for the infiltrate of mononuclear cells and eosinophils seen in this vessel.

Figure 5.20
Temporal (giant cell) arteritis

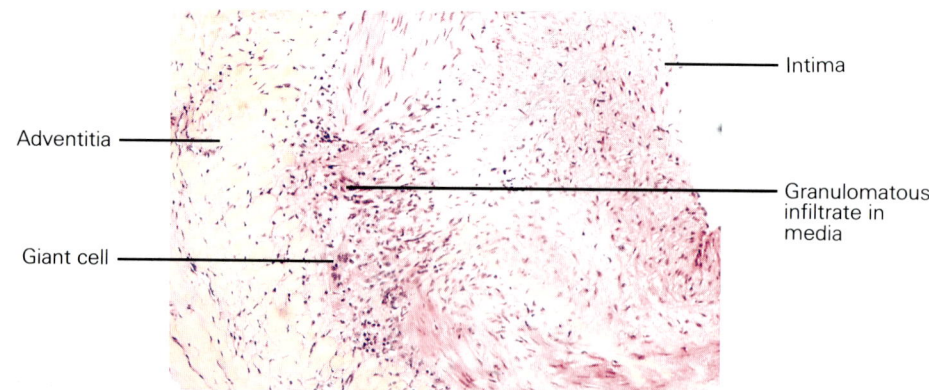

This is the most common form of vasculitis. Lesions are focal and may be missed on biopsy. Medium and small-sized cranial vessels are usually involved.

Figure 5.21
Polyarteritis nodosa (PAN)

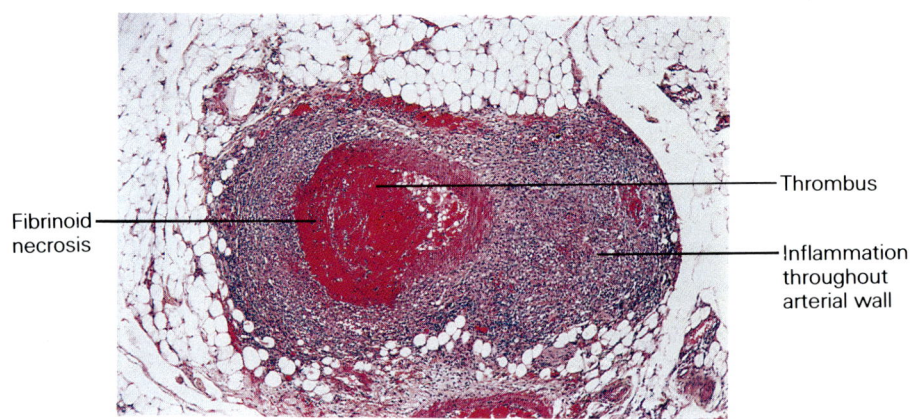

A medium-sized artery involved in PAN is shown here. A thrombus has formed over a severely affected portion of the vessel. Renal, cardiac, and hepatic arteries are commonly involved. One-third of cases have hepatitis B virus infection.

CHAPTER 6
PULMONARY PATHOLOGY

Figure 6.1
Lung

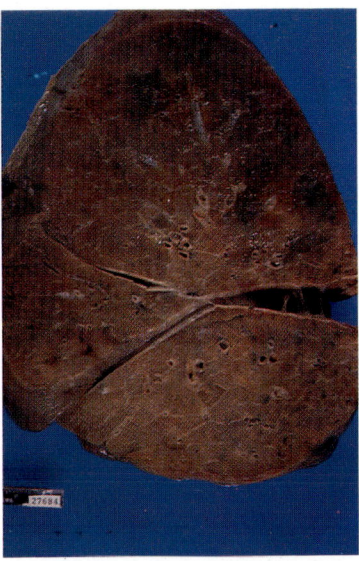

The upper lobe is congested. Normal weight: right (male, 455 g; female, 401 g) and left (male, 402 g; female, 345 g).

Figure 6.2A
Normal lung

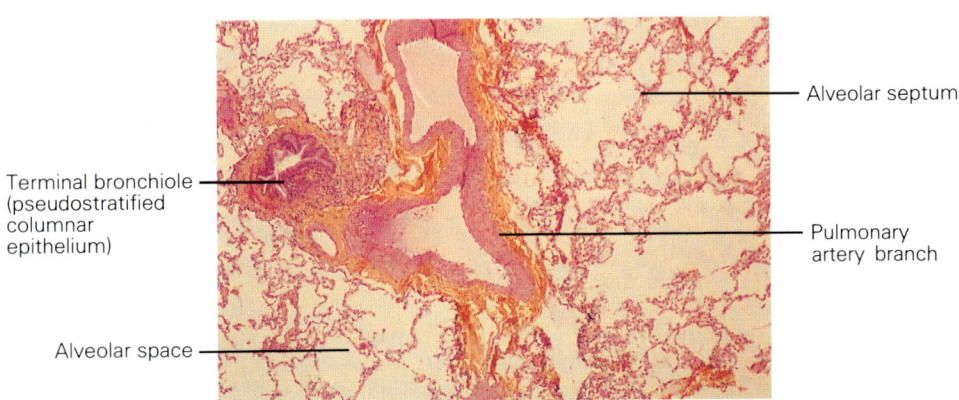

The low power microscopic examination of the lung assesses the relationship of pathologic lesions to alveoli, conducting airways, and vessels.

Figure 6.2B
Normal lung

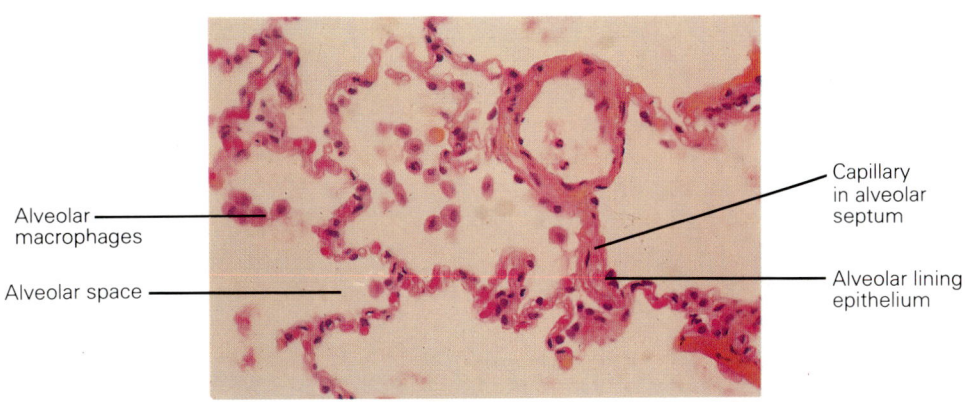

This field shows the normal microanatomy of alveoli.

Pulmonary Pathology

Figure 6.3
Respiratory system: major pathologic lesions

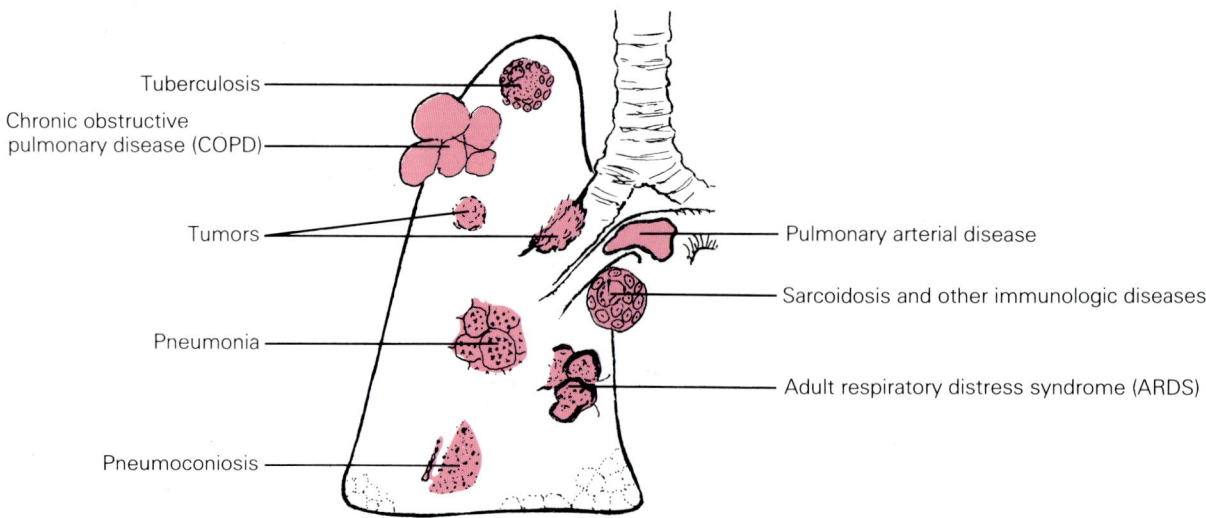

Tuberculosis includes primary tuberculosis (parenchymal Ghon focus and the Gohn complex, consisting of Ghon focus plus draining hilar lymph nodes), and secondary and late progressive pulmonary tuberculosis (apical caseating granulomas).

Chronic obstructive pulmonary disease (COPD) includes emphysema, chronic bronchitis, asthma, and bronchiectasis.

Tumors include bronchogenic carcinoma (squamous cell, adenocarcinoma, small cell, and large cell carcinoma), bronchioloalveolar carcinoma, bronchial carcinoids, and other miscellaneous tumors.

Pneumonia includes bronchopneumonia, lobar pneumonia, desquamative interstitial pneumonia (DIP), usual interstitial pneumonia (UIP), and other forms.

Pneumoconiosis is a disease of the lungs caused by inhalation of dusts. It includes asbestosis, coal workers' lung, silicosis, and berylliosis.

Pulmonary arterial disease: Prominent lesions include pulmonary artery thromboemboli with infarction and pulmonary vascular hypertension.

Sarcoidosis and other immunologic disorders: These disorders show evidence of immune-mediated damage in producing granulomas, parenchymal necrosis, or vasculitis. Examples include Goodpasture's disease and Wegener's granulomatosis.

Adult respiratory distress syndrome (ARDS): This clinical syndrome of respiratory insufficiency is associated with diffuse infiltrates on chest x-ray and hyaline membranes, alveolar hemorrhage, and interstitial edema. It may be due to infection, shock, and other conditions.

Figure 6.4
Pulmonary congestion

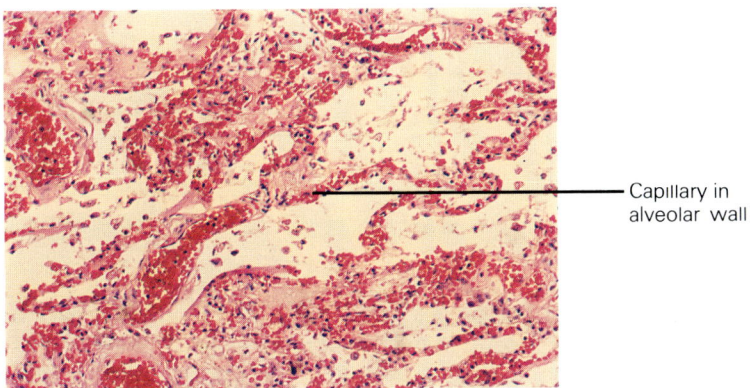

Lung of patient with left ventricular failure. Septal capillaries are engorged with blood.

Figure 6.5
Pulmonary edema

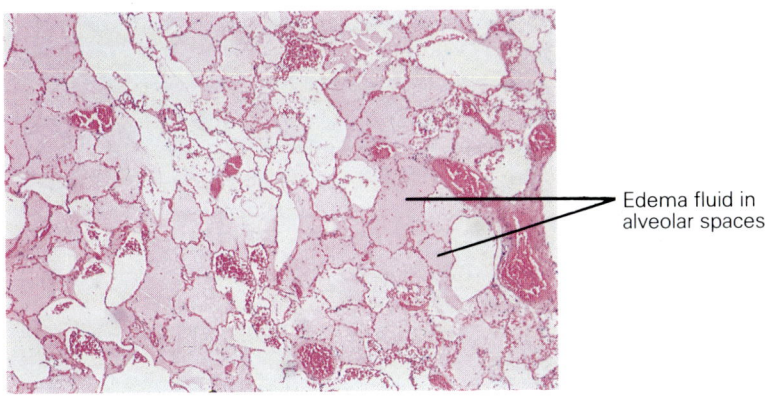

Lung with pulmonary edema from patient with congestive heart failure.

Figure 6.6
"Heart failure" cells

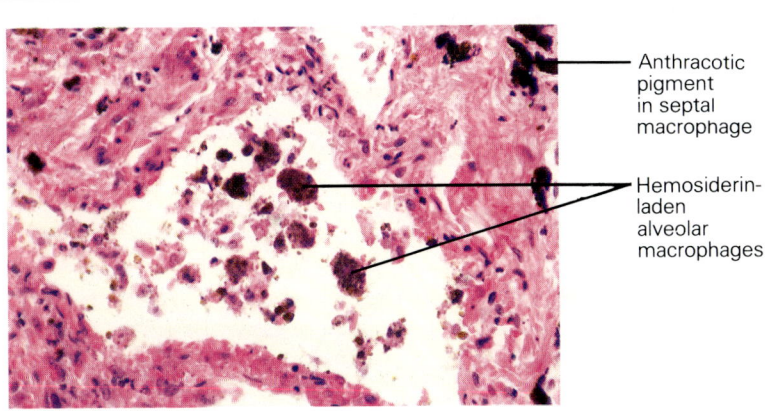

"Heart failure" cells (alveolar macrophages with hemosiderin) are seen in conditions of chronic pulmonary congestion (such as heart failure) or with recent alveolar hemorrhage.

Figure 6.7
Pulmonary embolus

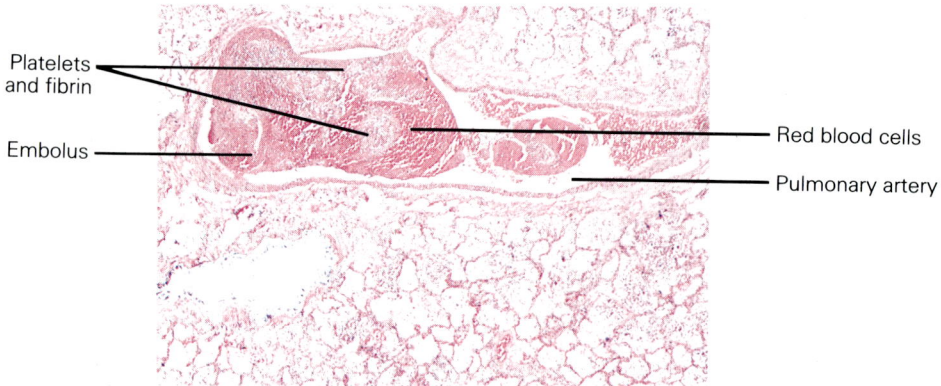

Pulmonary thromboemboli may arise in deep leg veins, pelvic veins, the inferior vena cava, or right side of heart. Less than 10 percent of emboli result in infarction.

Figure 6.8
Pulmonary infarct

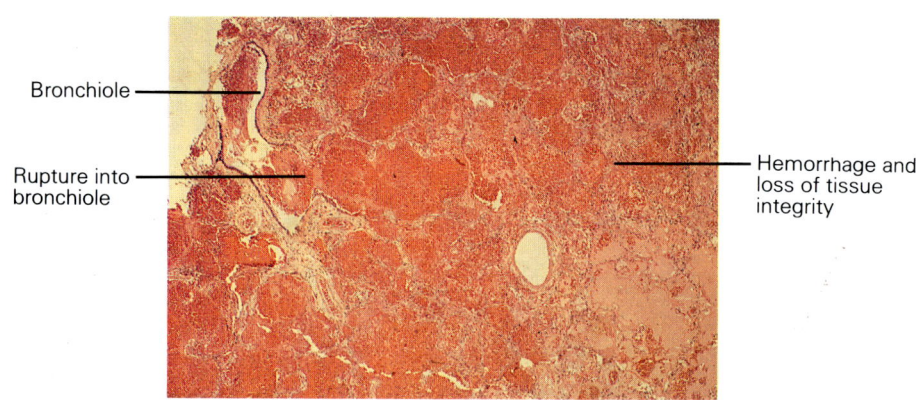

The pulmonary infarct shows breakdown of normal alveolar structures, hemorrhages, and loss of nuclear details throughout. This section demonstrates hemorrhage into a bronchiole, accounting for clinical hemoptysis.

Figure 6.9
Atelectasis

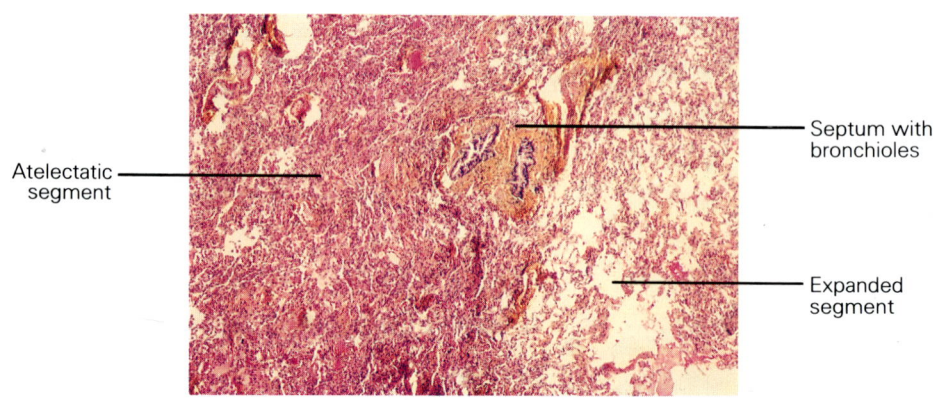

Collapse of lung tissue (atelectasis) may be due to airway obstruction, compression, fibrosis, or loss of surfactant.

Figure 6.10
Purulent bronchitis

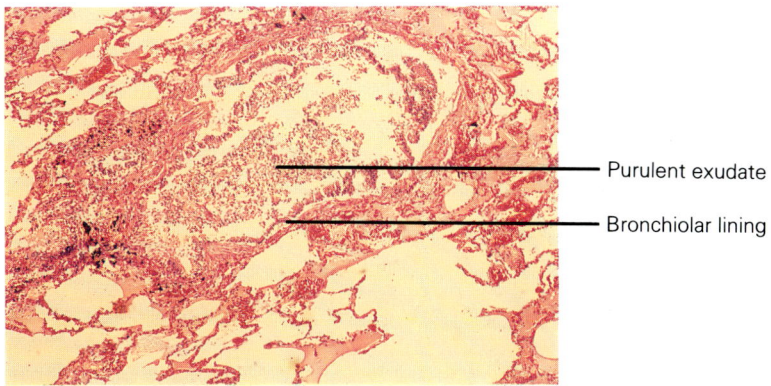

This condition is related to cigarette smoking, mucus hypersecretion, and hypertrophy of submucosal glands in the trachea and bronchi.

Figure 6.11
Chronic bronchitis

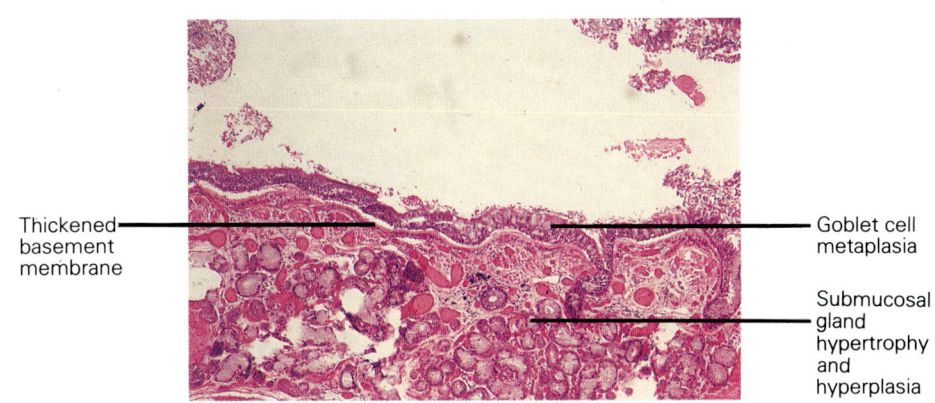

The changes shown here are associated with persistent cough and sputum production.

Figure 6.12
Emphysema

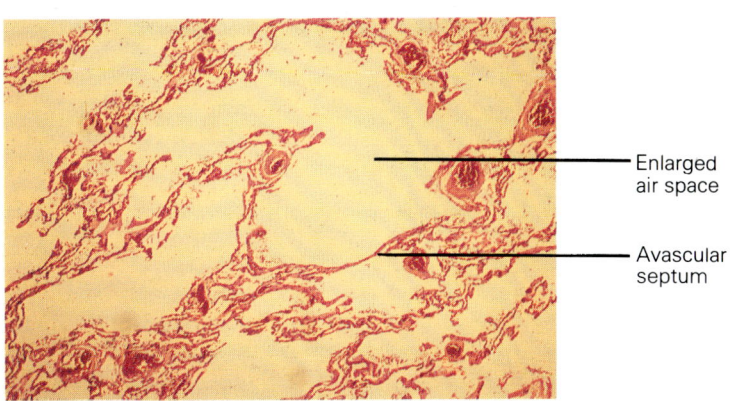

This condition is defined as enlargement of distal air spaces with destruction of their walls. Two major types, centrilobular (related to smoking) and panacinar (associated with alpha-1-antitrypsin deficiency), are based on the anatomic distribution of airway destruction.

Pulmonary Pathology

Figure 6.13
Diffuse alveolar damage (DAD)

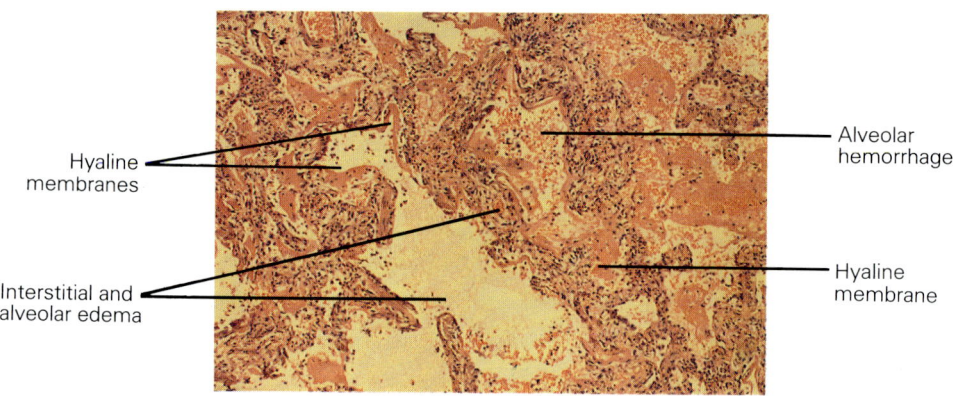

The histologic picture of DAD is associated with clinical adult respiratory distress syndrome (ARDS) due to infections, shock, radiation, and other causes.

Figure 6.14
Usual interstitial pneumonia (UIP)

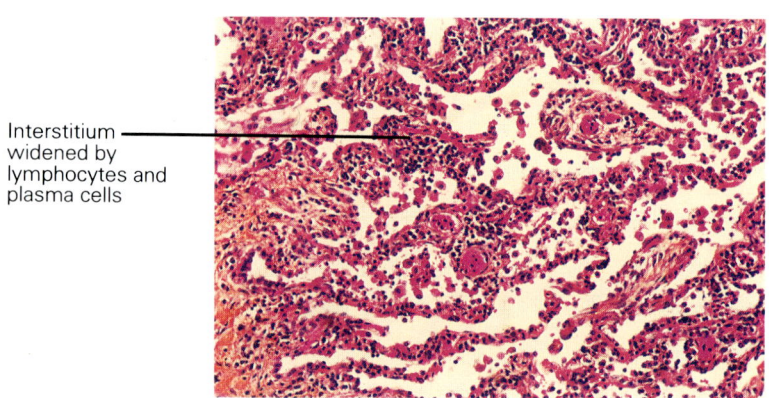

A patchy, interstitial pneumonia of uncertain etiology that pursues a chronic, progressive downhill course.

Figure 6.15
Desquamative interstitial pneumonia (DIP)

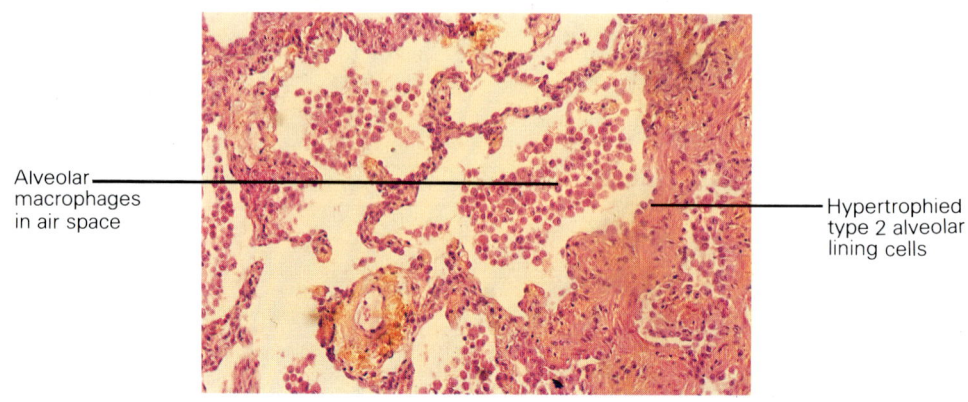

An interstitial pneumonia characterized by steroid responsiveness.

Figure 6.16
Bronchiolitis obliterans

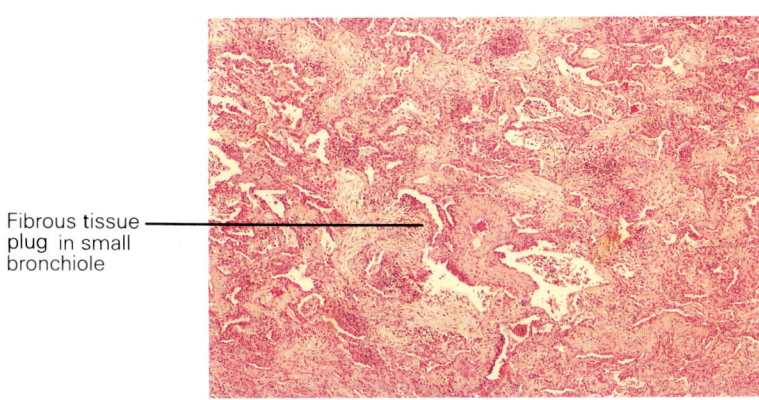

Terminal and respiratory bronchioles are plugged by polypoid masses of fibrous tissue in this pulmonary response to respiratory syncytial virus or adenovirus infection, silo filler's disease, or other insults.

Figure 6.17
Acute bronchopneumonia

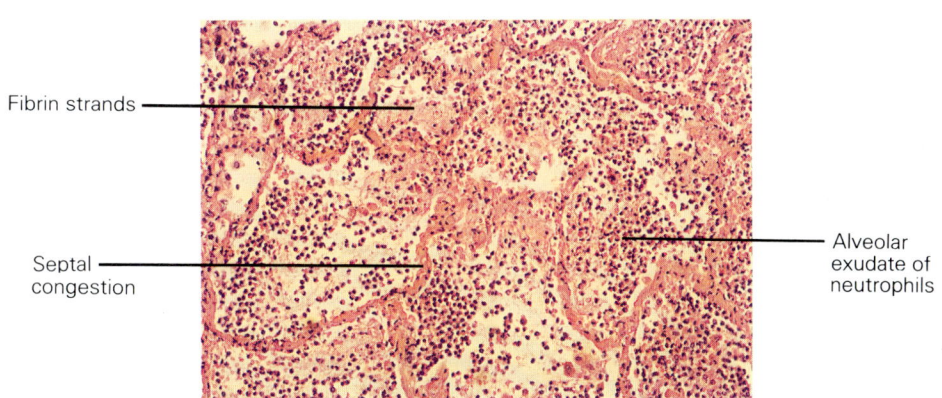

In bronchopneumonia, phases of red hepatization (alveolar neutrophils and extravasated red cells, septal congestion) and gray hepatization (alveolar fibrin, disintegrating neutrophils) are seen, usually followed by resolution.

Figure 6.18
Organizing pneumonia

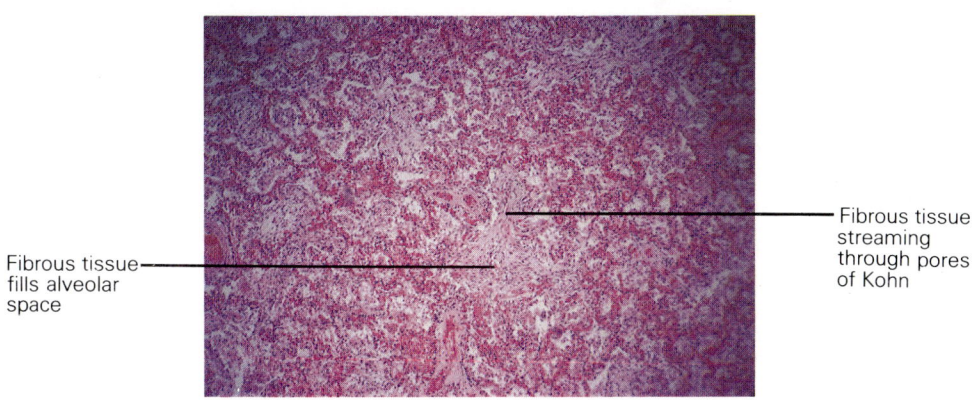

"Organization" of pneumonia represents a complication, by which lung parenchyma is converted to fibrous tissue scar.

Pulmonary Pathology

Figure 6.19
Pneumocystis pneumonia

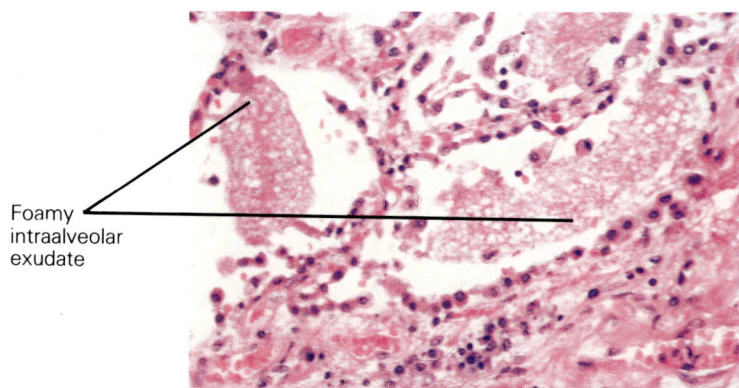

Pneumocystis organisms can be identified within the exudate on silver stains. This is the most common infection in patients with acquired immune deficiency syndrome (AIDS).

Figure 6.20
Cytomegalovirus (CMV) pneumonia

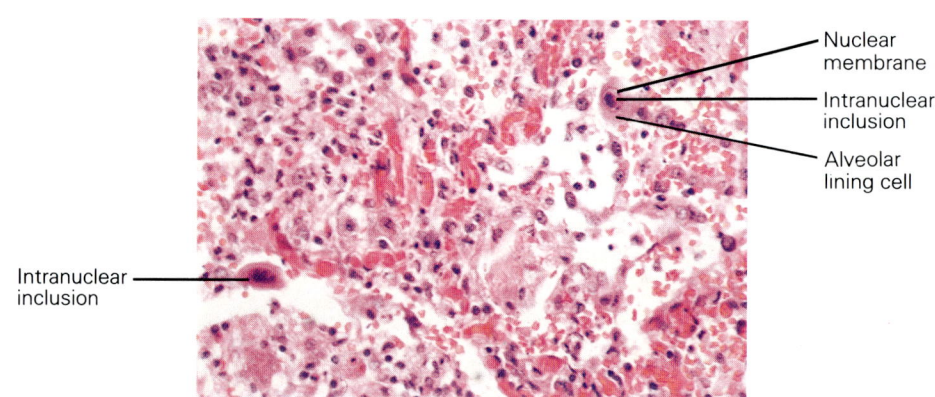

This lung section shows marked congestion in CMV pneumonia. Basophilic, intranuclear inclusions are seen in several cell types here. Smaller, basophilic cytoplasmic inclusions (see Figure 4.11) representing intracellular virions may also be seen.

Figure 6.21
Goodpasture's syndrome

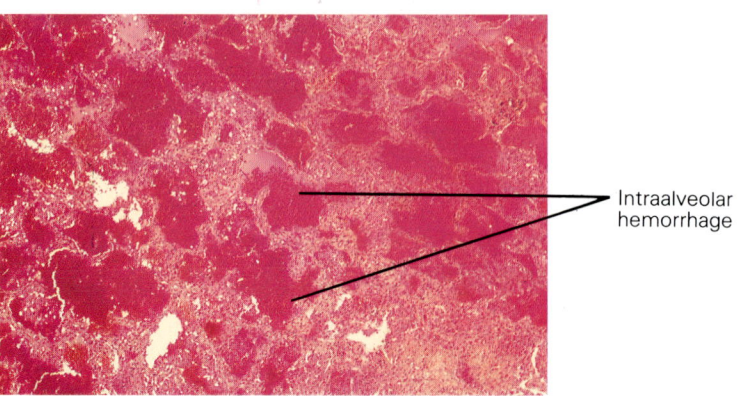

This necrotizing, hemorrhagic pneumonia is associated with rapidly progressive glomerulonephritis. Linear deposits of antibasement membrane antibodies are identified in lungs and kidneys.

Figure 6.22
Wegener's granulomatosis

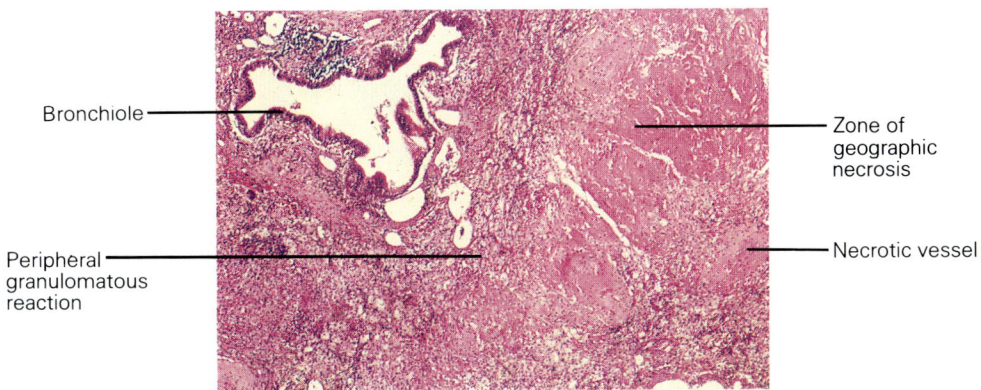

This disease of middle-aged adults combines necrotizing granulomatous pulmonary inflammation, upper respiratory tract vasculitis, and necrotizing glomerulonephritis.

Figure 6.23
Sarcoidosis

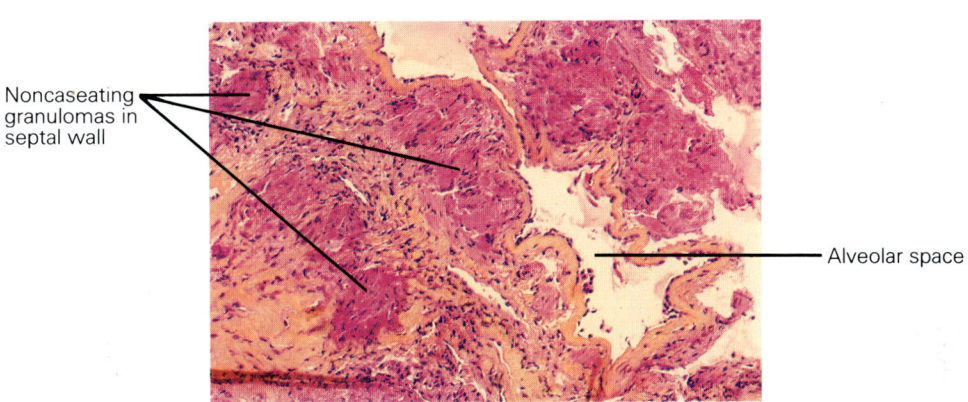

Common sites of involvement by sarcoid granulomas are hilar and mediastinal lymph nodes, lungs, and liver. Clinical findings include cutaneous anergy, positive Kveim test, and elevated serum angiotensin converting enzyme (ACE).

Figure 6.24
Pulmonary tuberculosis

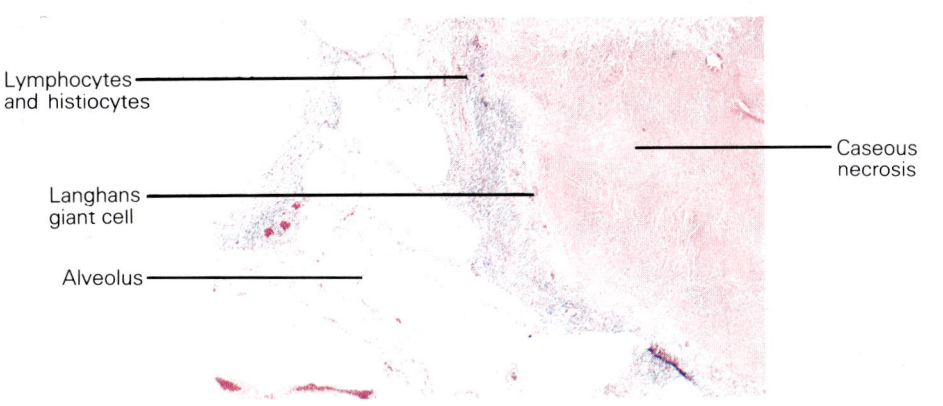

The tuberculous granuloma shown consists of a peripheral rim of lymphocytes, histiocytes, and Langhans' giant cells with central caseation necrosis.

Figure 6.25
Hamartoma of lung

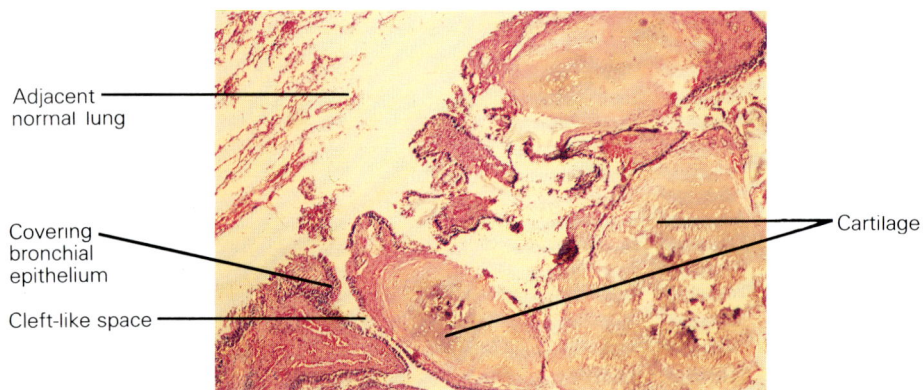

Hamartomas consist of normal tissues indigenous to an organ arranged abnormally in a mass. Lung hamartomas are several centimeter diameter benign cartilagenous masses seen as rounded densities on chest radiographs.

Figure 6.26
Squamous cell carcinoma with invasion

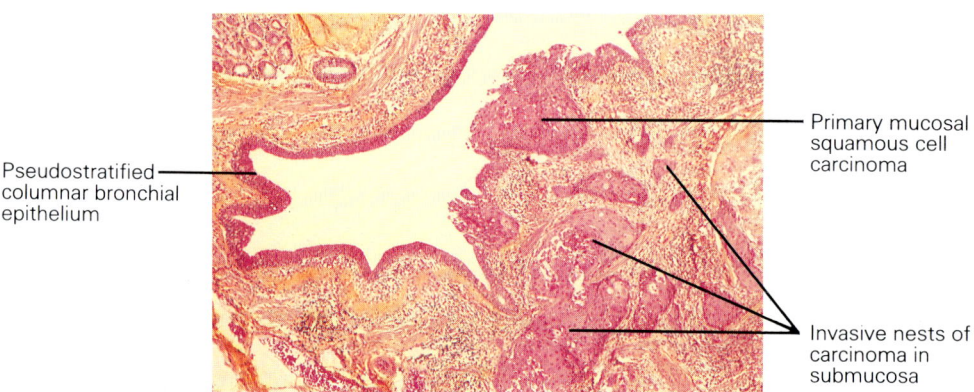

As the most common variety of bronchogenic carcinoma, this tumor arises in bronchial mucosa near the hilum. It is related to smoking.

Figure 6.27
Adenocarcinoma

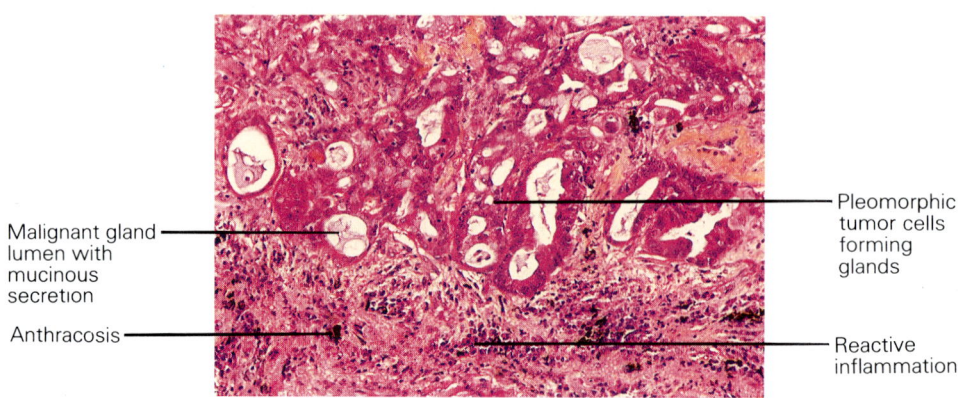

These tumors may arise peripherally in the lung. They are less frequently associated with a smoking history than are squamous carcinomas.

Figure 6.28
Bronchioloalveolar carcinoma

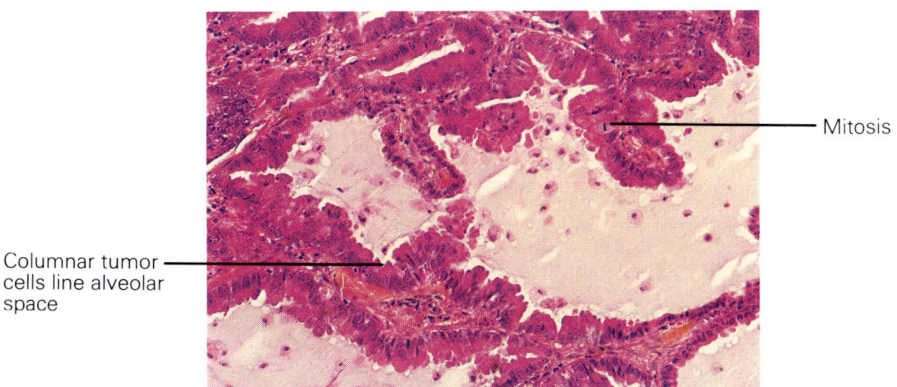

The tumor arises in terminal bronchioles and alveoli of the lung periphery, with growth of columnar tumor cells along the alveolar walls. Papillary projections into alveoli are formed.

Figure 6.29
Small cell ("oat cell") carcinoma

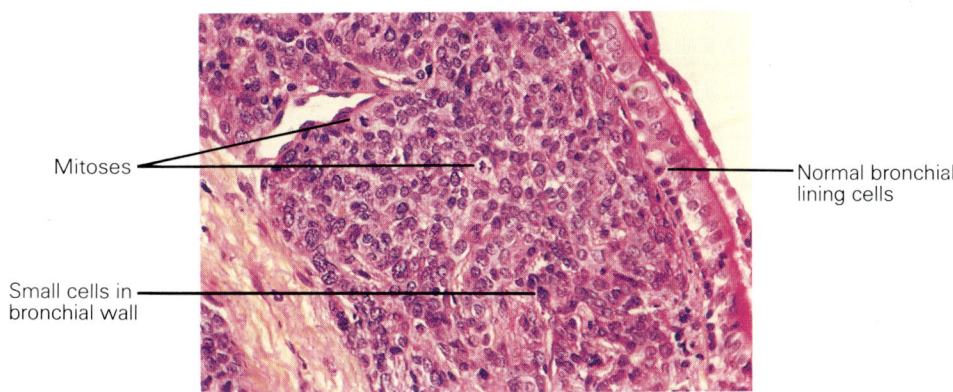

This highly malignant tumor consists of clusters of small, lymphocyte-like ("oat cell") tumor cells containing neurosecretory granules. It is the most common tumor associated with ectopic hormone production and is related to smoking.

Figure 6.30
Asbestosis

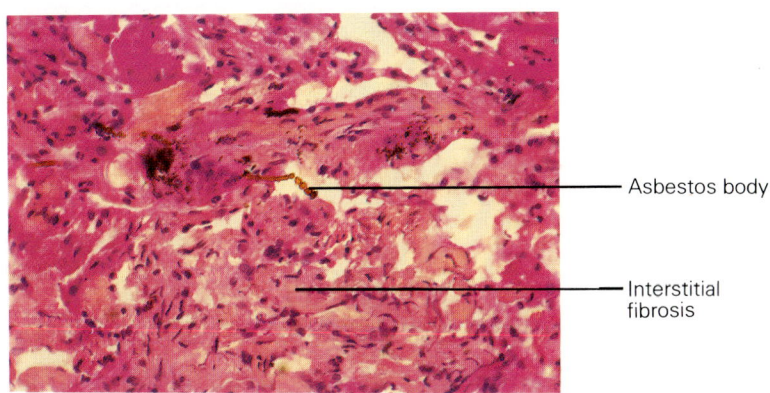

Asbestos bodies, within macrophages or in the interstitium, are associated with interstitial fibrosis, lung carcinoma, and pleural mesothelioma. Once coated with iron they are termed "ferruginous bodies."

Figure 6.31
Mesothelioma (malignant sarcomatoid type)

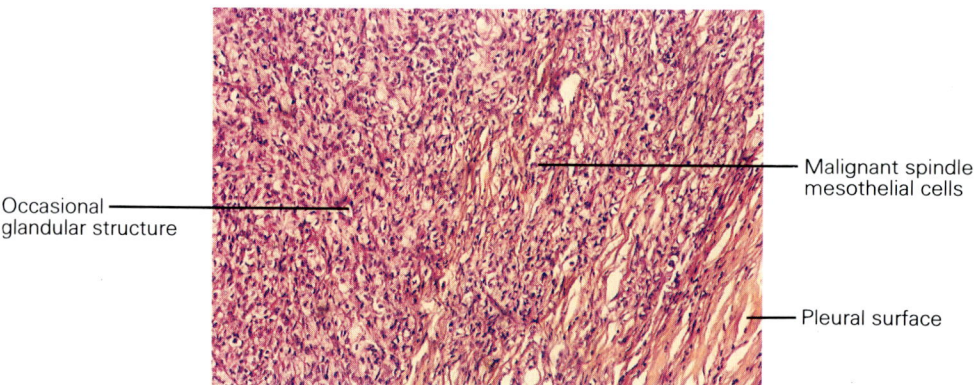

Mesotheliomas may be benign and localized or malignant and associated with invasion and pleural effusions. Fibrous (sarcomatoid) and epithelial types exist. The tumor is associated with asbestosis.

Figure 6.32
Vocal cord polyp ("singer's node")

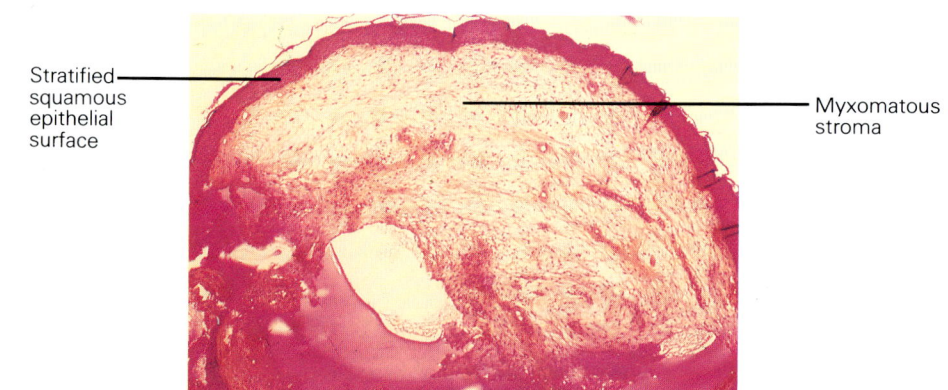

These small, benign polypoid nodules of the larynx are seen in smokers and singers. They usually occur on the true vocal cords and produce hoarseness.

Figure 6.33
Papilloma of larynx

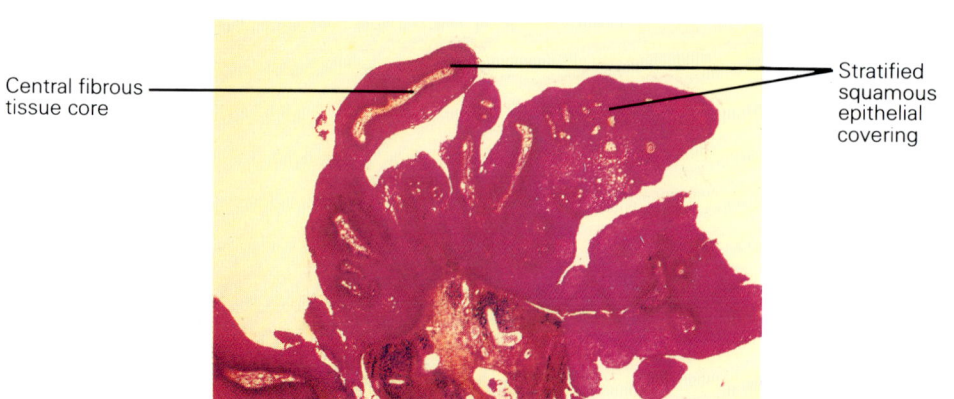

This is a small, benign, squamous neoplasm caused by human papillomavirus II infection. The laryngeal surface is thrown into papillary projections with central fibrous tissue cores.

Figure 6.34
Invasive squamous cell carcinoma of larynx

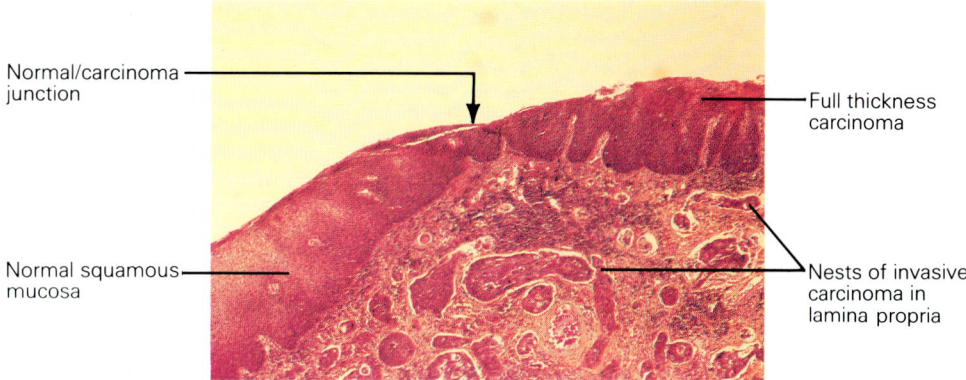

Note the lack of maturation of cells toward the surface in the full thickness mucosal carcinoma at right, compared to normal maturation at left.

Figure 6.35
Nasopharyngeal carcinoma

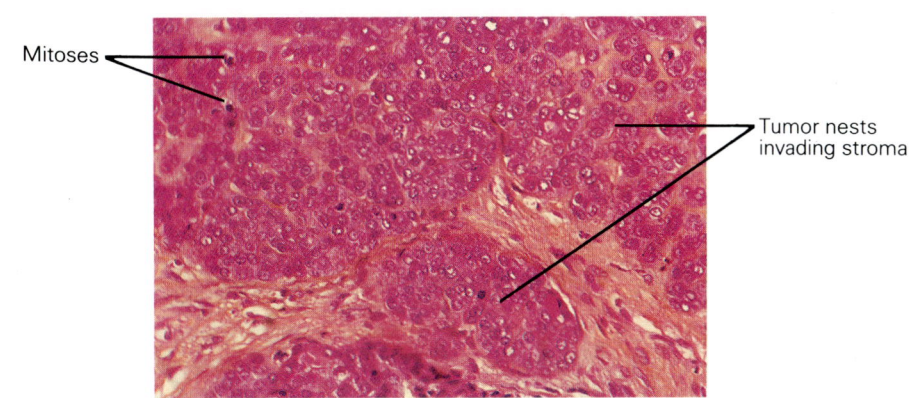

The tumor shown here consists of poorly differentiated, nonkeratinizing squamous cell carcinoma. Epstein-Barr virus infection is pathogenetically related to this lesion.

CHAPTER 7
HEMATOPATHOLOGY

Figure 7.1
Normal bone marrow

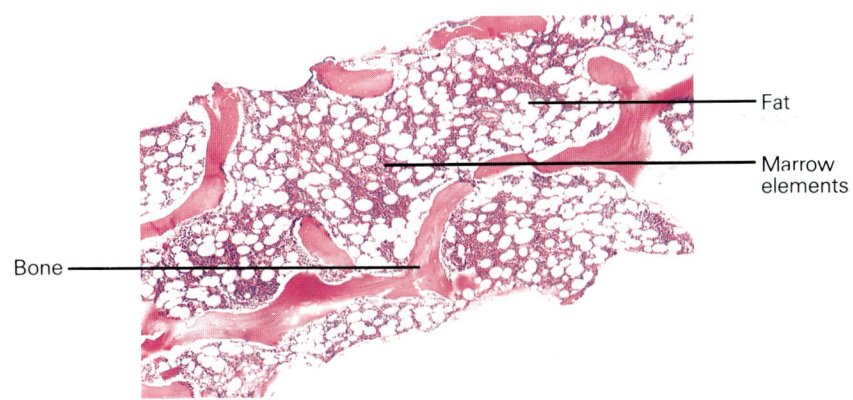

The bone marrow normally contains 50 percent marrow cells and 50 percent fat.

Figure 7.2
Normal bone marrow

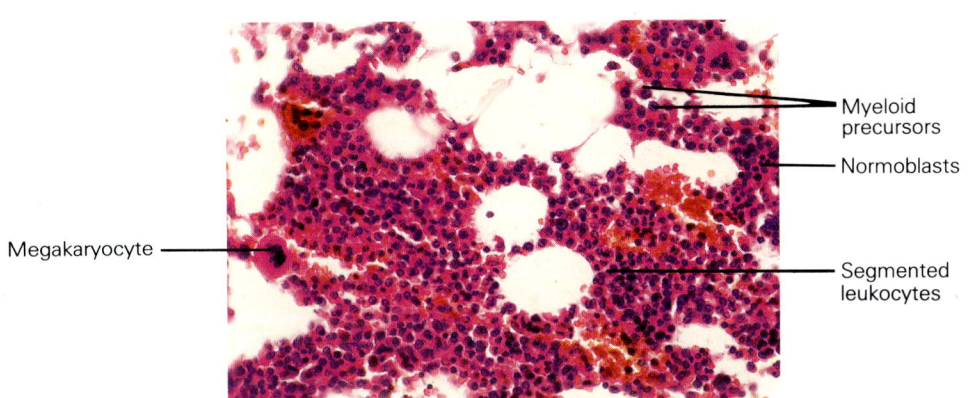

Representatives of all hematopoietic elements should be present in the normal marrow.

Figure 7.3
Bone marrow granulocytosis

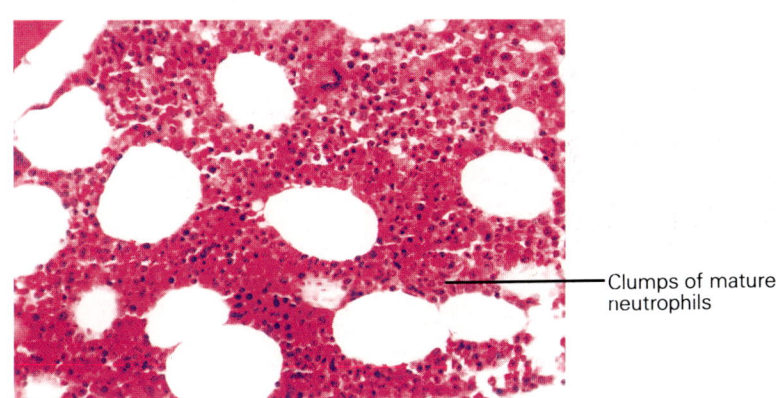

Granulocytosis is associated with peripheral blood leukocytosis and systemic infections.

Figure 7.4
Hematopoietic system: major pathologic lesions

Red blood cells

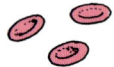

Anemia
   Blood loss
   Increased destruction (e.g., sickle cell disease)
   Decreased production (e.g., iron deficiency anemia, megaloblastic anemia, and marrow stem cell failure)

White blood cells

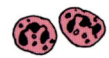

Leukopenia
Leukocytosis
Leukemoid reaction
Leukemia

Platelets

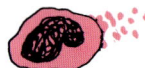

Thrombocytopenia
Thrombocytosis

Bone marrow

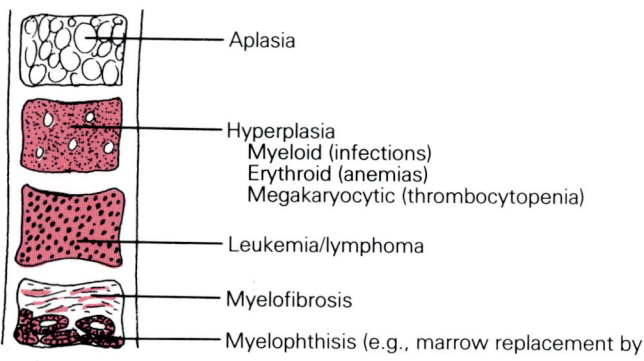

Aplasia

Hyperplasia
   Myeloid (infections)
   Erythroid (anemias)
   Megakaryocytic (thrombocytopenia)

Leukemia/lymphoma

Myelofibrosis

Myelophthisis (e.g., marrow replacement by carcinoma)

Lymph nodes

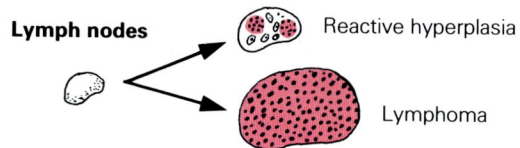

Reactive hyperplasia

Lymphoma

Spleen

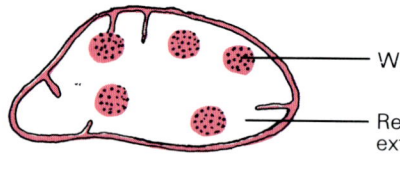

White pulp disease (reactive hyperplasia, lymphoma)

Red pulp disease (congestion, infarcts, sepsis, extramedullary hematopoiesis, hemosiderosis, leukemia)

Figure 7.5
Aplastic anemia

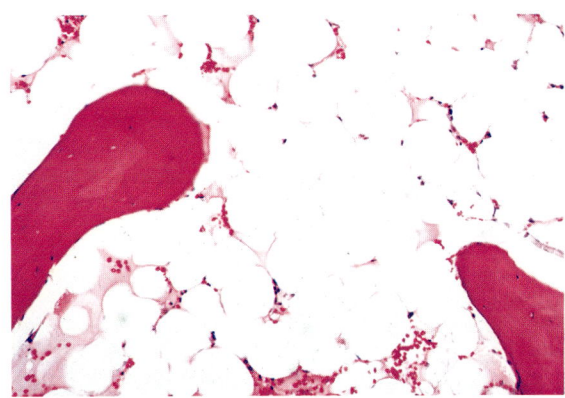

The marrow is devoid of cellular elements and shows fat and scattered small capillaries. This is associated with chemical or drug exposure, whole body irradiation, and non-A, non-B hepatitis.

Figure 7.6
Sickle cell anemia

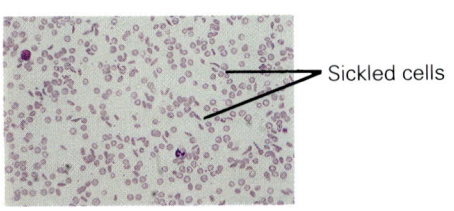

Peripheral smear.

Figure 7.7
Iron deficiency anemia

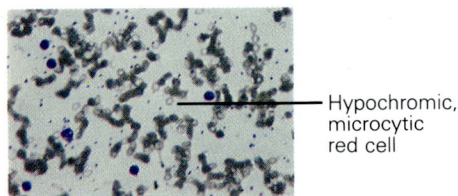

Peripheral smear.

Megaloblastic Anemia

Figure 7.8
Marrow aspirate

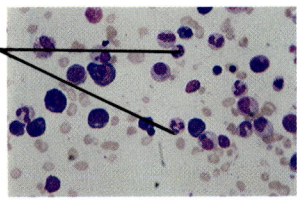

Figure 7.9
Marrow biopsy

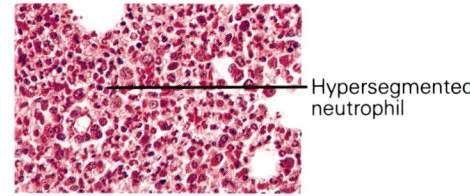

Megaloblastic anemia, due to pernicious anemia (B_{12} deficiency) or folate deficiency, results in impaired cell maturation and division. Erythrocytes, their precursors, and white blood cell forms show enlargement with increased nuclear size and lobation. Neutrophilic leukocytes show as many as five lobes or more in their nuclei.

Hematopathology

Figure 7.10
Bone marrow hemosiderosis

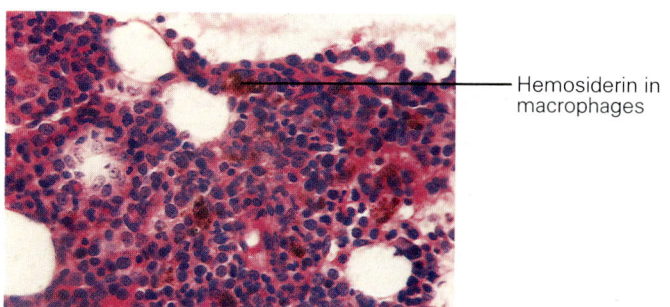

Ineffective utilization of storage iron results in excess hemosiderin marrow stores.

Figure 7.11
Gaucher's disease

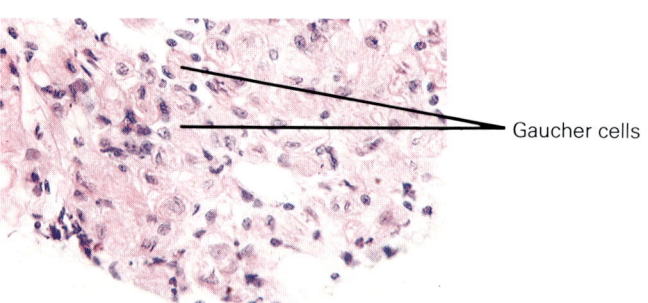

The marrow is infiltrated by Gaucher cells (macrophages). On this periodic acid-Schiff (PAS) stain, the cytoplasmic glucocerebroside appears as "wrinkled tissue paper" or striations.

Figure 7.12
Bone marrow granuloma

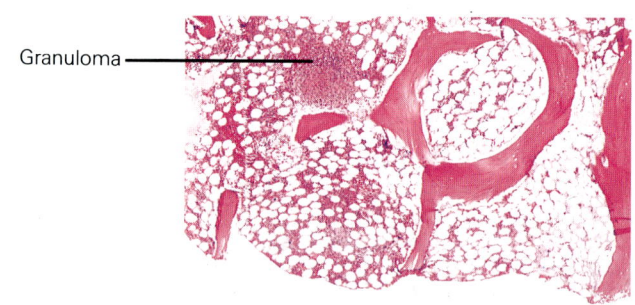

Causes of bone marrow granulomas include tuberculosis, sarcoidosis, drug reactions, and fungal infections.

Figure 7.13
Lymphoid aggregate in aging

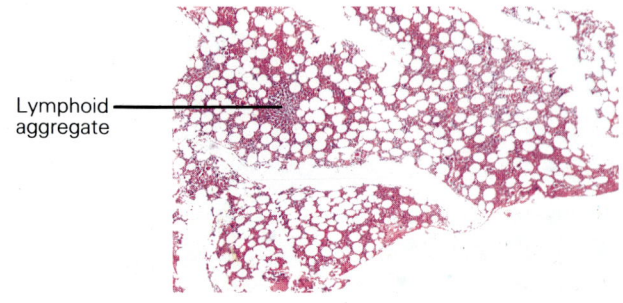

Rare, scattered lymphoid aggregates may be seen in bone marrow specimens from the elderly.

LEUKEMIAS

Figure 7.14
Leukemia in bone marrow biopsy

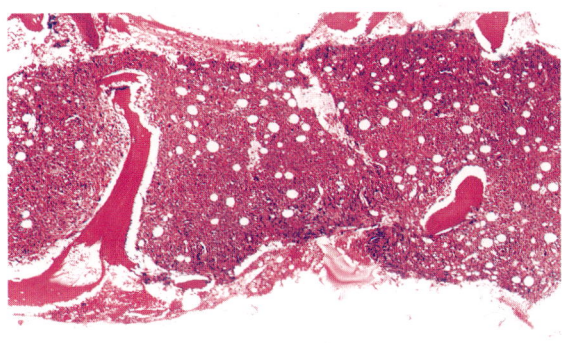

The marrow hypercellularity is due to infiltration by leukemic cells. Note reduction in fat, compared to Figure 7.1. Leukemias are defined as malignant proliferations of white blood cell precursors.

Acute Lymphocytic Leukemia (ALL)

Figure 7.15
Acute lymphocytic leukemia in bone marrow

Figure 7.16
Acute lymphocytic leukemia in peripheral smear

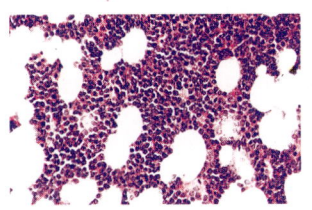
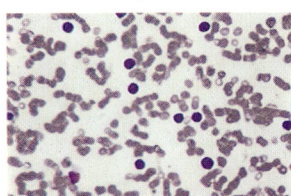

Leukemic lymphocytes infiltrate the marrow spaces and are seen in the peripheral blood. The majority of these cells express common ALL (CALLA) antigen on their surfaces.

Acute Myelogenous Leukemia (AML)

Figure 7.17
Acute myelogenous leukemia in bone marrow

Figure 7.18
Acute myelogenous leukemia in peripheral smear

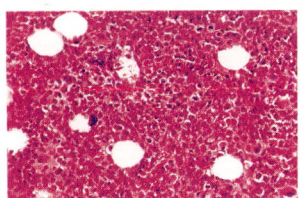
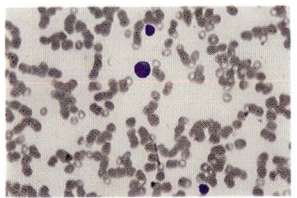

The leukemic marrow infiltrate consists of immature myeloid cells. Auer rods (red cytoplasmic rods) derived from myeloid cell granules can be identified in AML.

Chronic Lymphocytic Leukemia (CLL)

Figure 7.19
Chronic lymphocytic leukemia in bone marrow

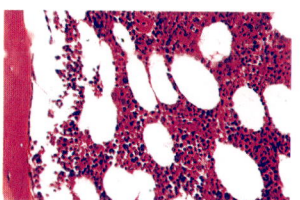

Figure 7.20
Chronic lymphocytic leukemia in peripheral smear

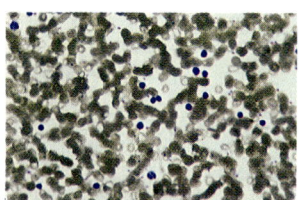

Leukemic infiltrates in CLL appear as homogeneous, small lymphocytes.

Figure 7.21
Chronic lymphocytic leukemia in lymph node

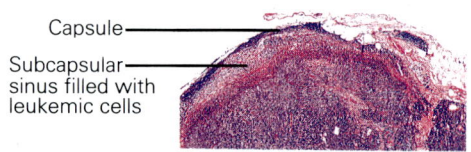

Capsule
Subcapsular sinus filled with leukemic cells

Figure 7.22
Chronic lymphocytic leukemia in liver

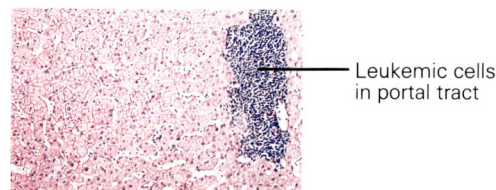

Leukemic cells in portal tract

Involvement of lymph nodes by CLL is histologically indistinguishable from well differentiated lymphocytic lymphoma. In the liver, CLL infiltrates are seen within portal tracts.

Chronic Myelogenous Leukemia (CML)

Figure 7.23
Chronic myelogenous leukemia in bone marrow

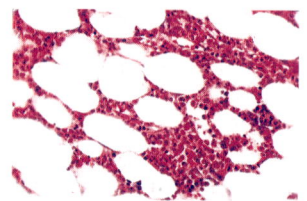

Figure 7.24
Chronic myelogenous leukemia in peripheral smear

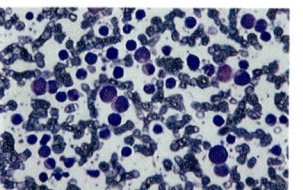

CML infiltrates characteristically show morphologically diverse immature myeloid forms. Splenomegaly is most prominent in CML.

Hairy Cell Leukemia

Figure 7.25
Peripheral smear

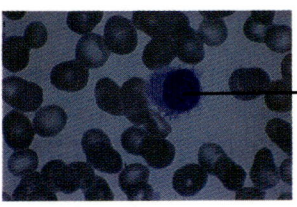
Leukemic cell with "hairy" cytoplasmic processes

Figure 7.26
Liver involvement

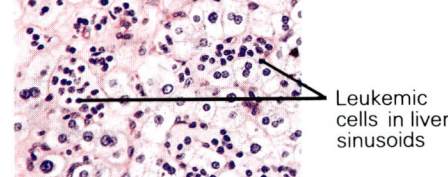
Leukemic cells in liver sinusoids

This leukemia is characterized by the distinctive "hairy" appearance of the neoplastic cells which stain positively for tartrate-resistant acid phosphatase (TRAP), pancytopenia, and splenomegaly. In the liver section above, note that many leukemic cells appear separated from the sinusoidal wall by an empty space or halo due to the cytoplasmic processes (which are poorly seen without oil immersion).

Erythroleukemia

Figure 7.27
Bone marrow

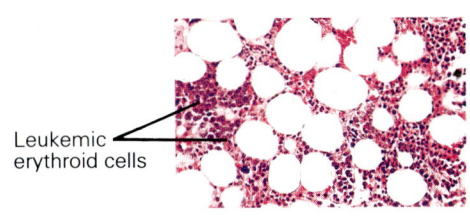
Leukemic erythroid cells

Figure 7.28
Peripheral smear

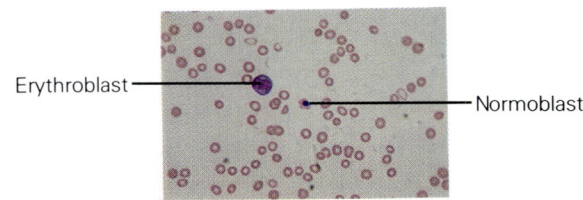
Erythroblast — Normoblast

Acute erythroleukemia (Di Guglielmo's syndrome) is classified as the M6 variant of acute myelogenous leukemia in the French-American-British (FAB) system.

MYELOID METAPLASIA WITH MYELOFIBROSIS

Figure 7.29
Marrow myelofibrosis

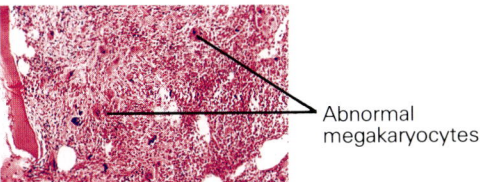
Abnormal megakaryocytes

Figure 7.30
Marrow reticulin stain

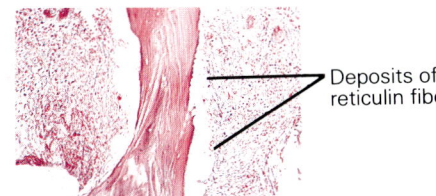
Deposits of reticulin fibers

Myeloid metaplasia with myelofibrosis is one of the myeloproliferative syndromes (which also include chronic myelogenous leukemia, polycythemia vera, and idiopathic thrombocythemia). The marrow undergoes fibrosis (with characteristic excess fiber demonstrated on reticulin stain) and may contain abnormal megakaryocytes. Extramedullary hematopoiesis develops in distant sites such as the spleen.

Hematopathology

MULTIPLE MYELOMA

Figure 7.31
Bone marrow

Figure 7.32
Russell bodies

Multiple myeloma, a monoclonal neoplastic proliferation of plasma cells, is associated with monoclonal (M) protein immunoglobulin spikes on serum electrophoresis, bony lytic lesions, and marrow infiltrates of both mature and immature plasma cell forms. Engorged immunoglobulin within plasma cells may appear as round, balloon-like red inclusions (Russell bodies) in myeloma cells and in normal plasma cells.

Figure 7.33
Waldenström's macroglobulinemia

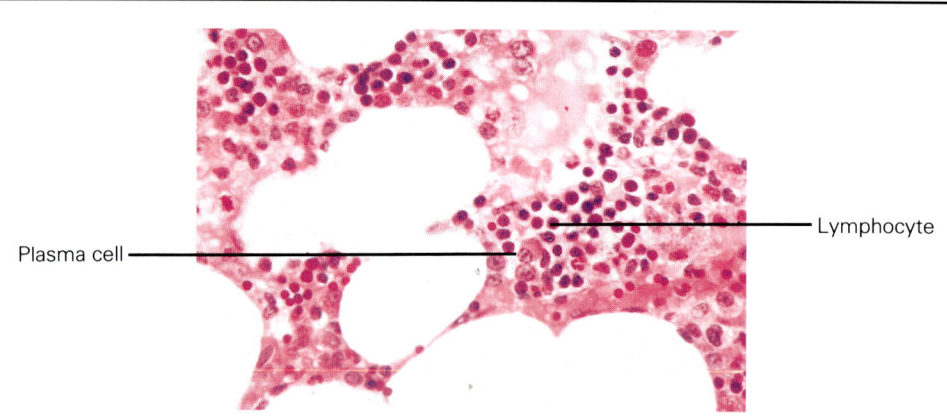

This is a lymphocyte-plasma cell malignancy of the bone marrow associated with a monoclonal IgM protein peak in serum.

Figure 7.34
Myelophthisis of bone marrow

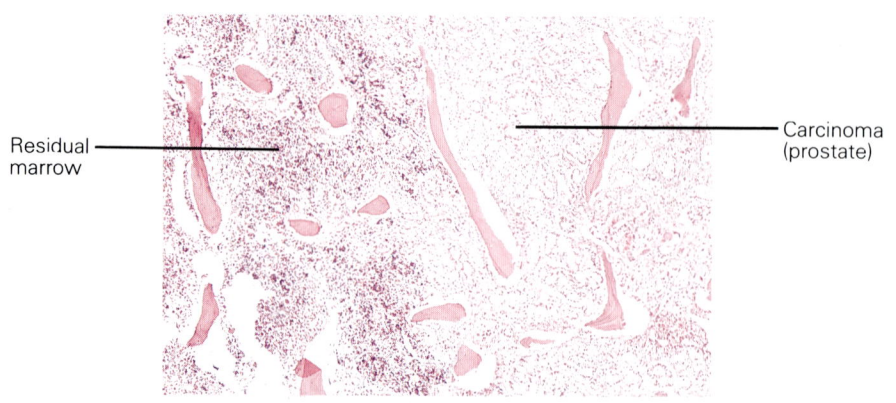

In myelophthisis, replacement of marrow by nonhematopoietic elements (such as the adenocarcinoma shown here) results in anemia, leukopenia, and/or thrombocytopenia.

Figure 7.35
Normal lymph node

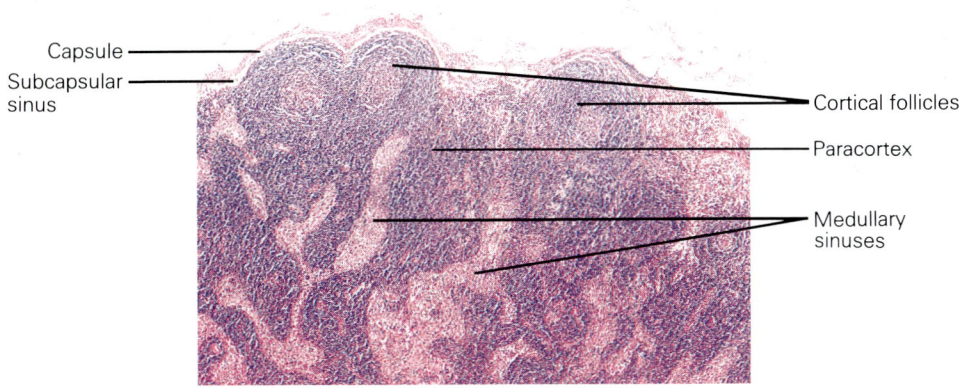

On low magnification, note the capsule, cortical follicles, and medullary sinuses.

Figure 7.36
Follicular hyperplasia

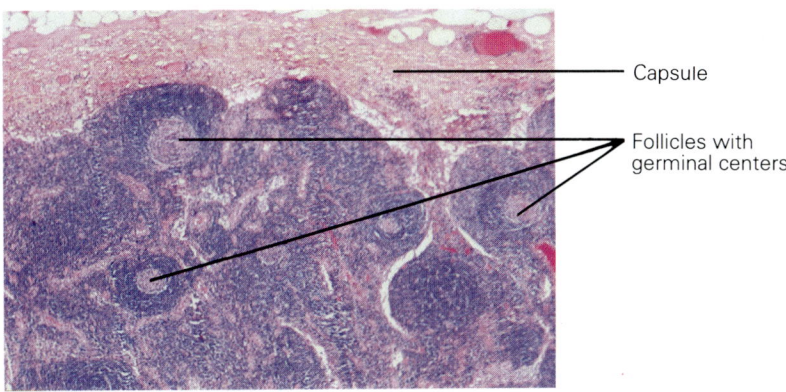

Increased number and size of cortical follicles is seen in antigenic stimulation of these B-cell areas, as in rheumatoid arthritis and syphilis.

Figure 7.37
Sinus histiocytosis

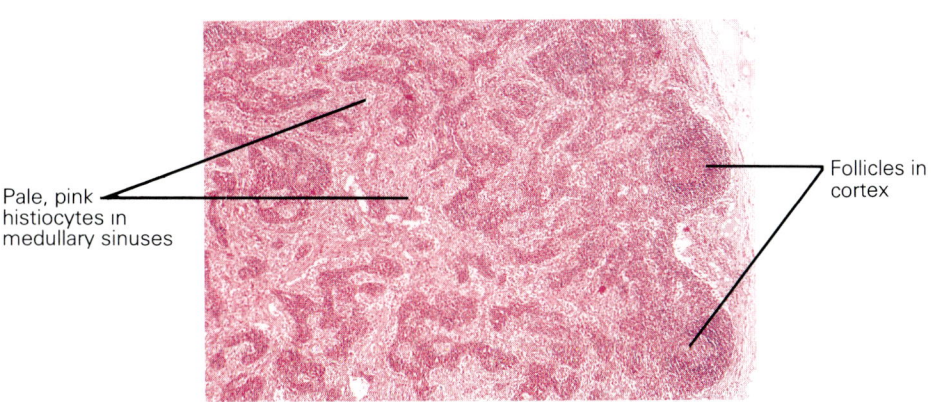

This change is common in nodes draining the extremities and in nodes near carcinoma.

Figure 7.38
Angioimmunoblastic lymphadenopathy

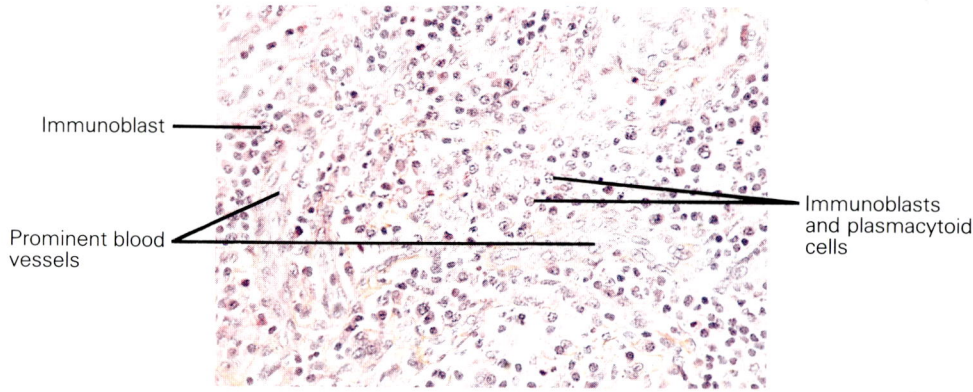

This disorder of elderly individuals shows lymph node effacement by a proliferating immunoblast and plasma cell population with abundant blood vessels. Mortality is related to severe infections or malignant transformation.

Figure 7.39
Lymphoid-depleted lymph node in AIDS

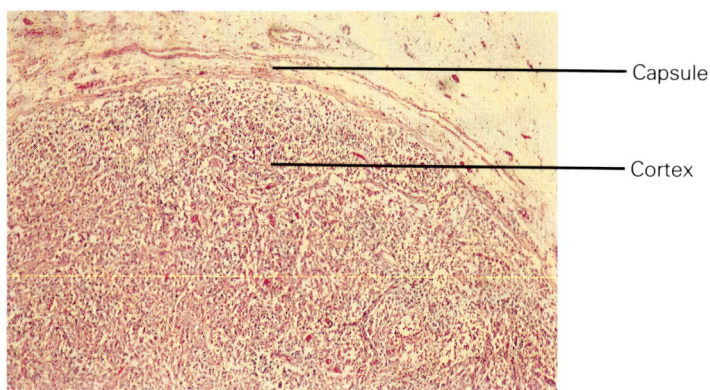

Lymph nodes in the late stages of lymphoid depletion in acquired immune deficiency syndrome show loss of cortical and paracortical lymphocytes, leaving an "open"-appearing underlying vascular and connective tissue framework.

LYMPHOMAS

Figure 7.40
Classification of lymphomas

Malignant lymphomas
Monoclonal neoplasms of lymphoid cells (including lymphocytes, histiocytes, and their precursors and derivatives)

- Hodgkin's lymphoma (HL)
  - Diagnostic Reed-Sternberg cell
  - Rye classification
    - Nodular sclerosing
    - Mixed cellularity
    - Lymphocyte-predominant
    - Lymphocyte-depleted

- Non-Hodgkin's lymphoma (NHL)
  - Nodal architecture
    - Follicular (nodular)
    - Diffuse
  - Working formulation for clinical usage
    - Low grade
      - Small lymphocytic
      - Follicular, small cleaved cell
      - Follicular, small and large cleaved cell
    - Intermediate grade
      - Follicular, large cell
      - Diffuse, small cleaved cell
      - Diffuse, large cell
    - High grade
      - Large cell, immunoblastic
      - Lymphoblastic
      - Small noncleaved cell
    - Miscellaneous

Figure 7.41
Malignant lymphoma (gross)

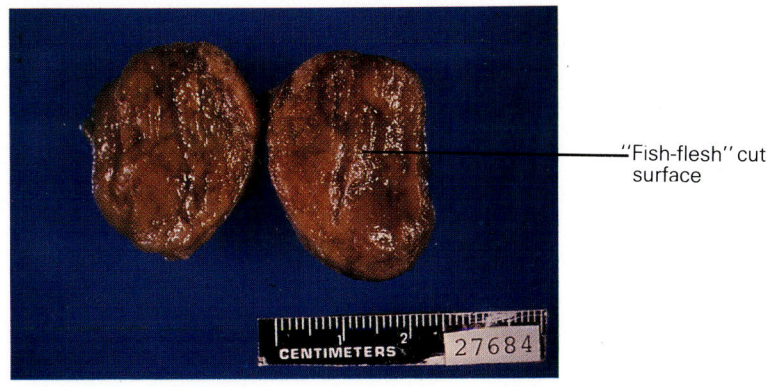

"Fish-flesh" cut surface

Lymph nodes in lymphoma are enlarged and show a rubbery, pale, "fish-flesh" cut surface.

Hematopathology

Figure 7.42
Diffuse non-Hodgkin's lymphoma

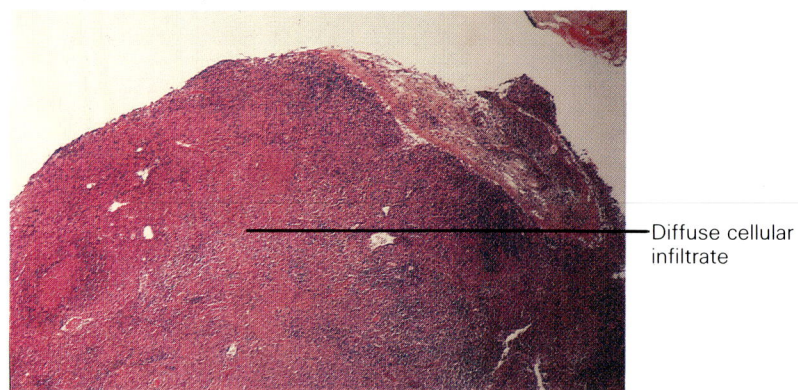

The nodal architecture is obliterated by a diffuse, homogeneous sea of cells.

Figure 7.43
Follicular (nodular) non-Hodgkin's lymphoma

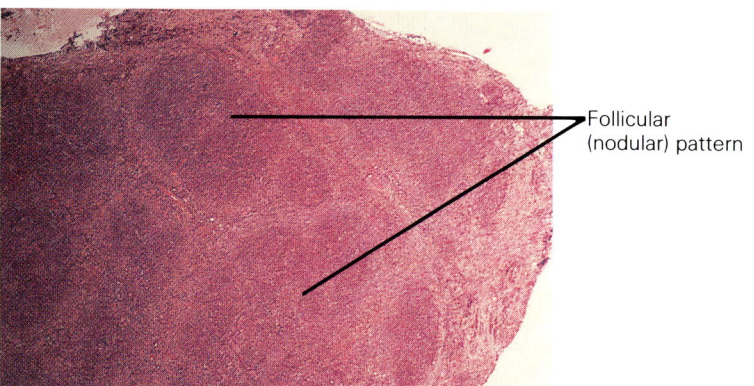

The nodal architecture is obliterated by neoplastic lymphocytes arranged in follicles.

Figure 7.44
Lymphoma extension into fat

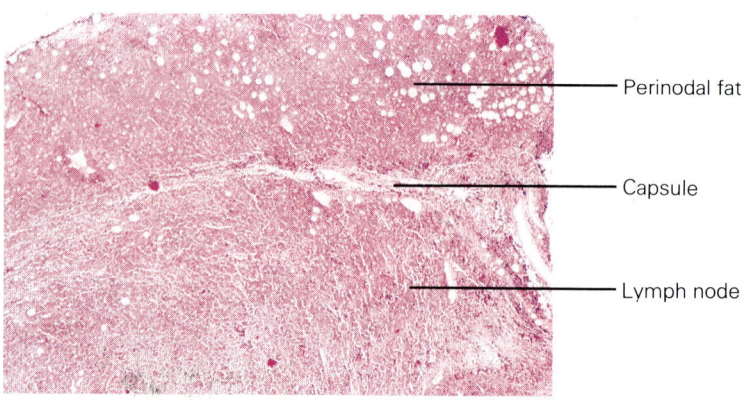

In addition to nodal architectural effacement, neoplastic cells may invade into the perinodal fat.

Figure 7.45
Lymphoma in bone marrow

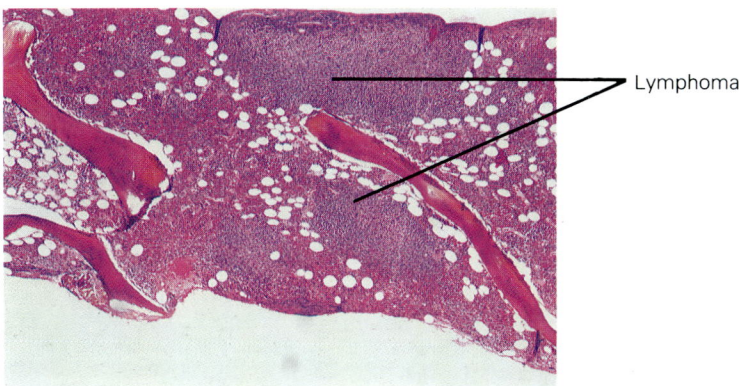

Areas of dense cellular infiltrate that replace marrow fat represent lymphoma.

Figure 7.46
Gastric lymphoma

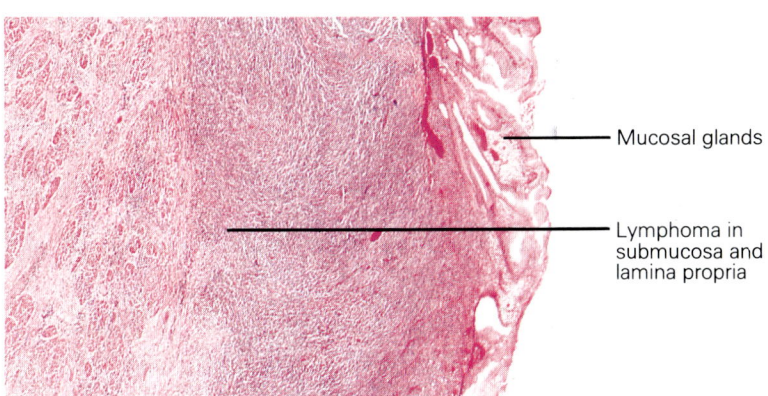

Although lymphomas may secondarily involve the gastrointestinal tract, they may arise primarily in its lymphoid tissue. Primary gastric lymphoma accounts for less than 5 percent of gastric malignancies.

Figure 7.47
Non-Hodgkin's lymphoma

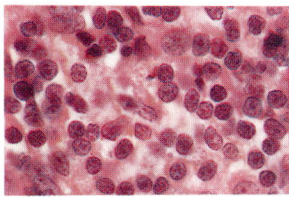

Small cell type.

Figure 7.48
Non-Hodgkin's lymphoma

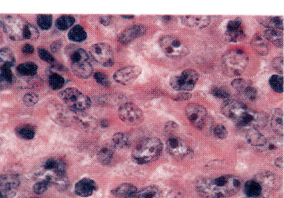

Large cell type.

Figure 7.49
Non-Hodgkin's lymphoma

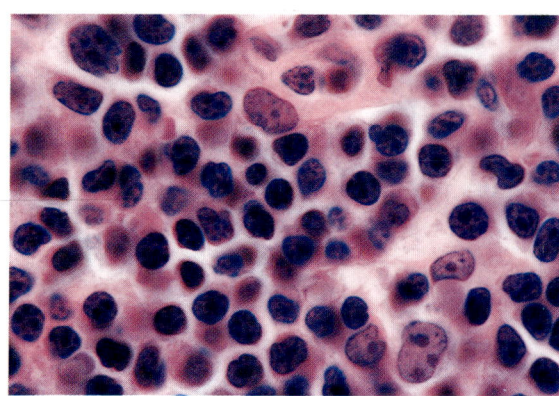

Mixed small cell/large cell type.

Figure 7.50
Non-Hodgkin's lymphoma

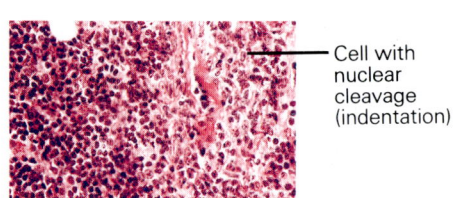

Small cell, cleaved type.

Figure 7.51
Non-Hodgkin's lymphoma

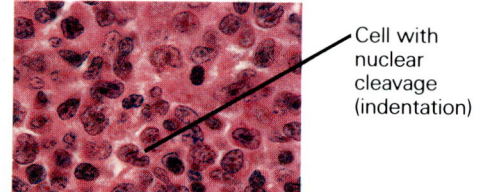

Large cell, cleaved type.

Figure 7.52
Burkitt's lymphoma

Figure 7.53
Burkitt's lymphoma

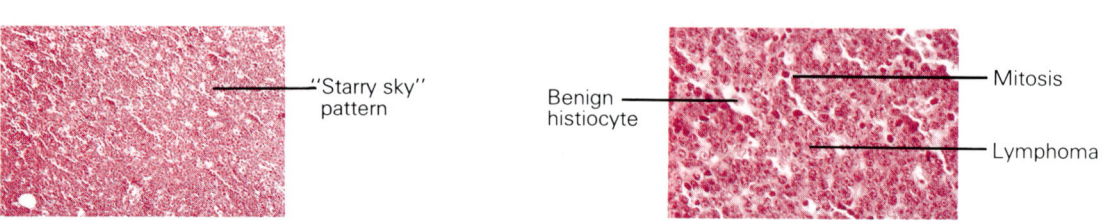

This is an undifferentiated, non-Hodgkin's lymphoma of B-cell origin. The "starry sky" pattern results from benign histiocytes with a surrounding clear space being interspersed among tumor cells. Evidence points to Epstein-Barr virus as the stimulus for B-cell proliferation. African (maxillary, mandibular) and American (abdominal tumors) forms are recognized.

80 *Histopathology of Disease*

Figure 7.54
Immunoblastic lymphoma

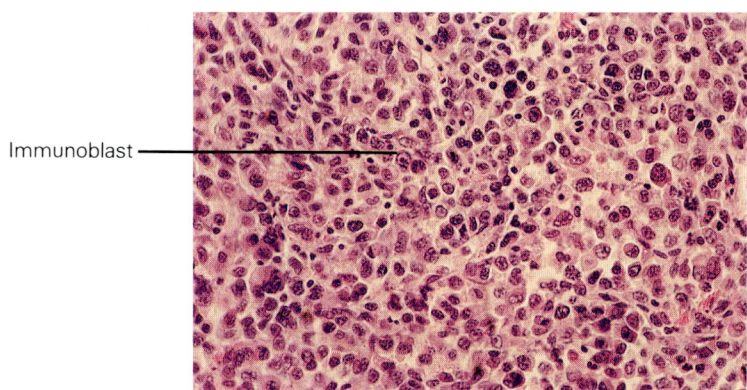

Tumor cells include immunoblasts with prominent central nuclei and others with plasmacytoid features.

Figure 7.55
Mycosis fungoides

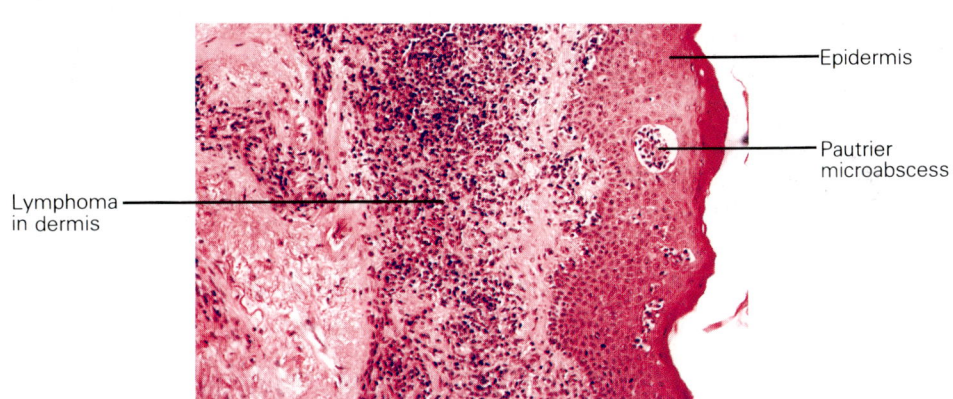

A T-cell lymphoma showing skin involvement and epidermal Pautrier microabscesses containing lymphoma cells.

Figure 7.56
Cutaneous T-cell lymphoma

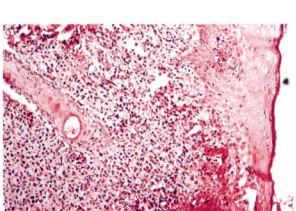

Dermal tumor infiltrate.

Figure 7.57
Cutaneous T-cell lymphoma

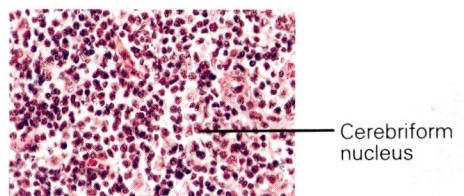

Tumor cells show cerebriform convolutions of their nuclei.

Figure 7.58
Hodgkin's lymphoma

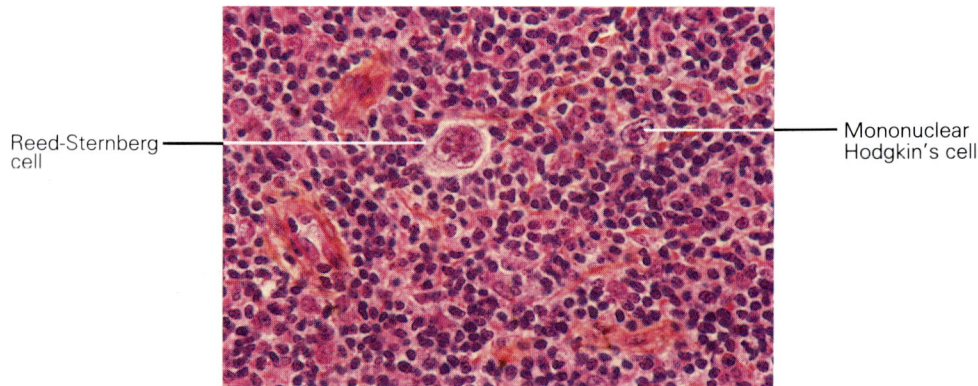

The diagnostic Reed-Sternberg (R-S) cell is large with a multilobated nucleus and prominent inclusion-like nucleoli. The R-S cell shown above is binuclear and with its prominent nucleoli has an "owl-eye" appearance. Although controversial, the R-S cell and variants such as mononuclear Hodgkin's cells and lacunar cells (not shown) are believed to be macrophages in origin.

Figure 7.59
Nodular sclerosing Hodgkin's lymphoma

Figure 7.60
Nodular sclerosing Hodgkin's lymphoma

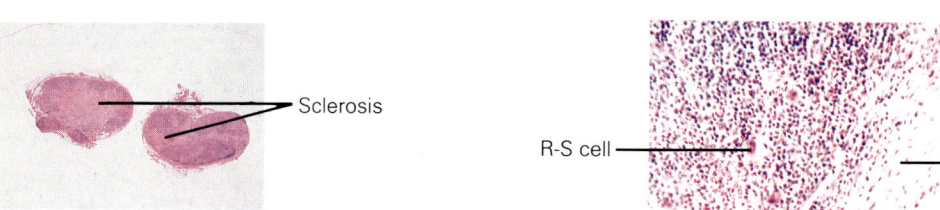

Figure 7.61
Mixed cellularity Hodgkin's lymphoma

Figure 7.62
Lymphocyte-predominant Hodgkin's lymphoma

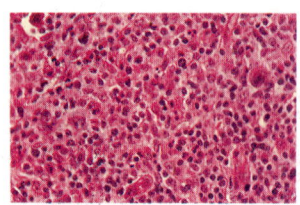
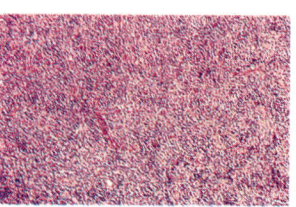

In addition to R-S cells, the background includes lymphocytes, plasma cells, and eosinophils.

R-S cells are scarce in this form which shows abundant lymphocytes.

82 *Histopathology of Disease*

Figure 7.63
Lymphocyte-depleted Hodgkin's lymphoma

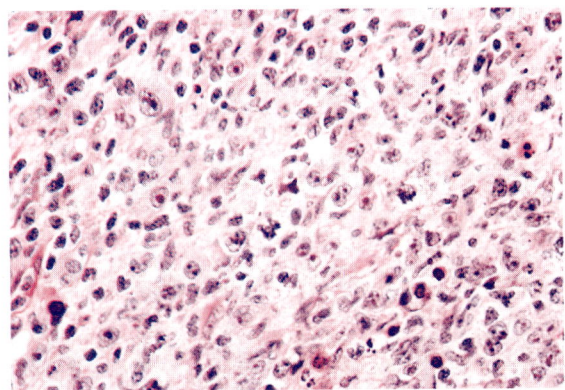

This form shows abundant R-S cells and their variants, with few lymphocytes. This type has the worst prognosis.

Figure 7.64
Normal spleen

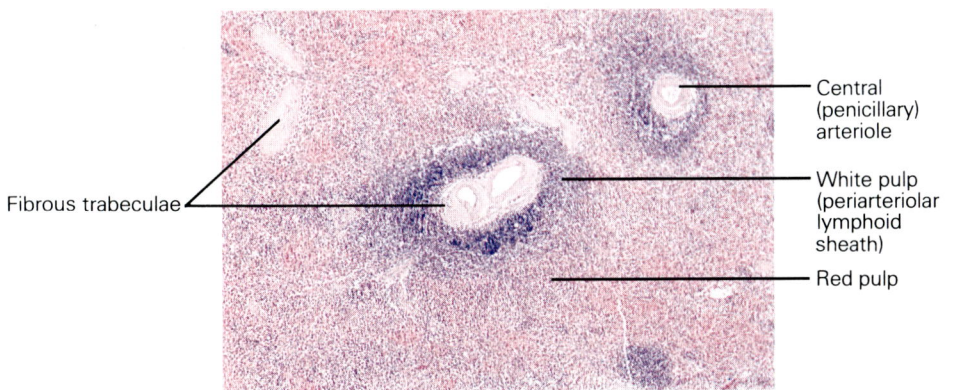

Histopathologic examination of spleen sections begins with overall evaluation of white pulp and red pulp architecture. The normal weight is 150 g.

Figure 7.65
Congestive splenomegaly

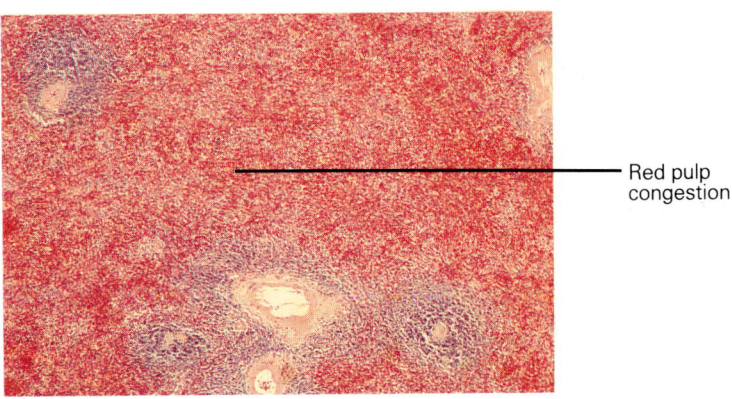

Common causes include portal hypertension due to cirrhosis and right-sided heart failure.

Figure 7.66
Acute splenitis (septic spleen)

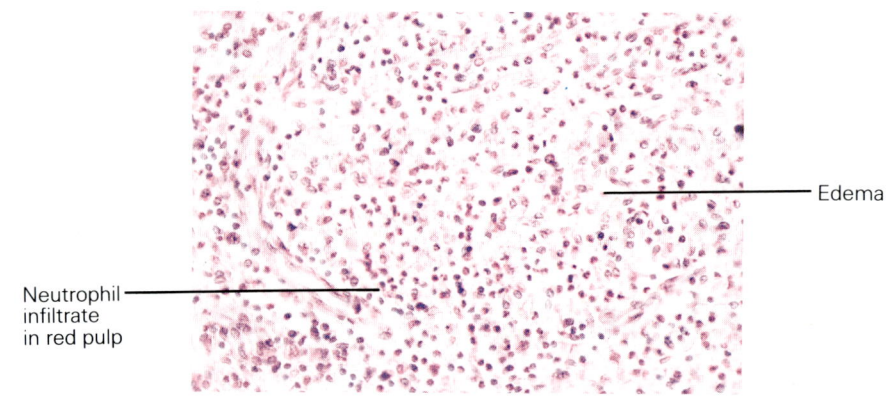

The spleen is grossly boggy, friable, and diffluent due to red pulp edema and inflammation. Neutrophils are scattered throughout the red pulp. This is seen in patients with septicemia.

Figure 7.67
Extramedullary hematopoiesis (EMH) in spleen

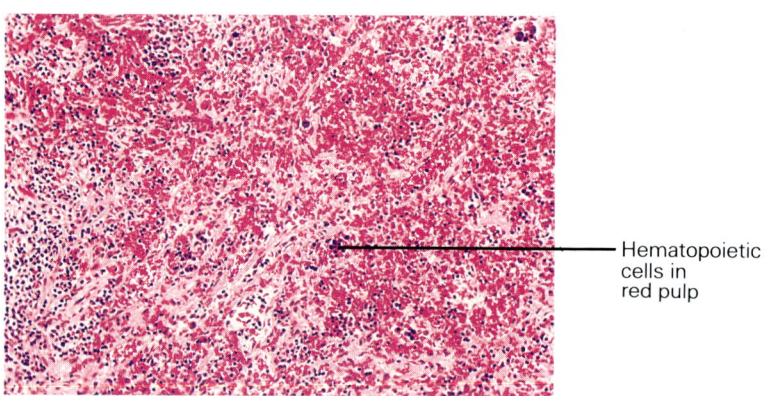

Splenic EMH is characterized by clumps of hematopoietic precursors, as well as solitary megakaryocytes, within the red pulp.

Figure 7.68
Lymphoma in spleen

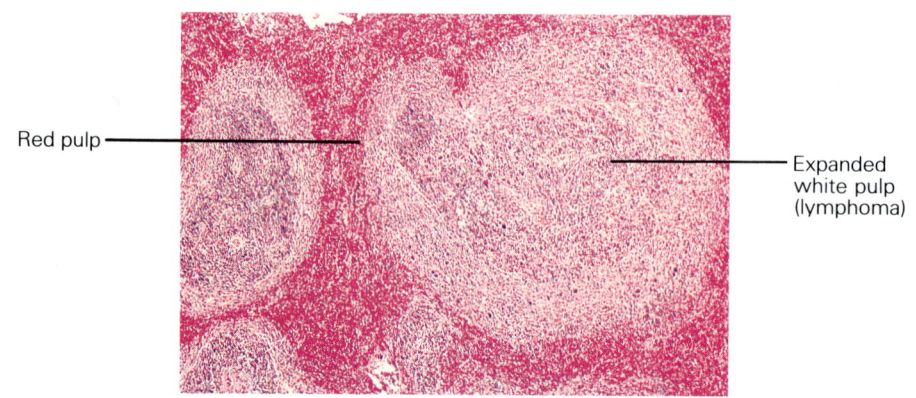

Splenic involvement by lymphoma characteristically shows enlargement of white pulp, often visible on gross examination.

Figure 7.69
Normal thymus

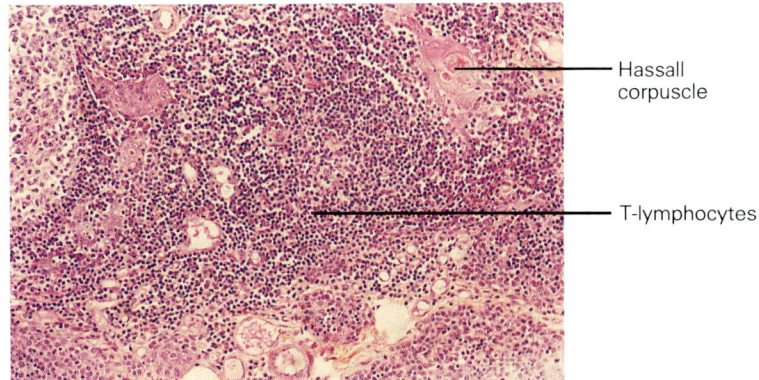

The major lesions affecting the thymus include agenesis, atrophy with aging, hyperplasia, and thymoma.

Figure 7.70
Thymoma

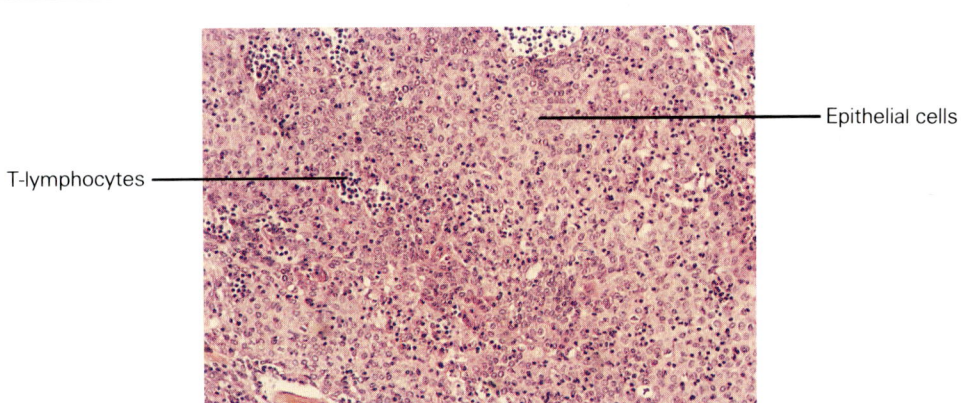

This tumor is composed of thymic epithelial cells admixed with T-lymphocytes. The majority are benign and in less than one-third of cases there is an associated clinical condition such as myasthenia gravis.

Figure 7.71
Chronic tonsillitis

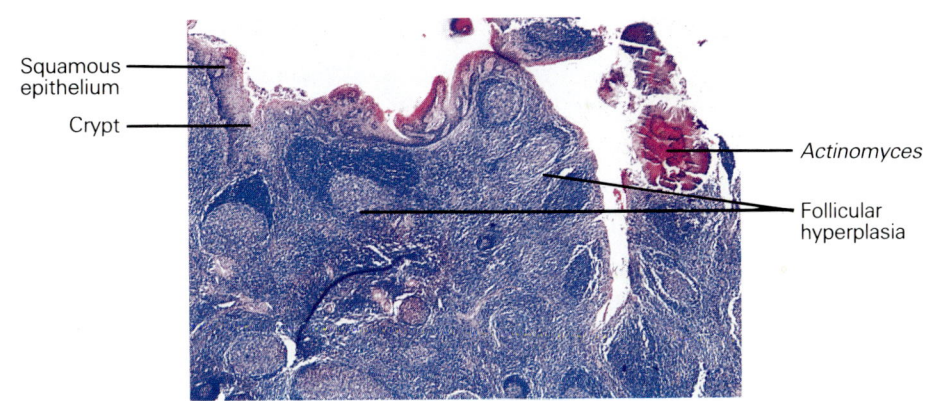

Chronically inflamed and clinically enlarged tonsils show hyperplastic lymphoid follicles. Histologic sections often show associated colonies of *Actinomyces*, visible grossly as yellow "sulfur granules."

CHAPTER 8

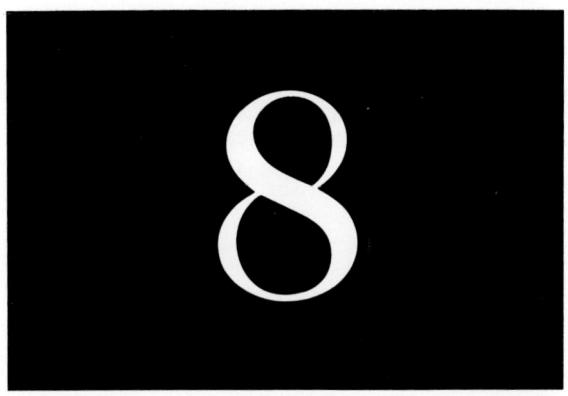

RENAL AND LOWER URINARY TRACT PATHOLOGY

Figure 8.1
Kidneys and bladder

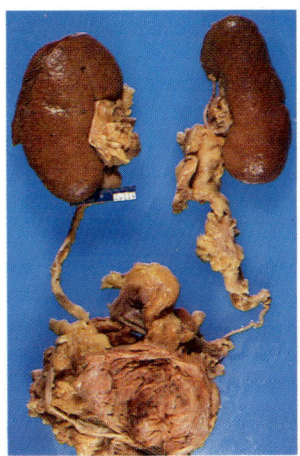

The kidneys here show a finely granular cortical surface due to benign nephro-arteriolosclerosis. The bladder has a trabecular mucosa due to muscle hypertrophy following prostatic hypertrophy (not shown). Normal weight: 150 g (each kidney).

Figure 8.2
Normal kidney

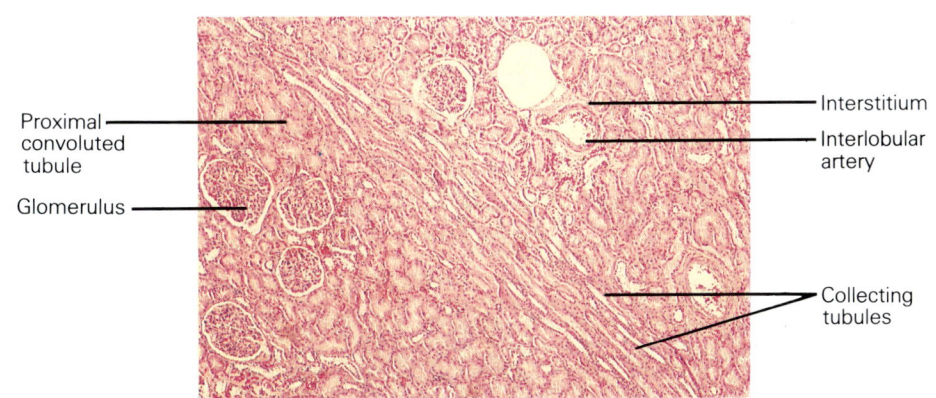

Four compartments (glomeruli, tubules, interstitium, and vessels) must be examined in the routine histopathologic assessment of renal tissue.

Figure 8.3
Normal kidney

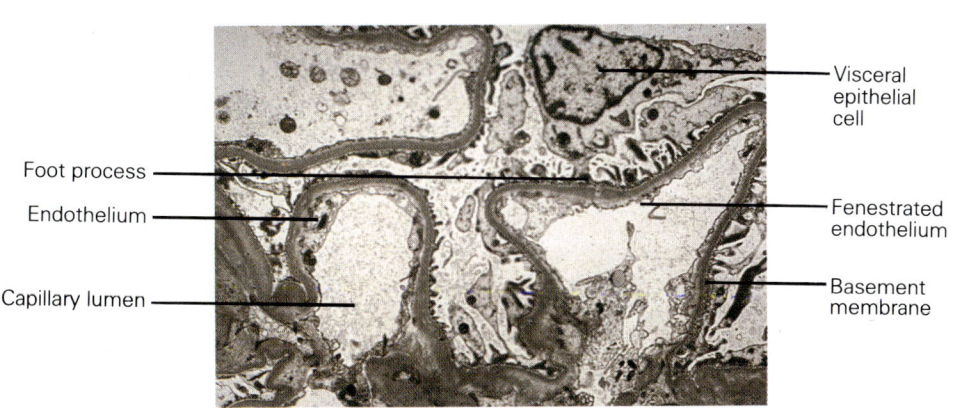

Transmission electron micrograph shows normal glomerular ultrastructure. The mesangium is not shown.

Renal and Lower Urinary Tract Pathology

Figure 8.4
Renal and lower urinary tract: major pathologic lesions

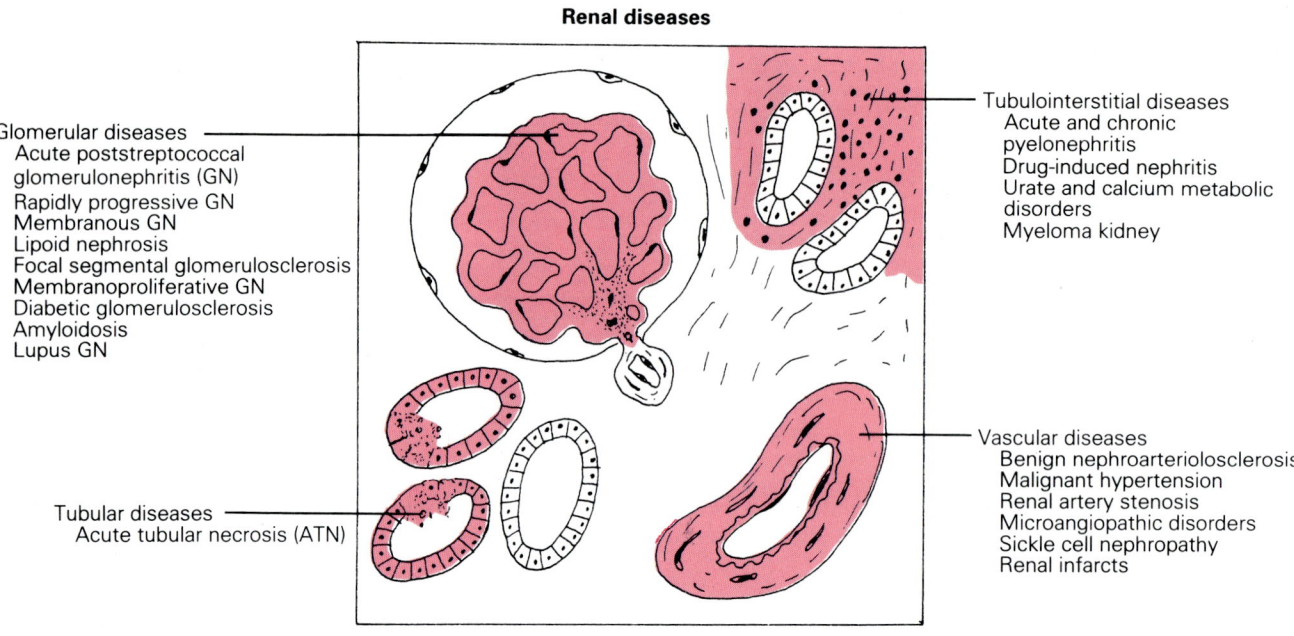

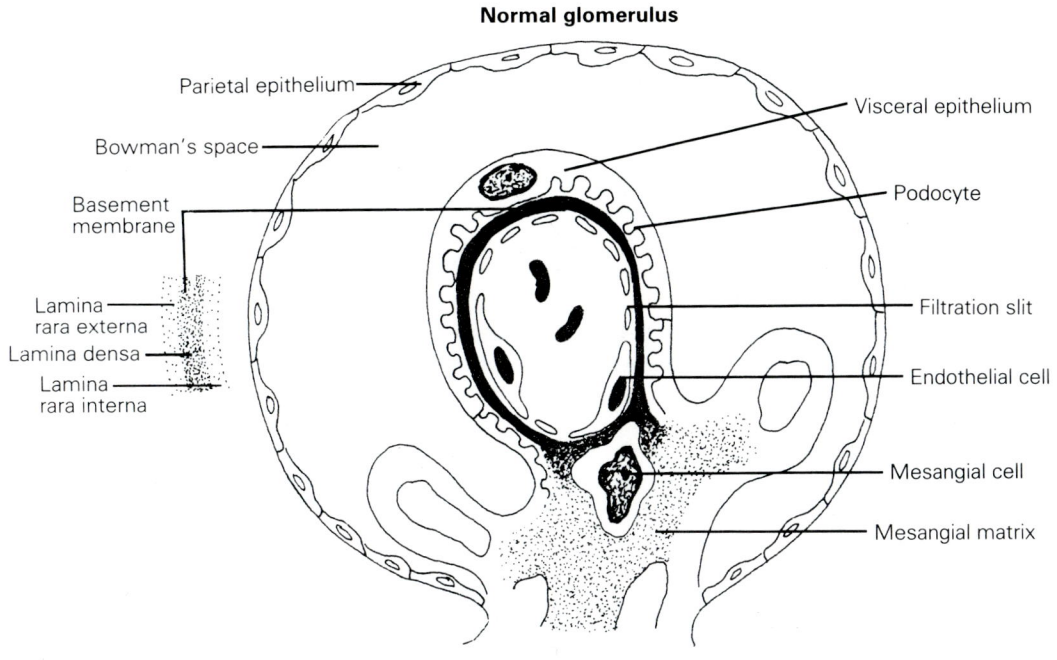
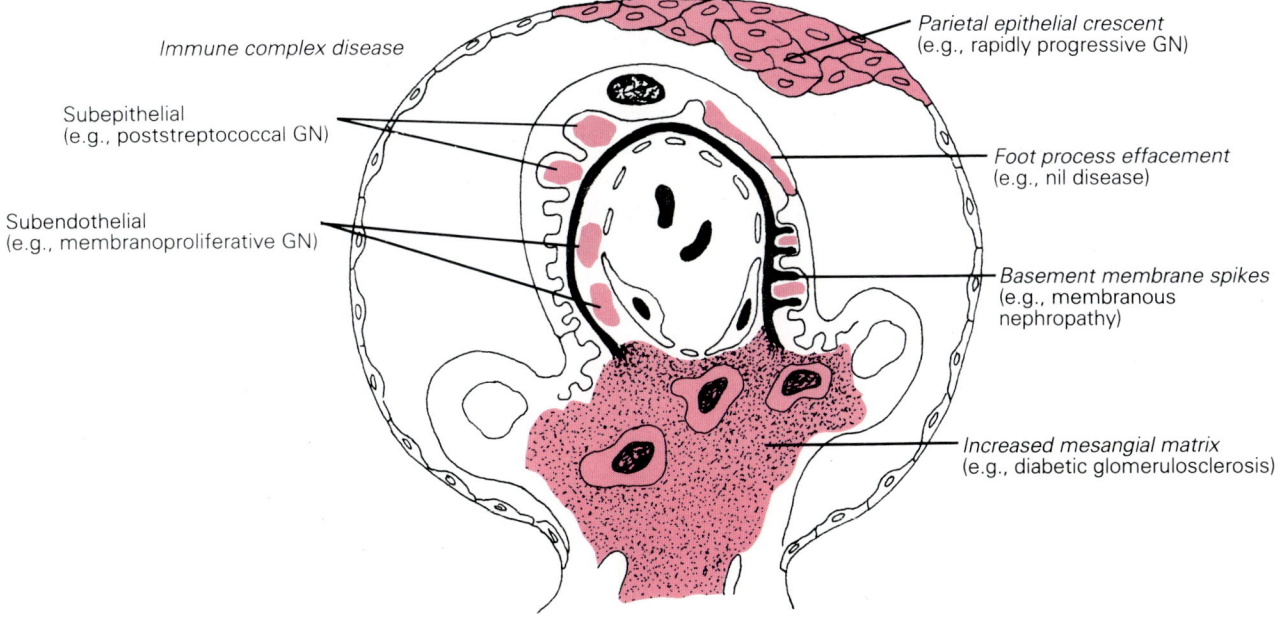

Figure 8.5
Acute poststreptococcal glomerulonephritis

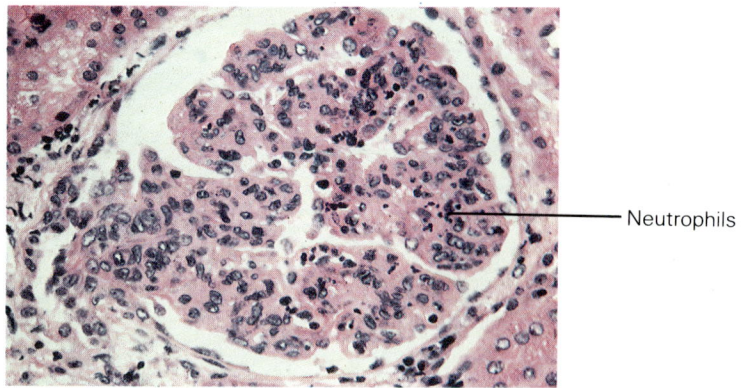

The glomerular hypercellularity is due to proliferation of endothelial and mesangial cells, with infiltration by segmented leukocytes.

Figure 8.6
Acute poststreptococcal glomerulonephritis

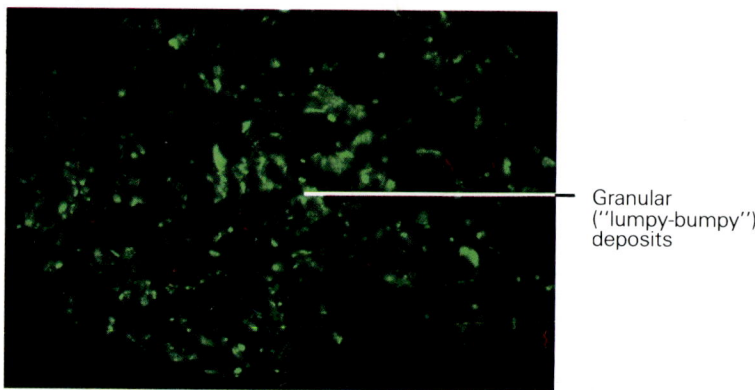

Immunofluorescence shows granular deposits of immunoglobulin (IgG) and complement in the mesangium and along the basement membrane.

Figure 8.7
Acute poststreptococcal glomerulonephritis

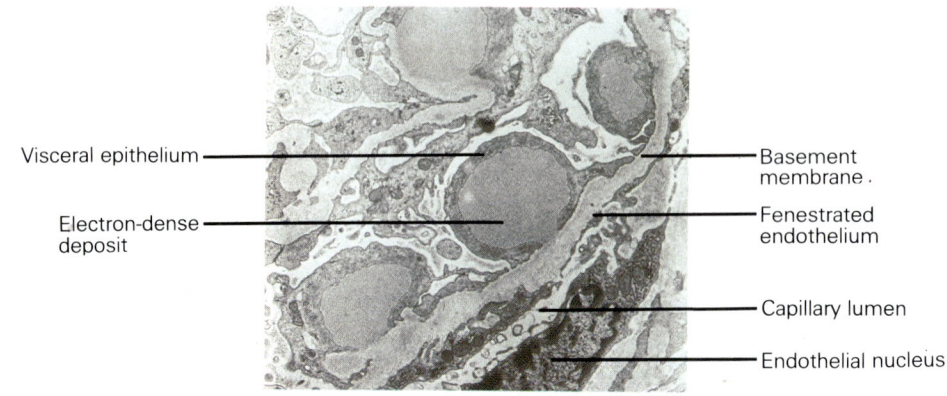

Subepithelial electron-dense, hump-like deposits are seen on electron microscopy.

Figure 8.8
Rapidly progressive glomerulonephritis

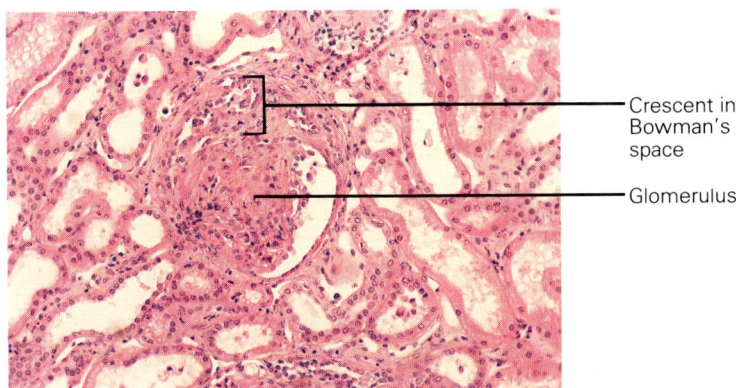

Proliferation of parietal epithelium and infiltration of macrophages produces the crescents in this syndrome. Seen in Goodpasture's syndrome, rare cases of poststreptococcal glomerulonephritis and other systemic diseases.

Figure 8.9
Rapidly progressive glomerulonephritis

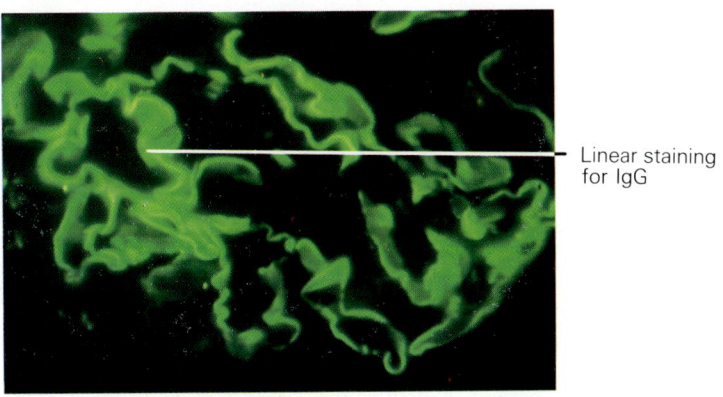

Anti-glomerular basement membrane antibodies stain in linear fashion on immunofluorescence.

Figure 8.10
Lipoid nephrosis (Nil disease)

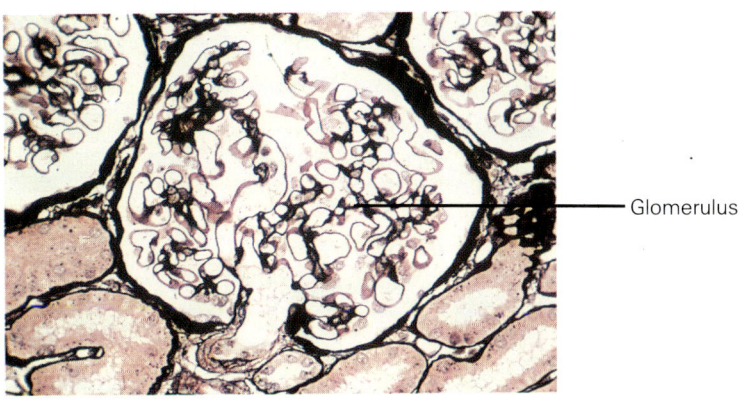

Silver stain shows normal appearing glomerulus in this most common cause of nephrotic syndrome in children.

Renal and Lower Urinary Tract Pathology

Figure 8.11
Lipoid nephrosis (Nil disease)

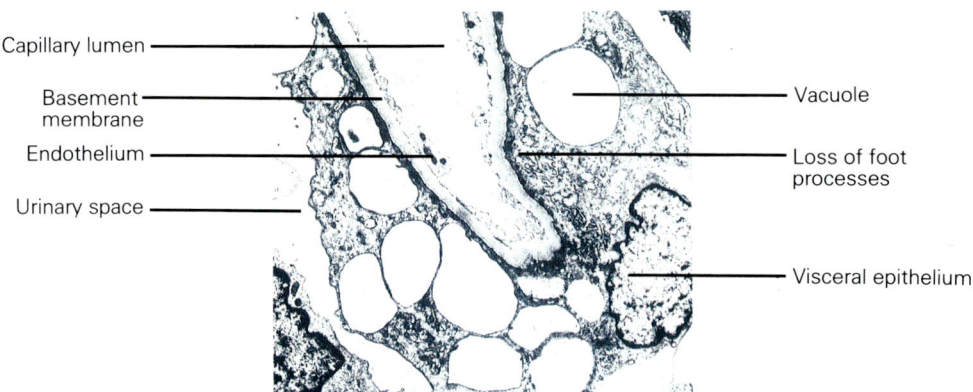

Electron microscopy shows diffuse loss (effacement) of visceral epithelial foot processes and vacuolization of these cells. Reduction in negative charge at this site is associated with albumin loss into urine.

Figure 8.12
Focal sclerosis (focal segmental glomerulosclerosis)

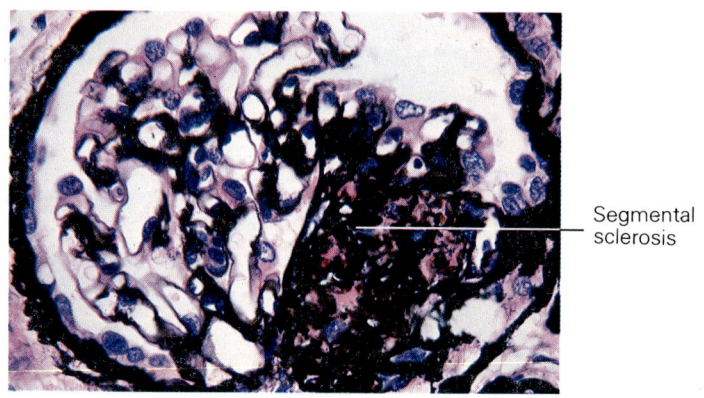

Silver stain shows segment of glomerulus with sclerosis due to entrapped plasma proteins and proliferation of mesangial matrix. The condition is believed to be a sequela of lipoid nephrosis.

Figure 8.13
Membranous glomerulonephritis (membranous nephropathy)

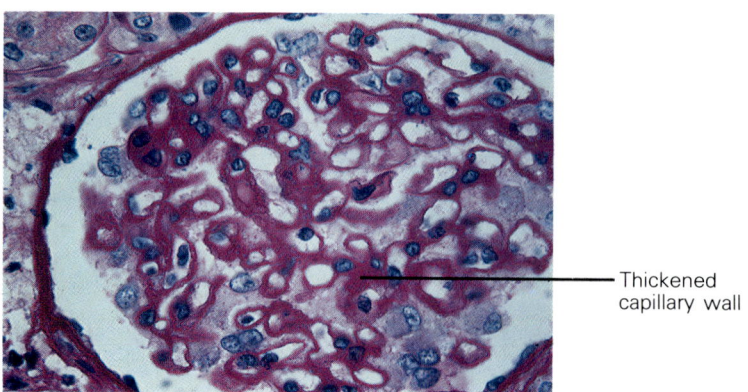

Periodic acid-Schiff (PAS) stain shows diffusely thickened glomerular capillary wall. Chronic antigen-antibody deposition in systemic lupus erythematosus, hepatitis B, gold therapy, and other conditions leads to electron-dense deposits and basement membrane proliferation.

Figure 8.14
Membranous glomerulonephritis (membranous nephropathy)

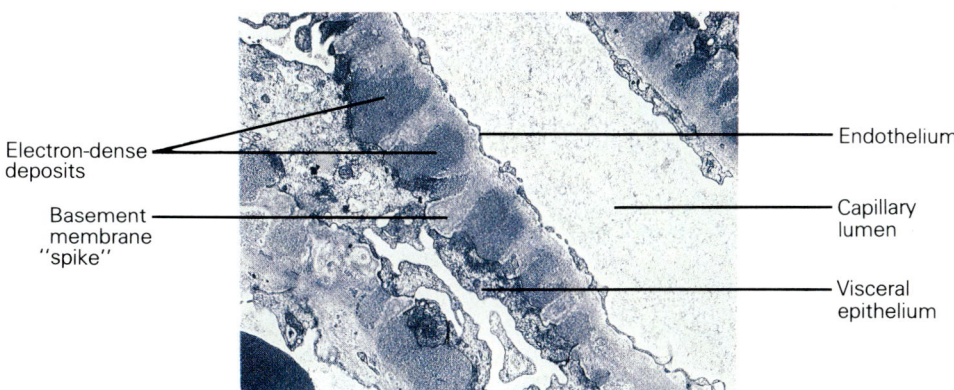

Electron microscopy shows subepithelial dense deposits (IgG and complement) and proliferation of basement membrane material as "spikes" between the deposits. Visceral epithelial foot processes are obliterated.

Figure 8.15
Membranoproliferative glomerulonephritis

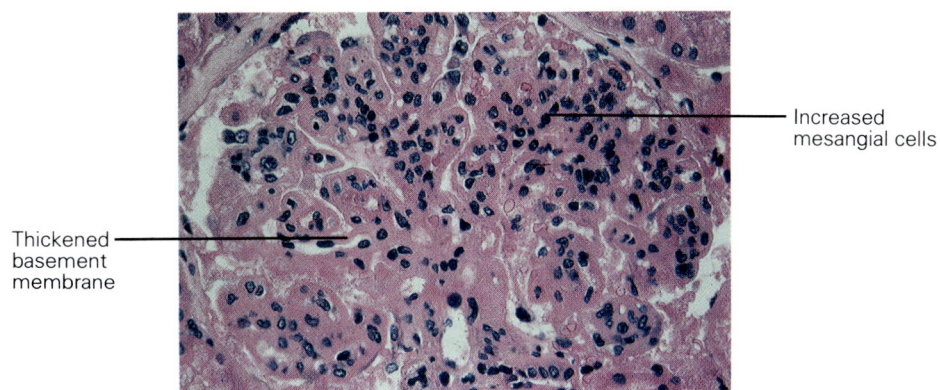

The glomerulus appears hypercellular, with increased mesangial cells and thickened basement membrane. Glomerular deposits of complement components are related to primary activation of complement or secondary to immune complex deposition.

Figure 8.16
Membranoproliferative glomerulonephritis

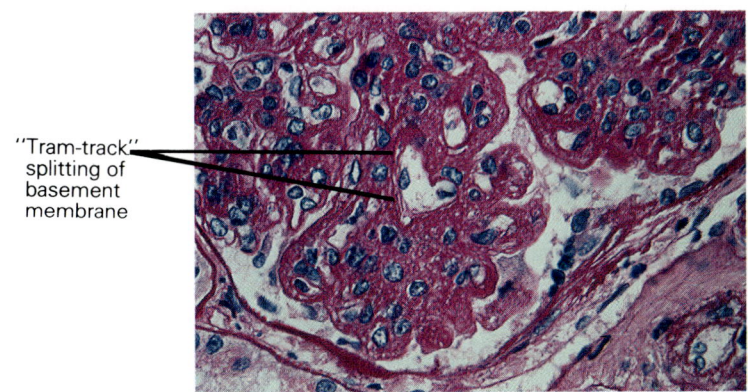

Periodic acid-Schiff (PAS) stain shows split ("tram-track") appearance of basement membrane where mesangial cell process interposition occurs.

Figure 8.17
Diffuse proliferative glomerulonephritis (systemic lupus erythematosus)

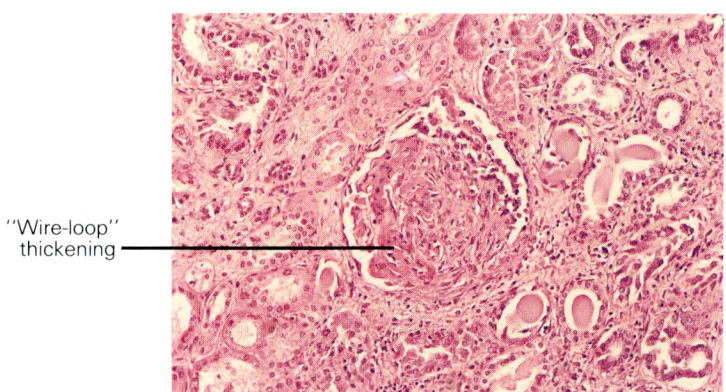

Mesangial proliferation and "wire-loop" thickening of the capillary wall (related to subendothelial deposits) characterize this most common form of lupus glomerulonephritis.

Figure 8.18
Acute tubular necrosis

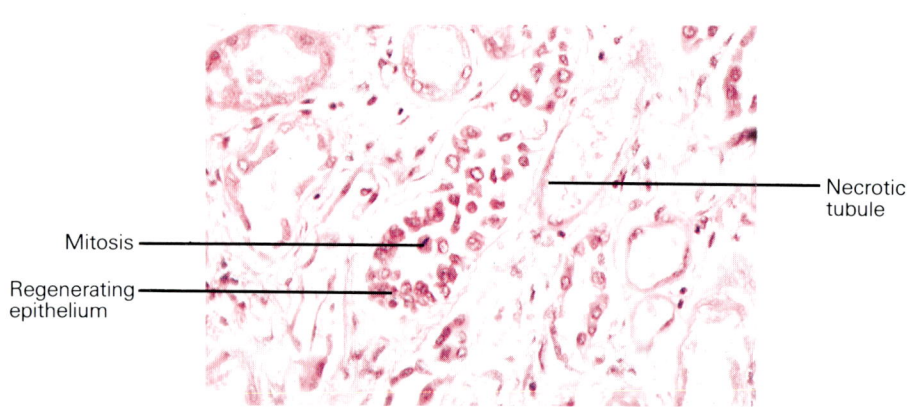

Ischemic or toxic damage (i.e., heavy metals, organic solvents, antibiotics) may produce this lesion. This field shows degenerating tubules admixed with regenerating tubules with hyperchromatic nuclei and occasional mitoses.

Figure 8.19
Urate nephropathy

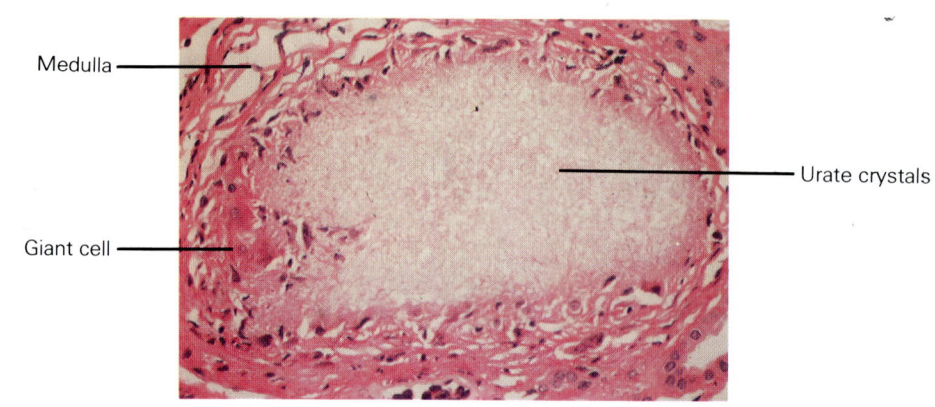

Urate crystals in the medullary interstitium have induced a local granulomatous lesion, with surrounding mononuclear and giant cells.

96   *Histopathology of Disease*

Figure 8.20
Acute pyelonephritis

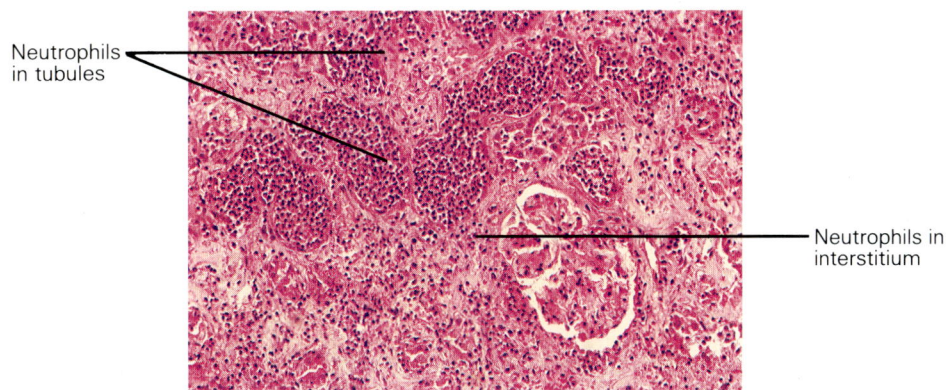

Bacterial infection from ascending or hematogenous spread produces this suppurative interstitial and tubular lesion.

Figure 8.21
Benign nephroarteriolosclerosis

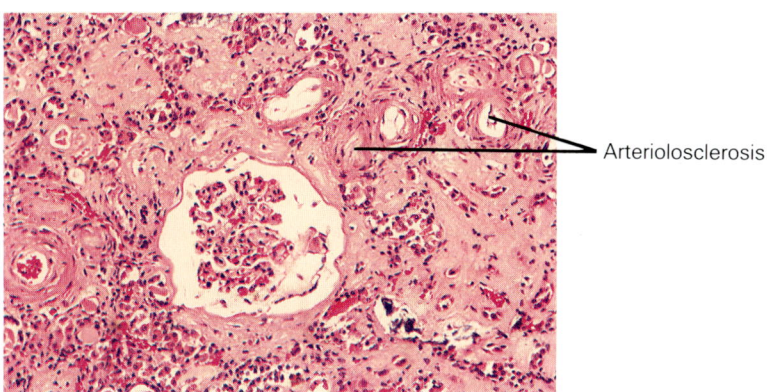

Interlobular arteries are thickened in this tissue correlate to systemic hypertension. The kidney cortical surface is grossly finely granular.

Figure 8.22
Polyarteritis nodosa (PAN)

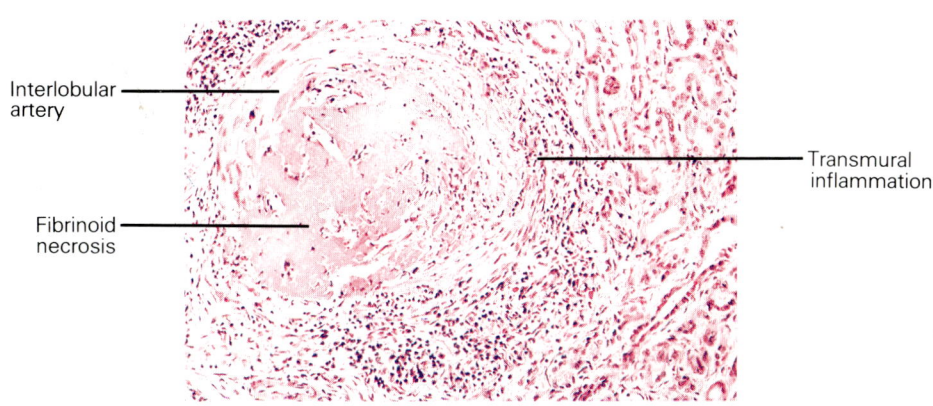

The kidneys are involved in the majority of cases of PAN. Fibrinoid necrosis seen here affects the intima and media, with near total obliteration of the vessel. The transmural inflammation includes lymphocytes and neutrophils.

Figure 8.23
Diabetic nodular glomerulosclerosis (Kimmelstiel-Wilson disease)

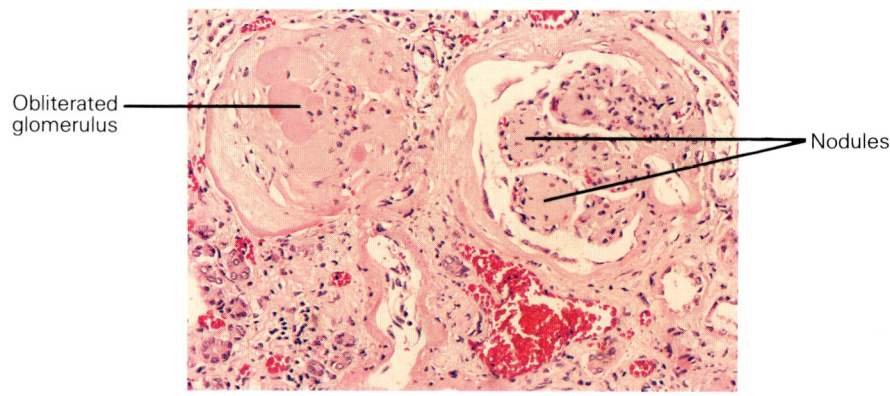

Hyaline nodules of mesangial matrix, lipid and fibrin are present in the glomerulus.

Figure 8.24
Diabetic diffuse glomerulosclerosis

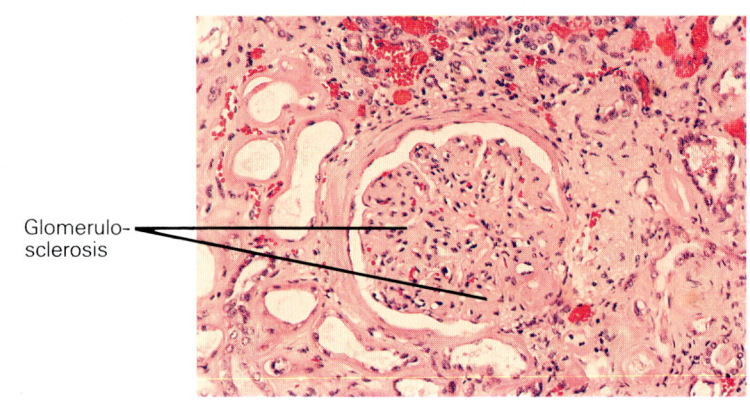

This diffuse alteration of the glomerular tuft results from mesangial matrix and cell proliferation with basement membrane thickening.

Figure 8.25
Renal amyloidosis

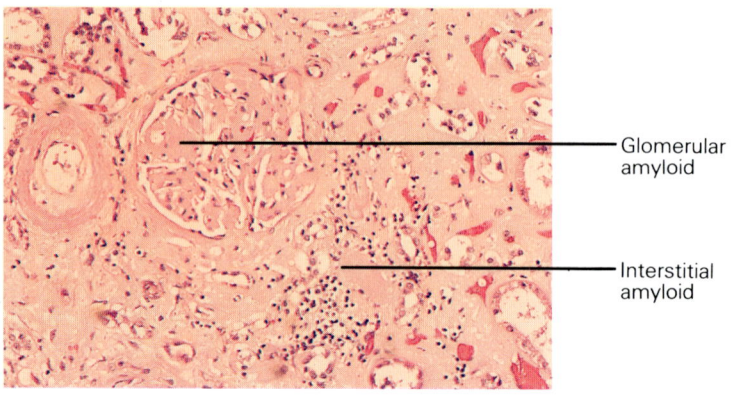

Primary (AL type) and secondary (AA type) amyloidosis involve several histologic sites in the kidney.

Figure 8.26
Renal amyloidosis (congo red stain)

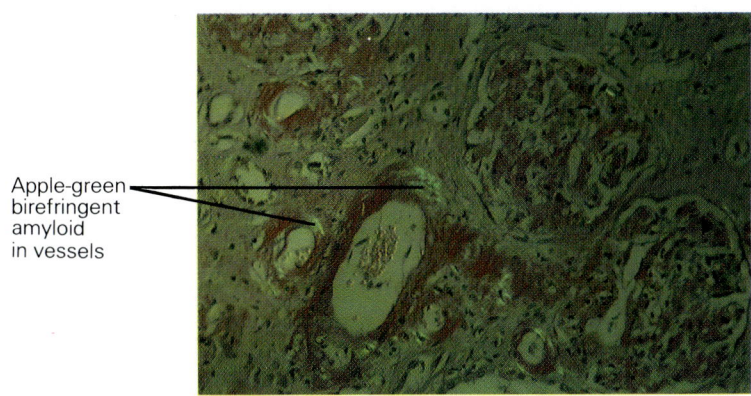

The β-pleated sheet configuration of amyloid confers an apple-green birefringence when stained with congo red and examined under polarized light.

Figure 8.27
Endstage kidney

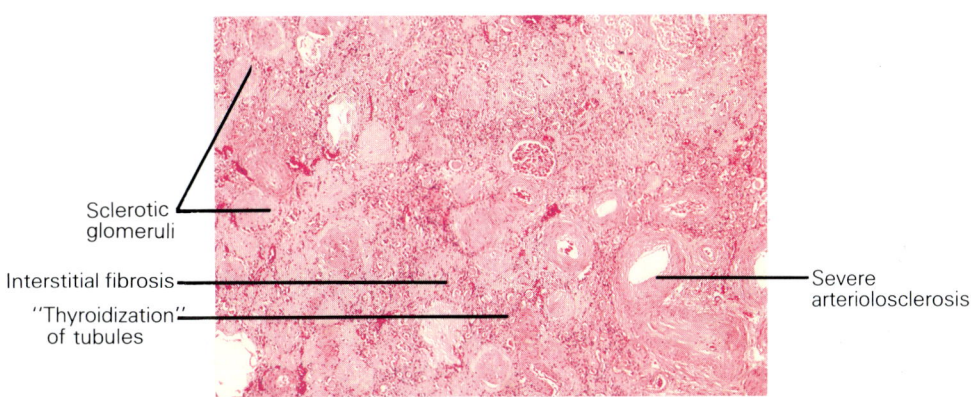

Chronic glomerulonephritis, vascular disease, or tubulointerstitial disease may eventuate in severe damage to all four renal compartments in the "endstage" kidney. Marked tubular atrophy results in features similar to thyroid follicles ("thyroidization").

Figure 8.28
Acute cellular rejection of renal transplant

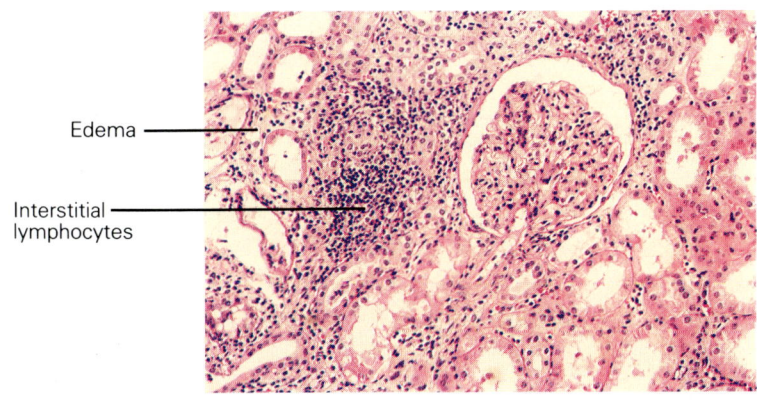

Acute cellular rejection within months of transplant is manifested by interstitial lymphocytes and edema.

Renal and Lower Urinary Tract Pathology

Figure 8.29
Renal cell (clear cell) carcinoma

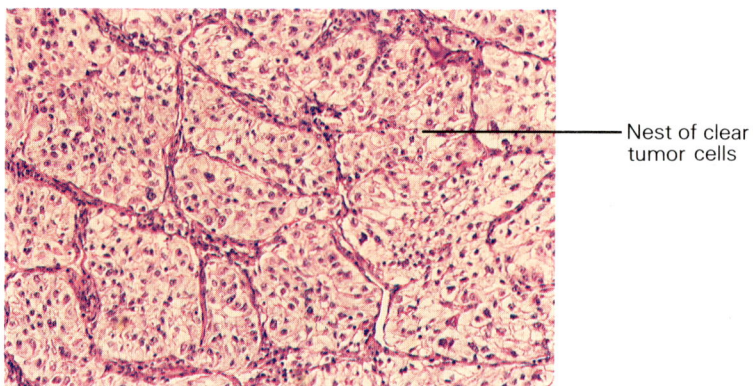

This is the most common form of renal cancer. Malignant cells shown here are clear (containing glycogen and lipid) and form closely packed nests.

Figure 8.30
Wilms' tumor (nephroblastoma)

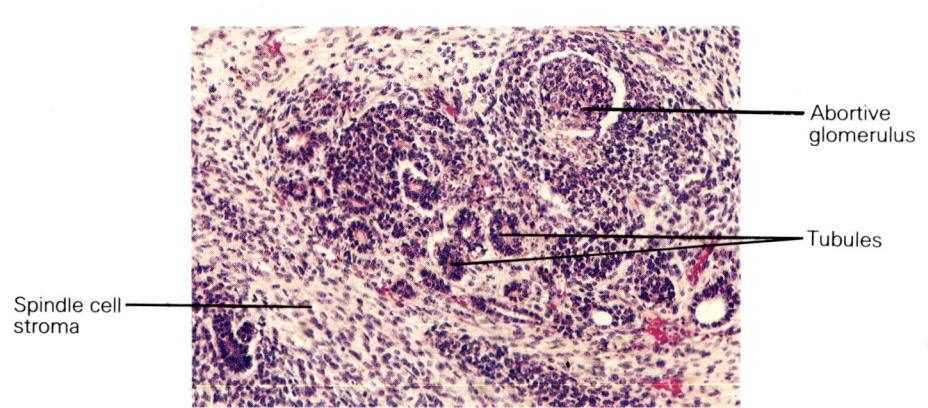

A common childhood malignancy (ages 1 to 4). The tumor is derived from mesonephric mesoderm and consists of tubules, abortive glomeruli, striated muscle, and spindle cell elements.

Figure 8.31
Cystitis cystica of urinary bladder

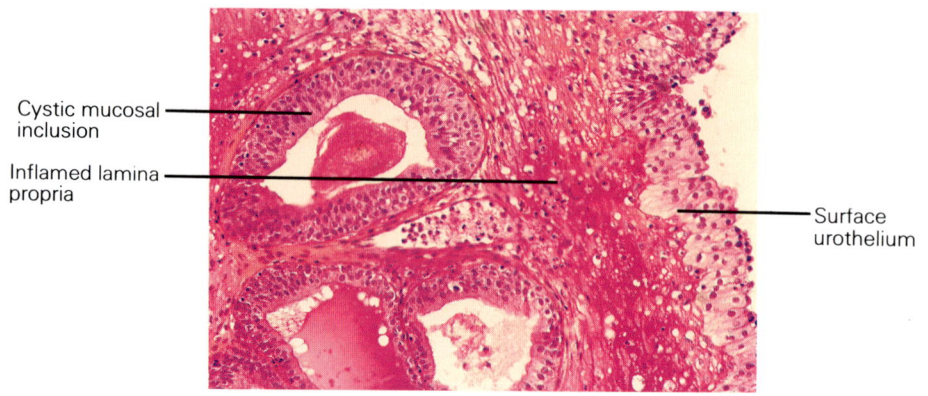

In this variant of cystitis (bladder inflammation), cystic portions of mucosa become buried within a lamina propria containing acute and chronic inflammatory cells.

Figure 8.32
Transitional cell carcinoma of urinary bladder

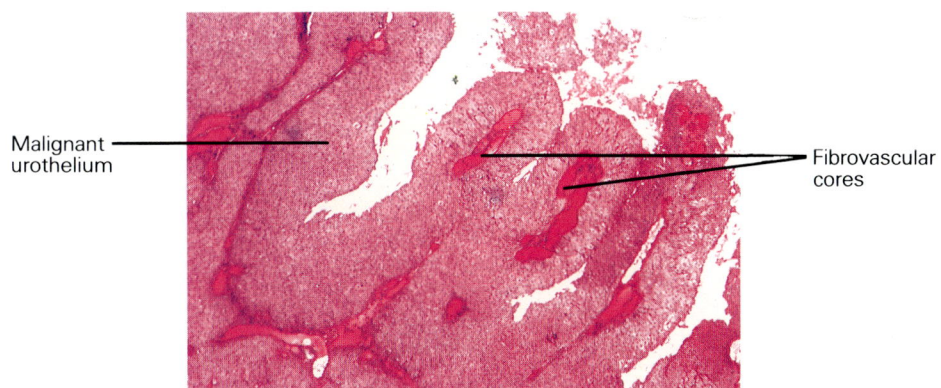

This field shows the most common form of bladder cancer, transitional cell carcinoma, growing in a papillary, exophytic pattern. Grade 1 tumors such as this cytologically resemble normal urothelium closely.

CHAPTER 9

GASTROINTESTINAL PATHOLOGY

Figure 9.1
Esophagus and stomach

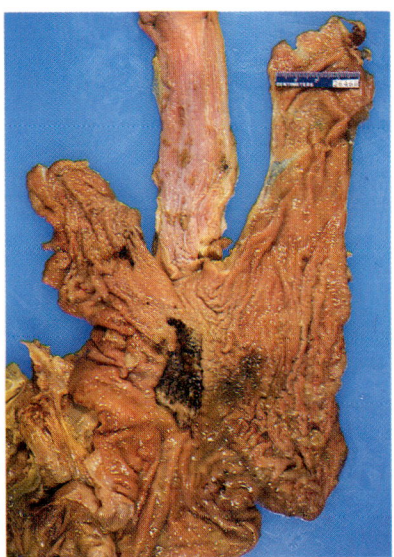

The esophagus and stomach opened show a large, hemorrhagic gastric ulcer on the lesser curvature. Normal lengths: esophagus, 25 cm; duodenum, 30 cm; small intestine, 550–650 cm; and colon, 150–170 cm.

Figure 9.2
Normal esophagus

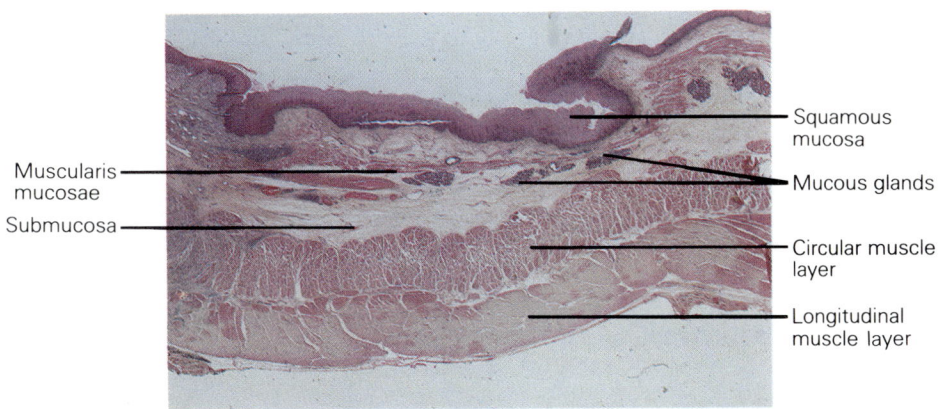

Figure 9.3
Normal stomach (antrum)

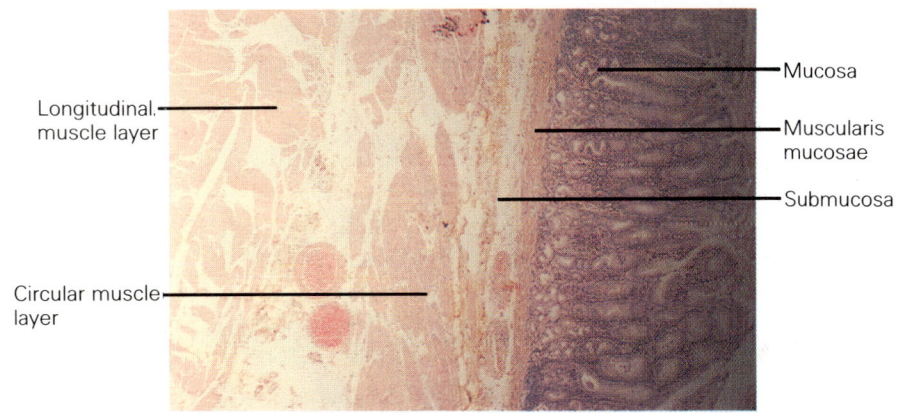

Gastrointestinal Pathology 105

Figure 9.4
Normal duodenum

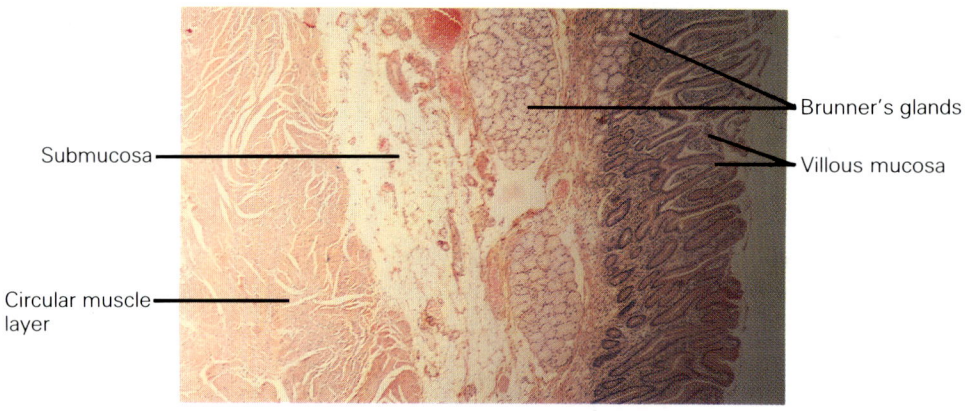

Figure 9.5
Normal small intestine (jejunum)

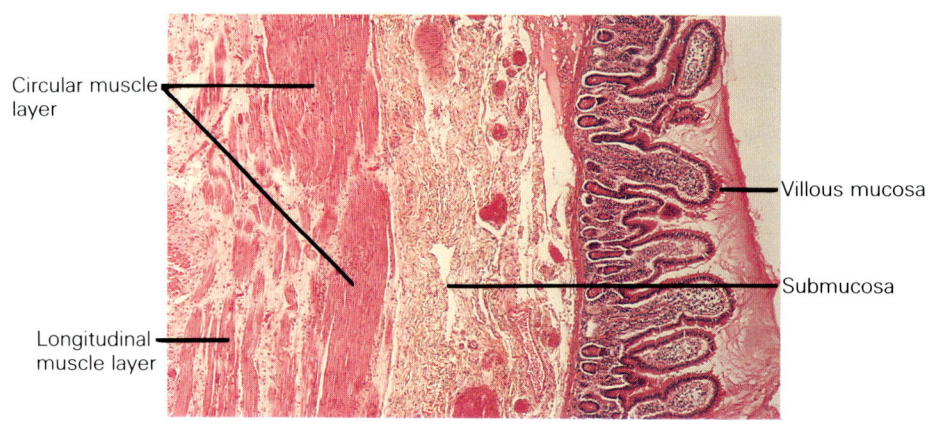

Figure 9.6
Normal colon

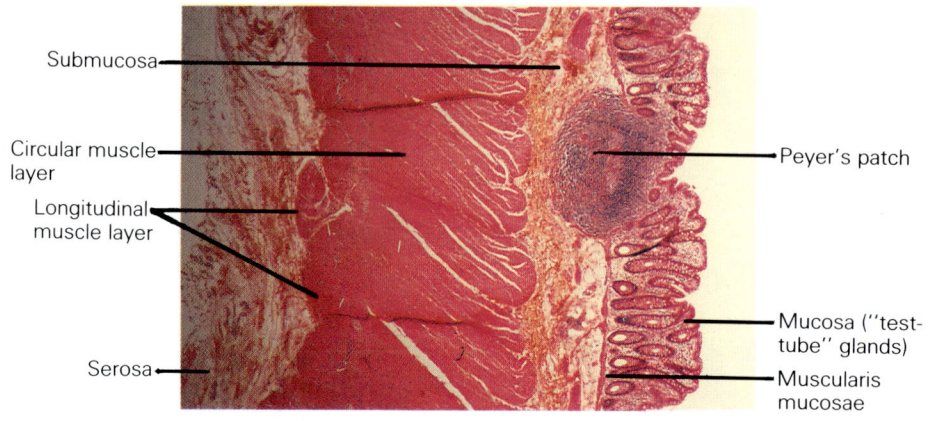

106 *Histopathology of Disease*

Figure 9.7
Gastrointestinal tract: major pathologic lesions

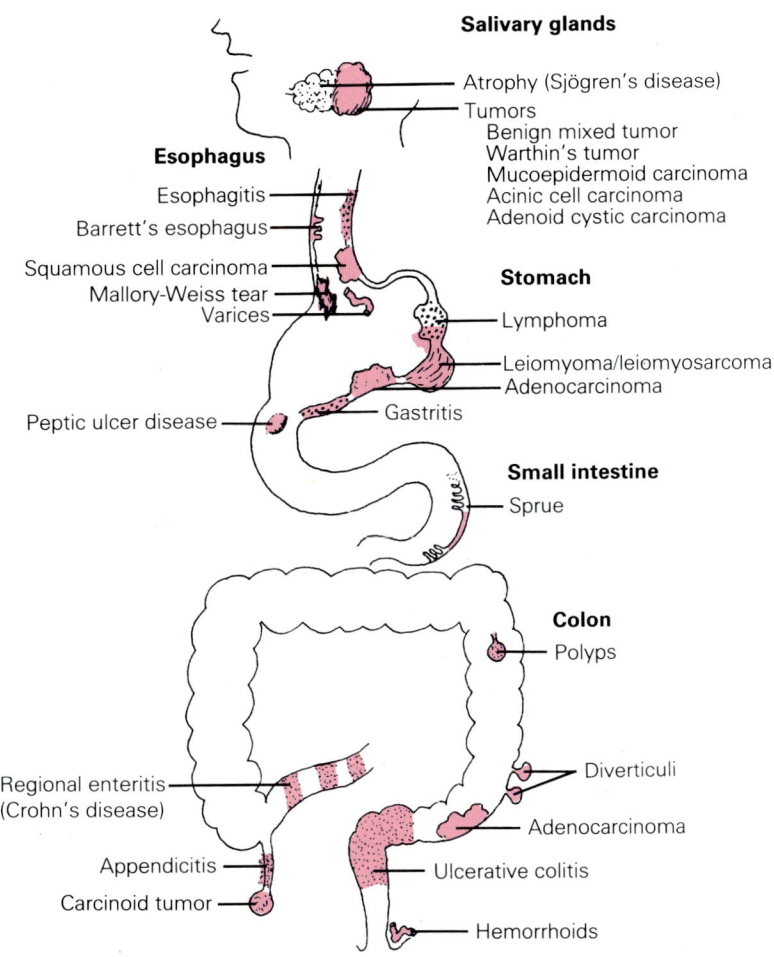

Figure 9.8
Esophagitis

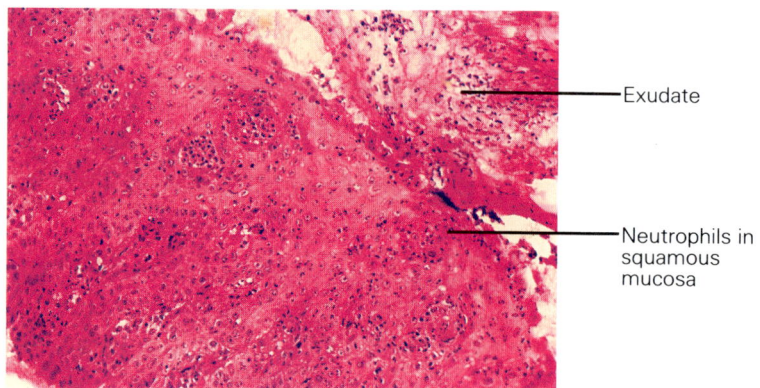

Acute inflammation of the esophagus may result from reflux of gastric contents, ingestion of irritants such as alcohol, or viral and fungal infections.

Figure 9.9
Barrett's esophagus (columnar metaplasia)

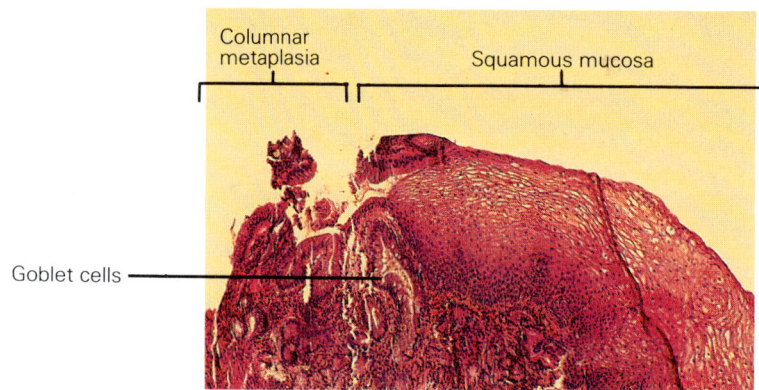

Chronic gastroesophageal reflux may cause the lower esophageal squamous mucosa to undergo columnar metaplasia, appearing as gastric-type or intestinal-type glands. This zone may become ulcerated and is associated with development of adenocarcinoma.

Figure 9.10
Esophageal varices

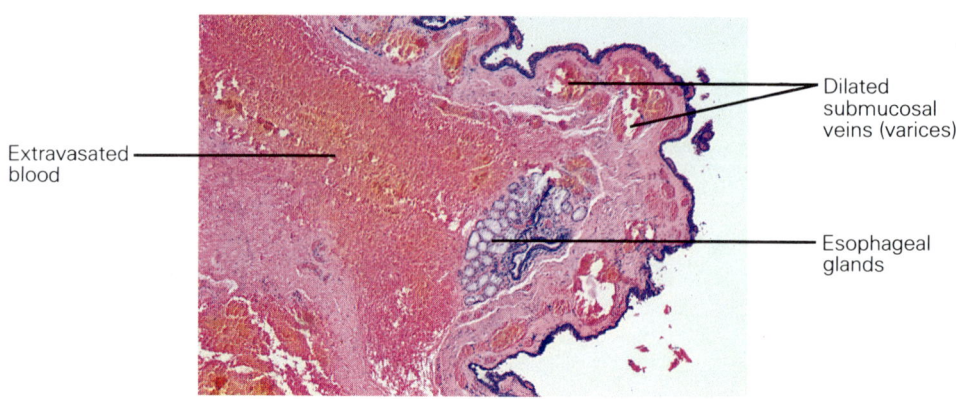

This postmortem section of esophagus was from an alcoholic with cirrhosis and varices. The dilated submucosal veins may rupture through the mucosa with resultant hematemesis.

Figure 9.11
Squamous cell carcinoma of esophagus

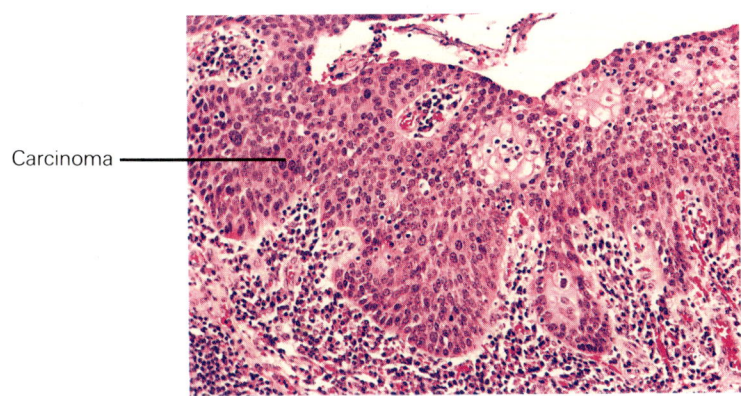

The full thickness of the mucosa is replaced by a poorly differentiated squamous carcinoma without obvious keratin production. The tumor is related to chronic ethanol and cigarette use.

Figure 9.12
Peptic ulcer

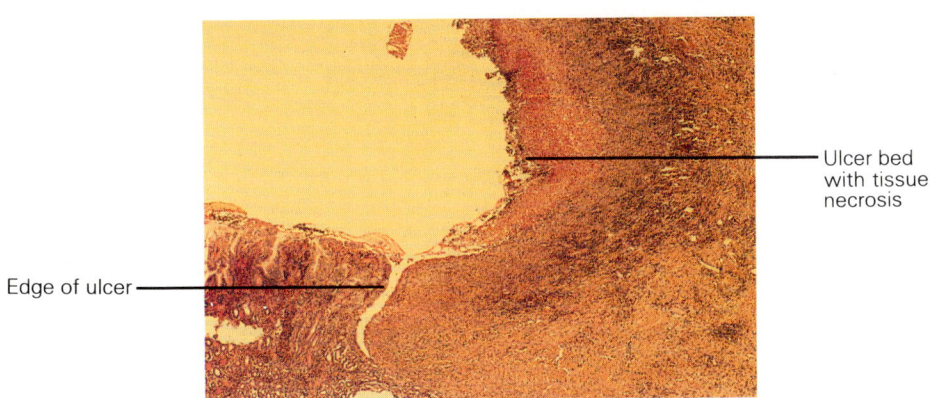

Tissue loss involving the entire mucosa through to the muscularis mucosae is seen in this ulcer. These are related to acid-pepsin hypersecretion and/or breakdown in mucosal defenses.

Figure 9.13
Chronic atrophic gastritis

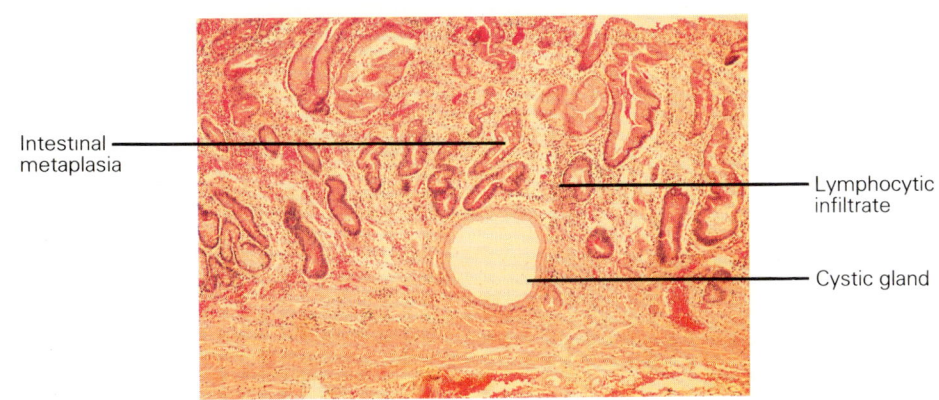

The mucosa is flattened, shows infiltrates of lymphocytes and glandular abnormalities such as cystic dilatation and metaplasia to intestinal-type glands with goblet cells.

Figure 9.14
Adenocarcinoma of stomach

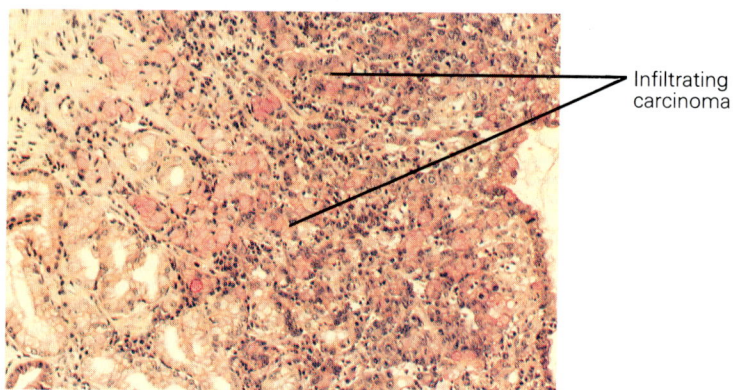

The entire mucosa is infiltrated by malignant glands and single "signet-ring" cells. The section was stained with mucicarmine to demonstrate mucinous secretion (pink).

Figure 9.15
Adenocarcinoma of stomach ("signet-ring" cells)

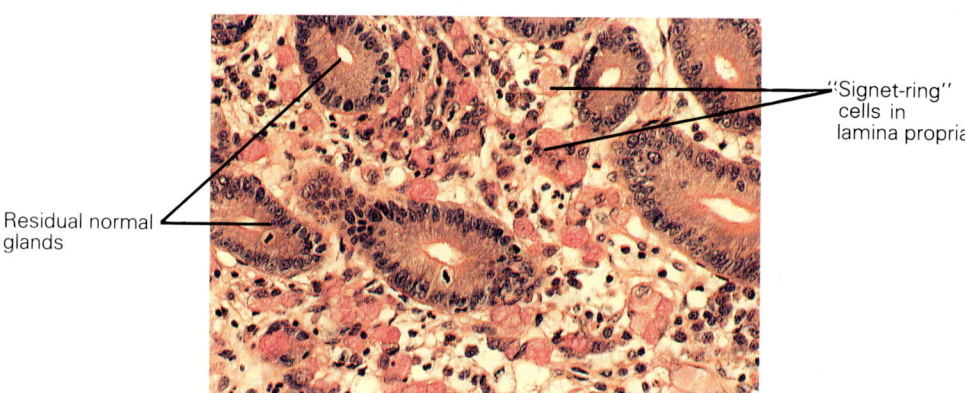

Mucicarmine stain showing morphology of "signet-ring" cells infiltrating the lamina propria. These contain a large cytoplasmic droplet of mucin compressing the nucleus to the periphery.

Figure 9.16
Gastric leiomyoma

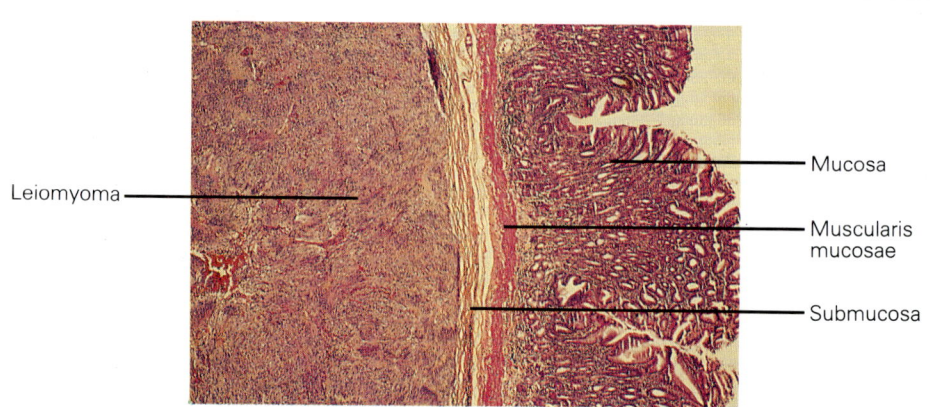

These benign tumors arise from the muscularis. They elevate the overlying mucosa and may eventually cause an umbilicated ulceration. Their malignant counterparts (leiomyosarcomas) ulcerate, infiltrate, and show necrosis and mitotic activity.

Figure 9.17
Celiac sprue (jejunum)

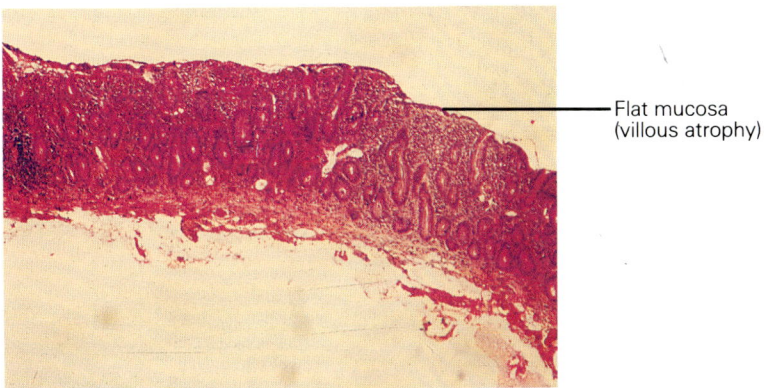

Also known as gluten-sensitive enteropathy, nontropical sprue, and celiac disease, the disorder consists of intestinal damage by the gliadin derivative in dietary gluten.

Figure 9.18
Celiac sprue (jejunum)

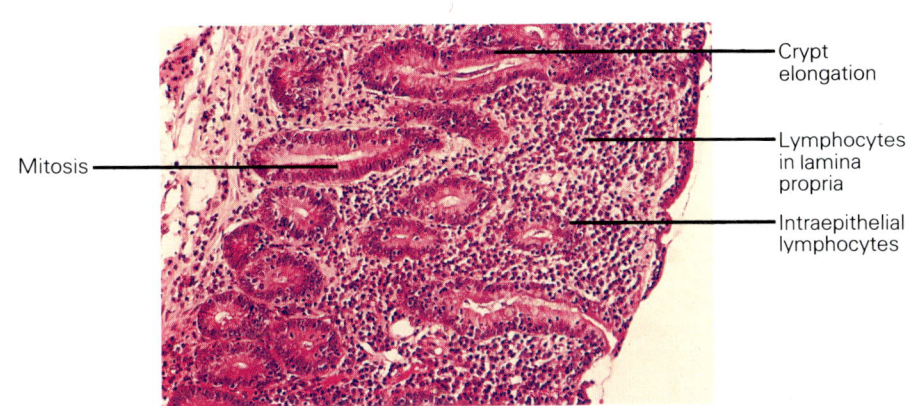

Higher magnification of Figure 9.17 shows flat mucosa, elongated crypts with increased mitotic activity, and a diffuse lymphocytic infiltrate.

Figure 9.19
Carcinoid tumor of ileum

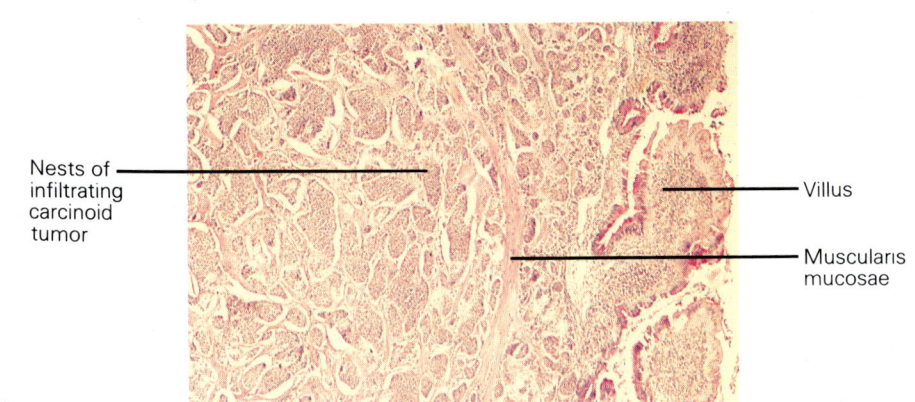

These Kulchitsky (enterochromaffin) cell-derived tumors invade locally within the intestinal wall and may metastasize to regional lymph nodes and liver. They are classified within the family of APUD (amine precursor uptake and decarboxylation) tumors.

Figure 9.20
Carcinoid tumor (Grimelius silver stain)

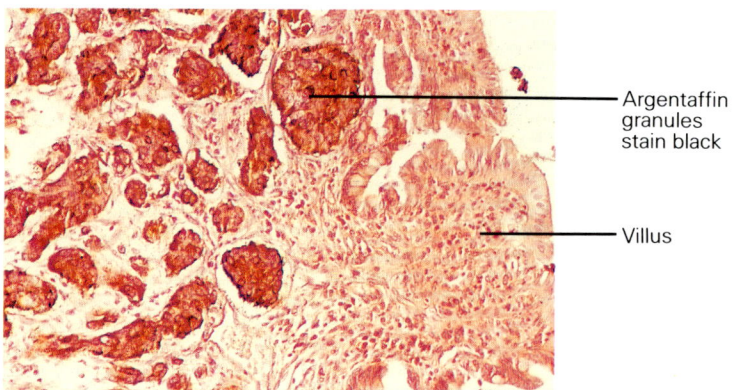

Deposits of silver stain (black) mark the presence within these carcinoid tumor cells of secretory (neuroendocrine) granules.

Figure 9.21
Carcinoid tumor of appendix

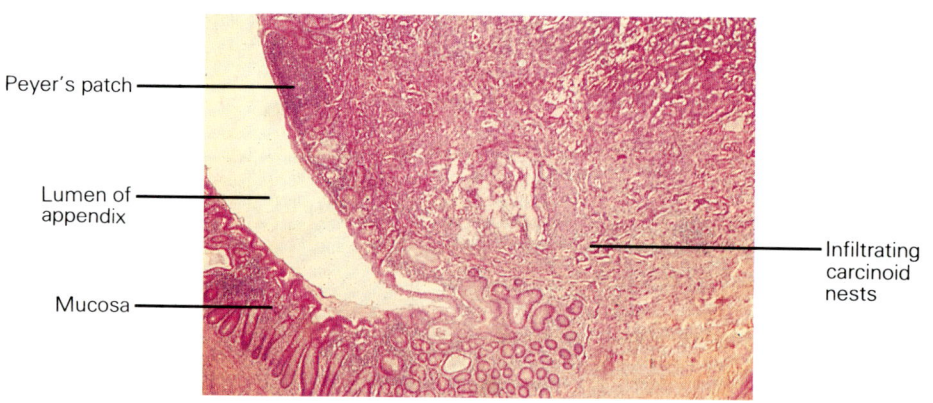

Carcinoid tumors in decreasing order of frequency develop in the appendix, small intestine, lungs and bronchi, rectum and rectosigmoid, colon, esophagus, and stomach.

Figure 9.22
Acute appendicitis

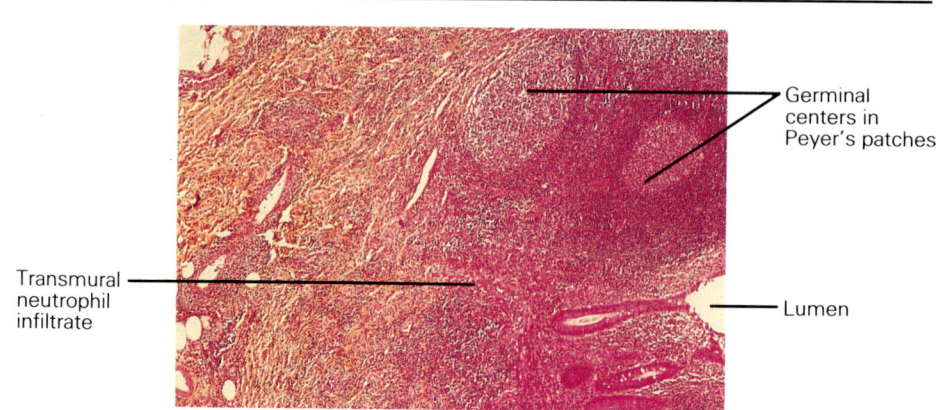

Appendiceal obstruction, usually by a fecalith, results in suppurative inflammation of the wall of the appendix. Complications include gangrene and rupture.

112   *Histopathology of Disease*

Figure 9.23
Differential features of regional enteritis and ulcerative colitis

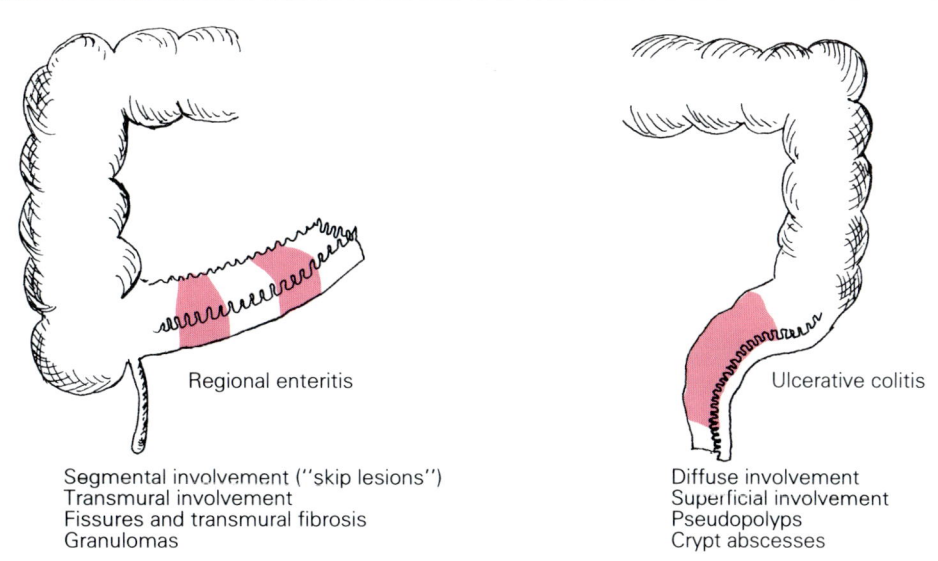

Regional enteritis
Segmental involvement ("skip lesions")
Transmural involvement
Fissures and transmural fibrosis
Granulomas

Ulcerative colitis
Diffuse involvement
Superficial involvement
Pseudopolyps
Crypt abscesses

Figure 9.24
Regional enteritis

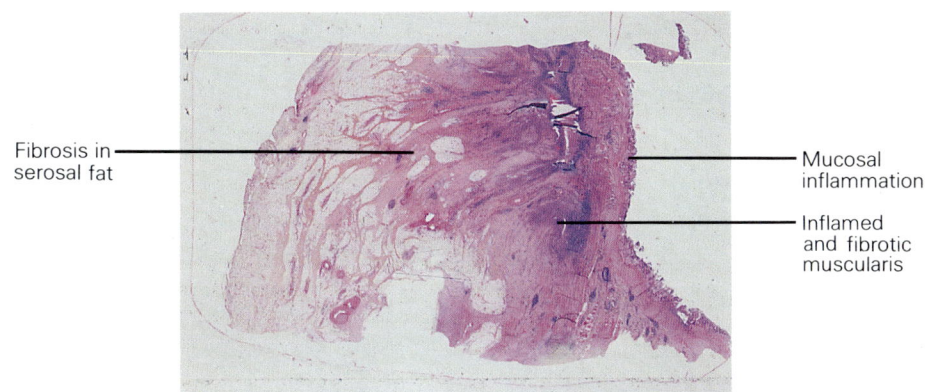

Transmural inflammation of segments of terminal ileum produces an inflexible, "rubber hose" wall and a narrow lumen ("string sign") on a radiograph.

Figure 9.25
Regional enteritis

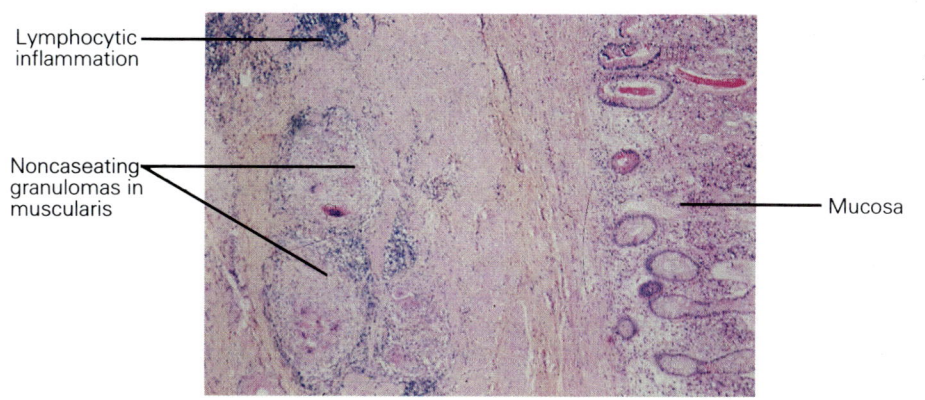

Characteristic features include transmural chronic inflammation and fibrosis with granulomas in approximately 60 percent of cases.

Figure 9.26
Ulcerative colitis

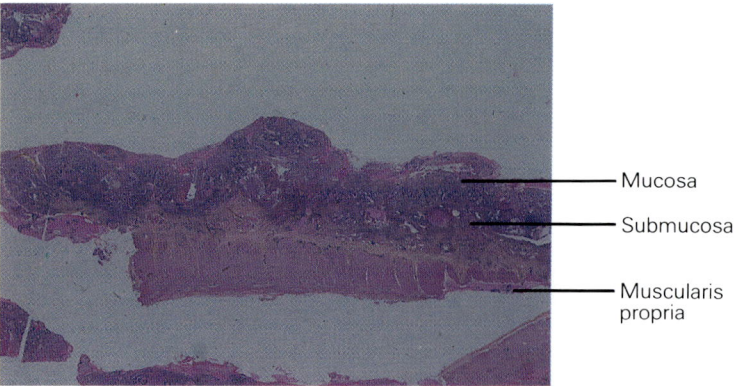

Lesions of ulcerative colitis characteristically show ulceration and inflammation without skip lesions that are superficial (confined to mucosa and submucosa).

Figure 9.27
Ulcerative colitis

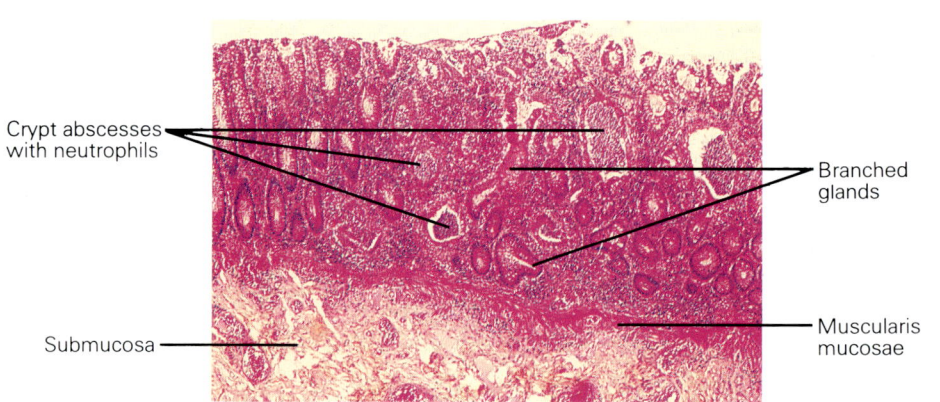

Section of colon with characteristic crypt abscesses, dense lymphocytic infiltrate in lamina propria, and scattered branched glands whose abnormal configuration reflects altered architecture following epithelial regeneration.

Figure 9.28
Pseudopolyps in ulcerative colitis

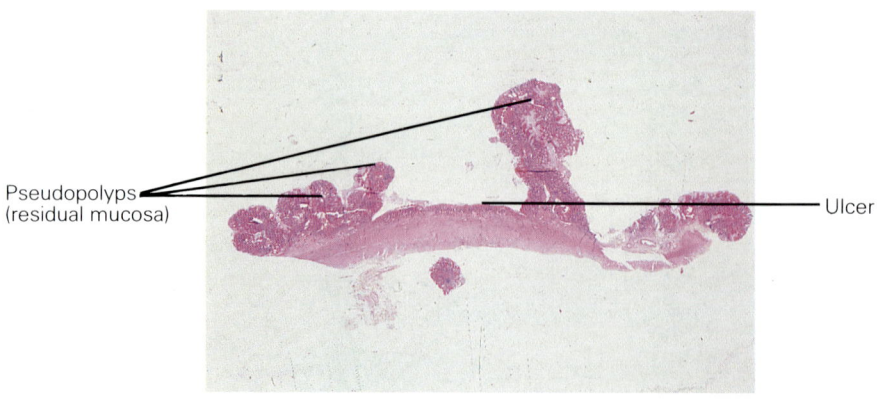

Residual polypoid mucosal surfaces project upward, surrounded by areas of ulceration.

Figure 9.29
Hyperplastic polyp

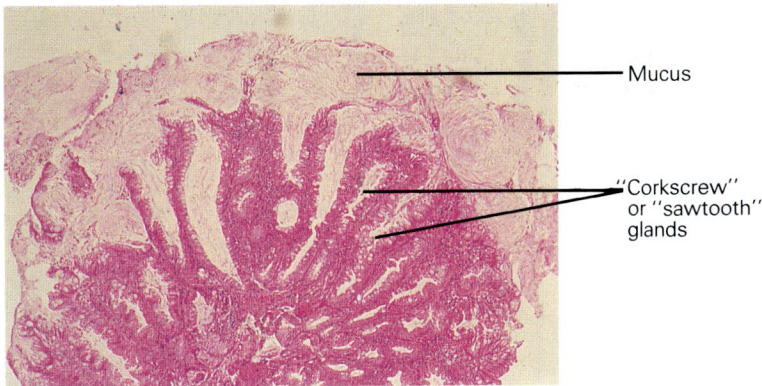

Polyps can be defined as protrusions of the surface mucosa, and the hyperplastic variety seen in the colon is the most common. The glands show abundant goblet cells and "corkscrew" or "sawtooth" configurations due to hyperplastic growth. These polyps are benign and not precancerous.

Figure 9.30
Adenomatous polyp (tubular, pedunculated type)

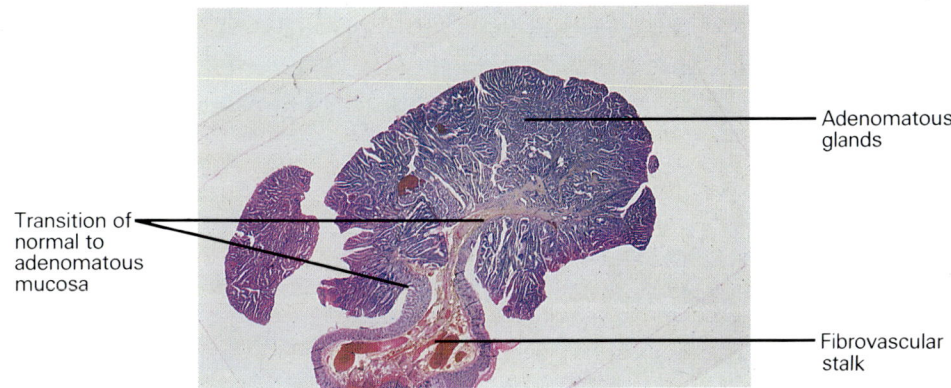

This pedunculated polyp was attached to the colon mucosa by a stalk. See Figures 9.32 and 9.33 for comparison of adenomatous to normal glands.

Figure 9.31
Villous adenoma

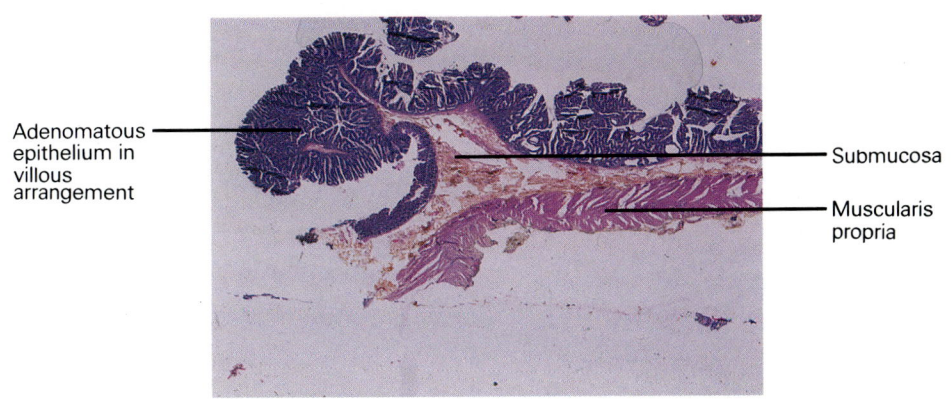

This was a broad-based, sessile mucosal lesion in the colon. The epithelium is adenomatous, as in the pedunculated polyp seen in Figure 9.30. Carcinomas are found in 25 to 50 percent of villous adenomas.

Gastrointestinal Pathology

Figure 9.32
Normal colon glands

Figure 9.33
Adenomatous glands

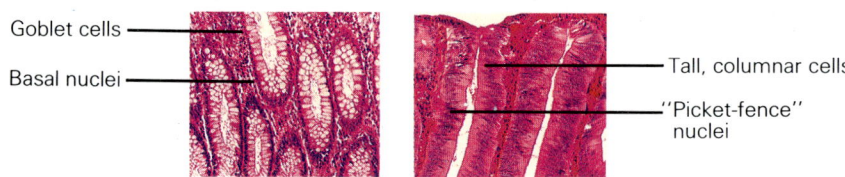

Compare the inconspicuous, basal nuclei of normal colonic glands to the tall, cigar-shaped hyperchromatic nuclei of adenomatous glands that show a "picket-fence" arrangement.

Figure 9.34
Dukes' staging system for colonic carcinoma

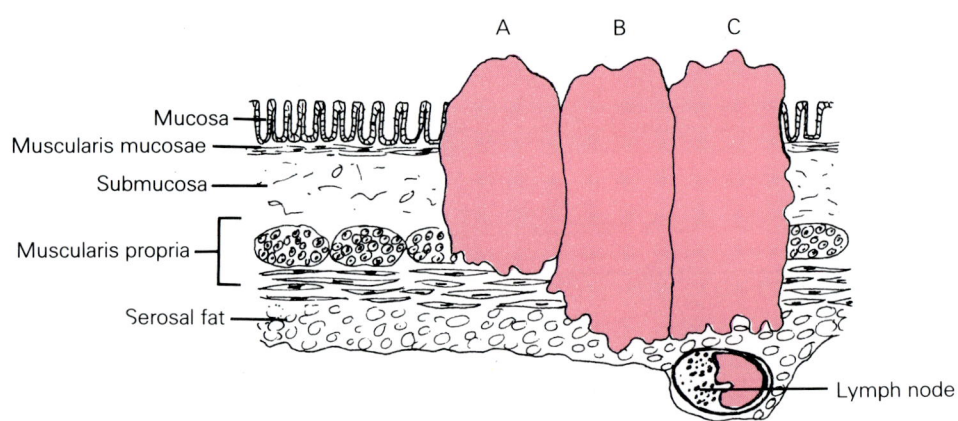

Dukes' A is carcinoma in the bowel wall but not beyond muscularis propria. Dukes' B is carcinoma beyond the muscularis propria into pericolic/perirectal tissues. Dukes' C is carcinoma through the bowel wall with lymph node involvement.

Figure 9.35
Dukes' A colon adenocarcinoma

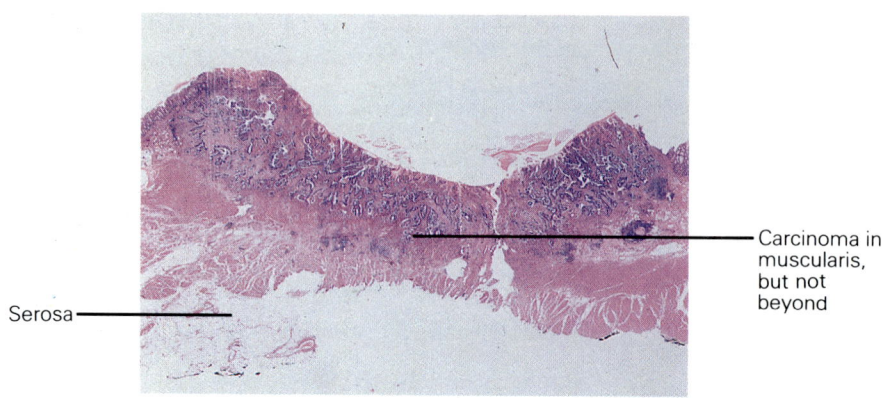

The mucosal surface is replaced by irregular carcinoma glands which extend into the muscularis propria (Dukes' A).

Figure 9.36
Diverticulosis

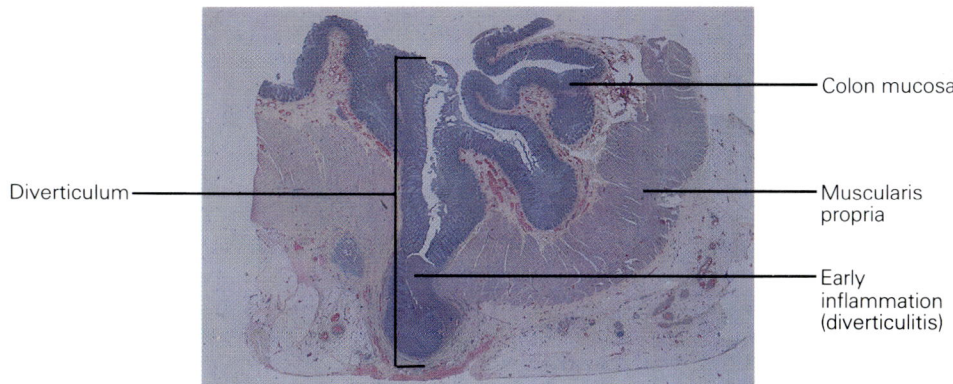

Diverticula are herniated outpouchings of mucosa through weakened or absent muscularis propria. Complications include inflammation (diverticulitis), fibrosis, and bleeding.

Figure 9.37
Melanosis coli

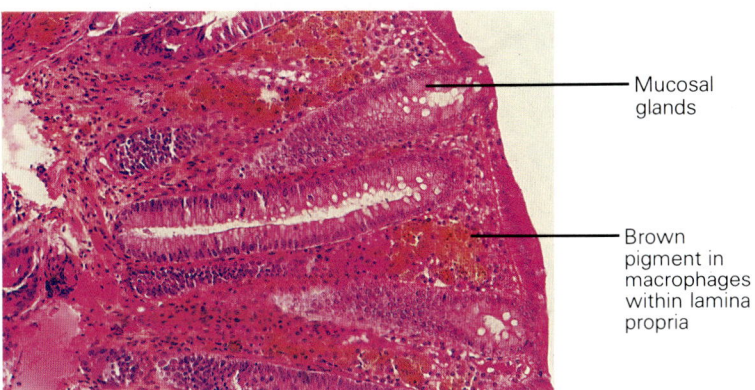

Use of cathartics such as cascara produces brown-black discoloration of the colon mucosa. The pigment (within lysosomes of lamina propria macrophages) is related to melanin and lipofuscin.

Figure 9.38
Hernia sac

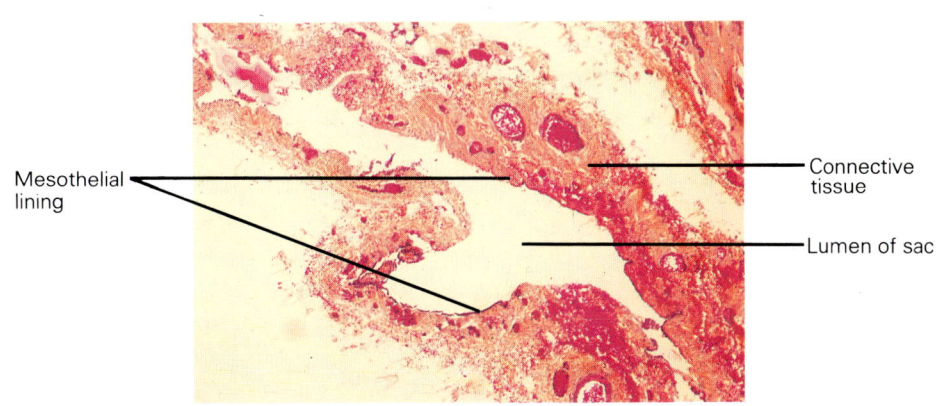

Abdominal wall weakness in the region of the inguinal and femoral canals, surgical wounds, or umbilicus may lead to protrusion of a mesothelium-lined sac. Loops of bowel may become incarcerated or strangulated within hernia sacs.

Figure 9.39
Hemangioma of buccal mucosa

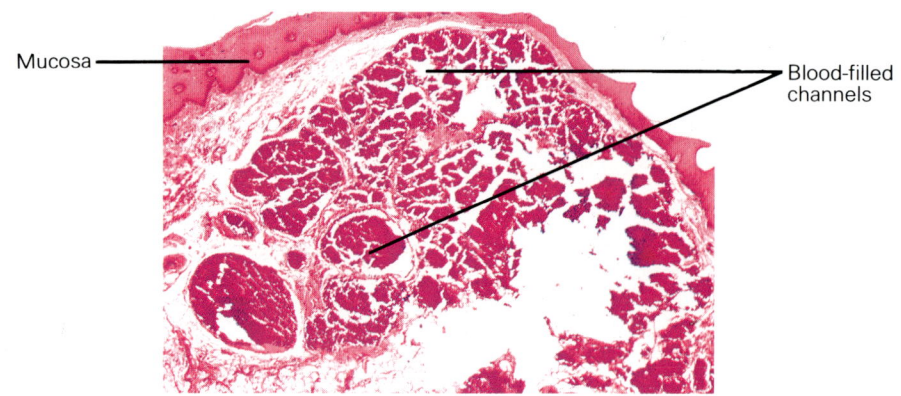

This benign tumor is a common lesion of the mouth.

Figure 9.40
Fibroma of palate

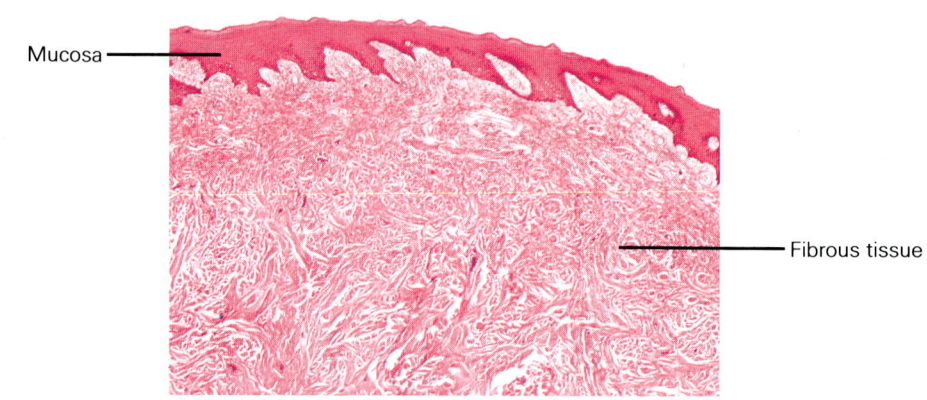

This common benign lesion is believed to be hamartomatous rather than a true tumor.

Figure 9.41
Ameloblastoma

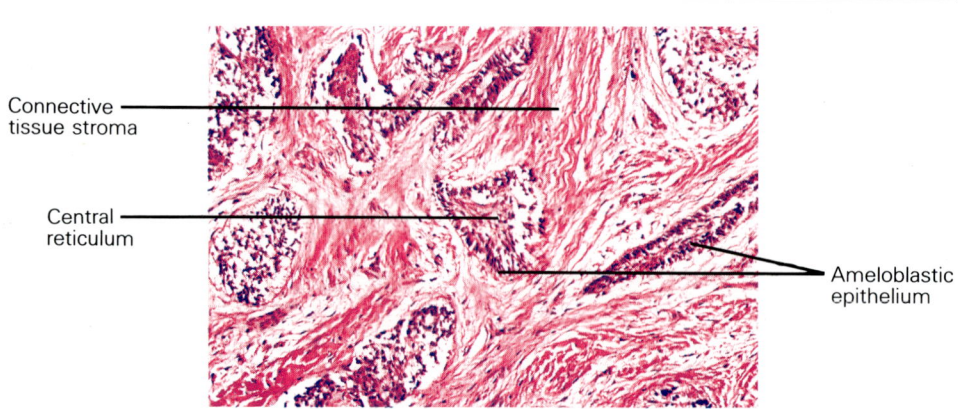

This locally invasive, destructive odontogenic tumor is seen most frequently in the mandible. It consists of nests of cuboidal to columnar ameloblastic epithelium with central stellate reticulum deposits growing within connective tissue stroma.

Figure 9.42
Sjögren's syndrome (salivary gland)

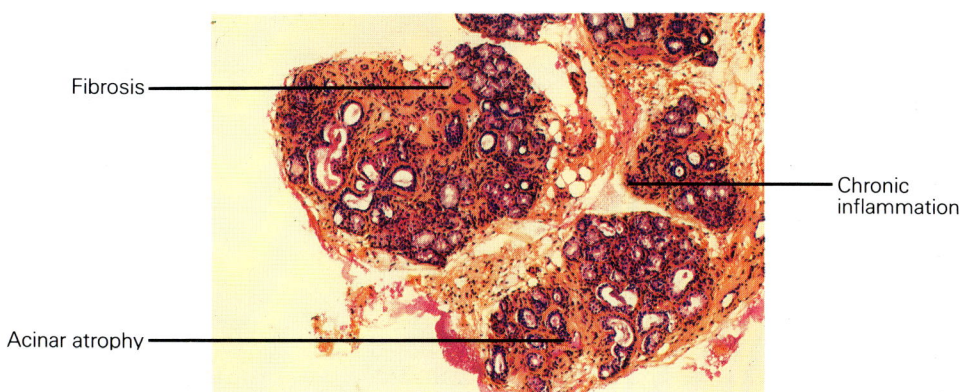

The minor salivary gland shown here has undergone fibrosis with atrophy of secretory acini and accompanying chronic inflammation.

Figure 9.43
Benign mixed tumor (pleomorphic adenoma)

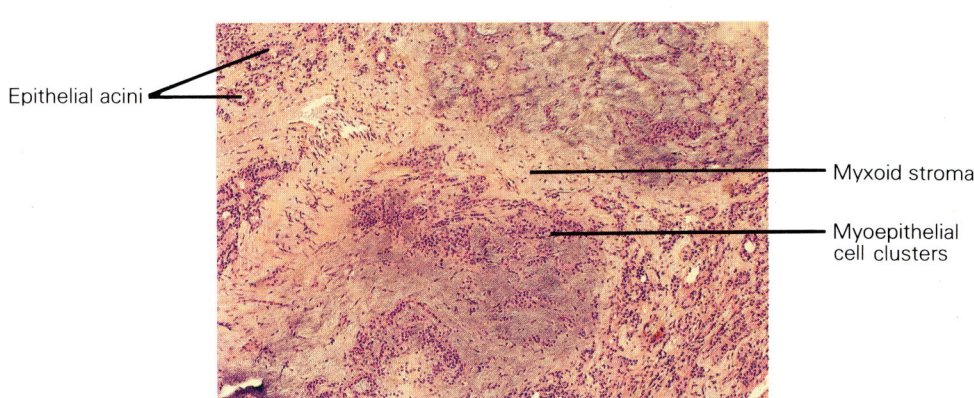

This histologically heterogeneous tumor contains a myxoid background in which nests and cords of epithelial and myoepithelial cells proliferate. This is the most common type of salivary gland tumor.

Figure 9.44
Warthin's tumor (adenolymphoma)

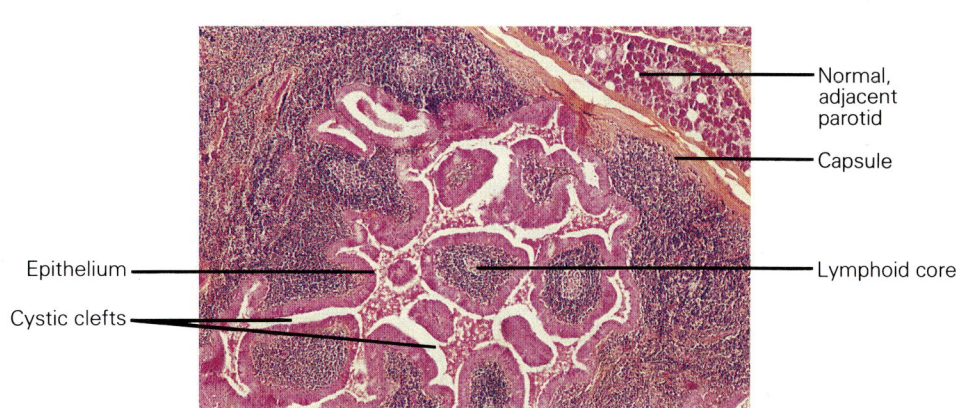

This is a benign, parotid gland tumor composed of epithelial lined papillary projections covering lymphoid tissue. The plump, acidophilic lining epithelial cells are oncocytic (i.e., contain numerous mitochrondria).

Figure 9.45
Mucoepidermoid carcinoma

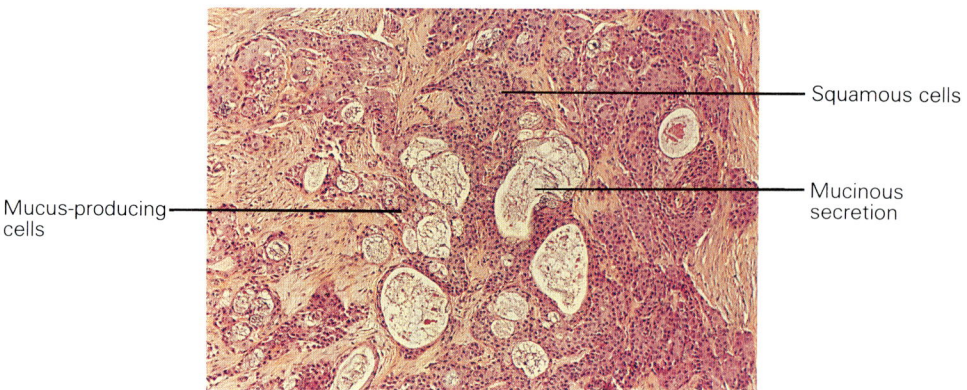

This malignant salivary gland tumor is composed of squamous, mucous, and intermediate cells in varied combinations.

Figure 9.46
Acinic cell carcinoma

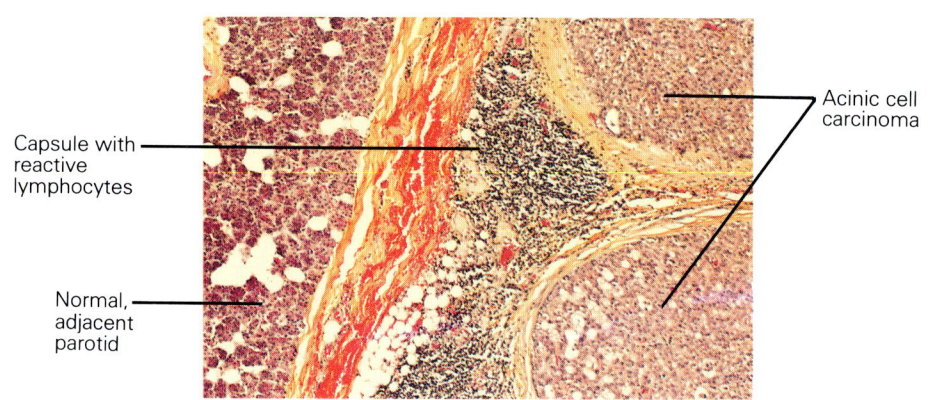

This salivary gland tumor is composed of tightly packed glands and cords of polyhedral acinar cells that contain secretory granules.

Figure 9.47
Adenoid cystic (cylindromatous) carcinoma

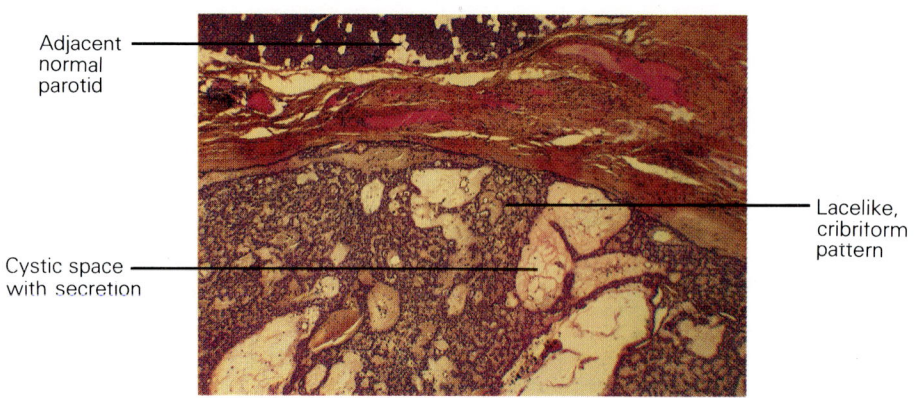

The epithelial cells in this malignant salivary gland tumor grow in anastomosing, lacelike, or cribriform arrangements with scattered cystic spaces.

CHAPTER 10
LIVER PATHOLOGY

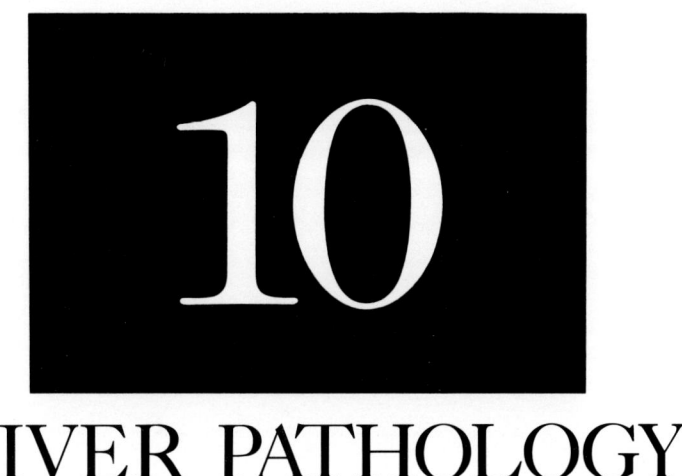

Figure 10.1
Normal liver

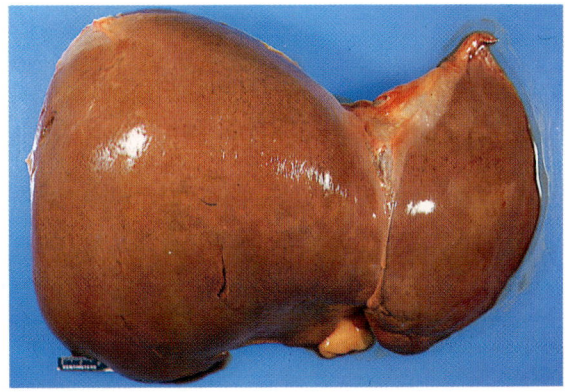

The normal anterior surface shows a smooth, glistening Glisson's capsule and red-brown parenchyma. Normal weight: 1400–1600 g.

Figure 10.2A
Normal liver

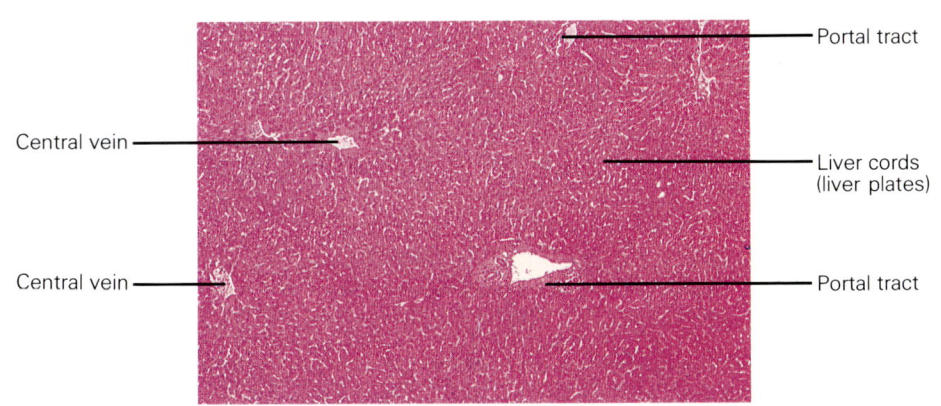

The lobular architecture consists of regularly spaced central veins and portal tracts with cords of hepatocytes radiating outward from centrilobular regions.

Figure 10.2B
Portal tract

Figure 10.2C
Centrilobular region (zone 3)

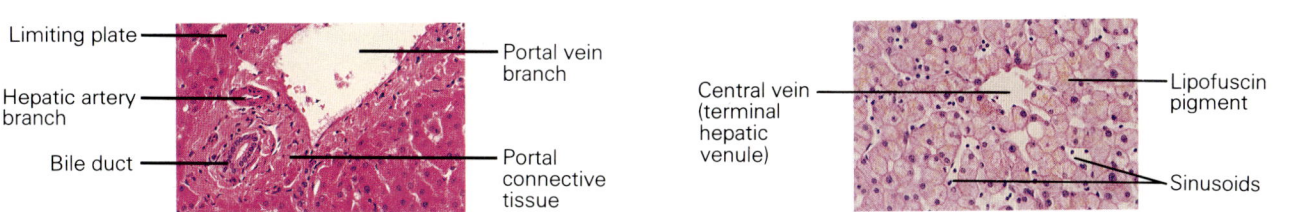

The normal portal and centrilobular structures are shown. The portal tract consists of connective tissue (with a distinct rim of hepatocytes comprising the limiting plate) and contains an interlobular bile duct and branches of the portal vein and hepatic artery. Central veins are surrounded by single-cell thick liver plates and intervening sinusoids. Lipofuscin ("wear and tear") lysosomal pigment is prominent in central hepatocytes.

Liver Pathology

Figure 10.3
Liver pathology: major pathologic lesions

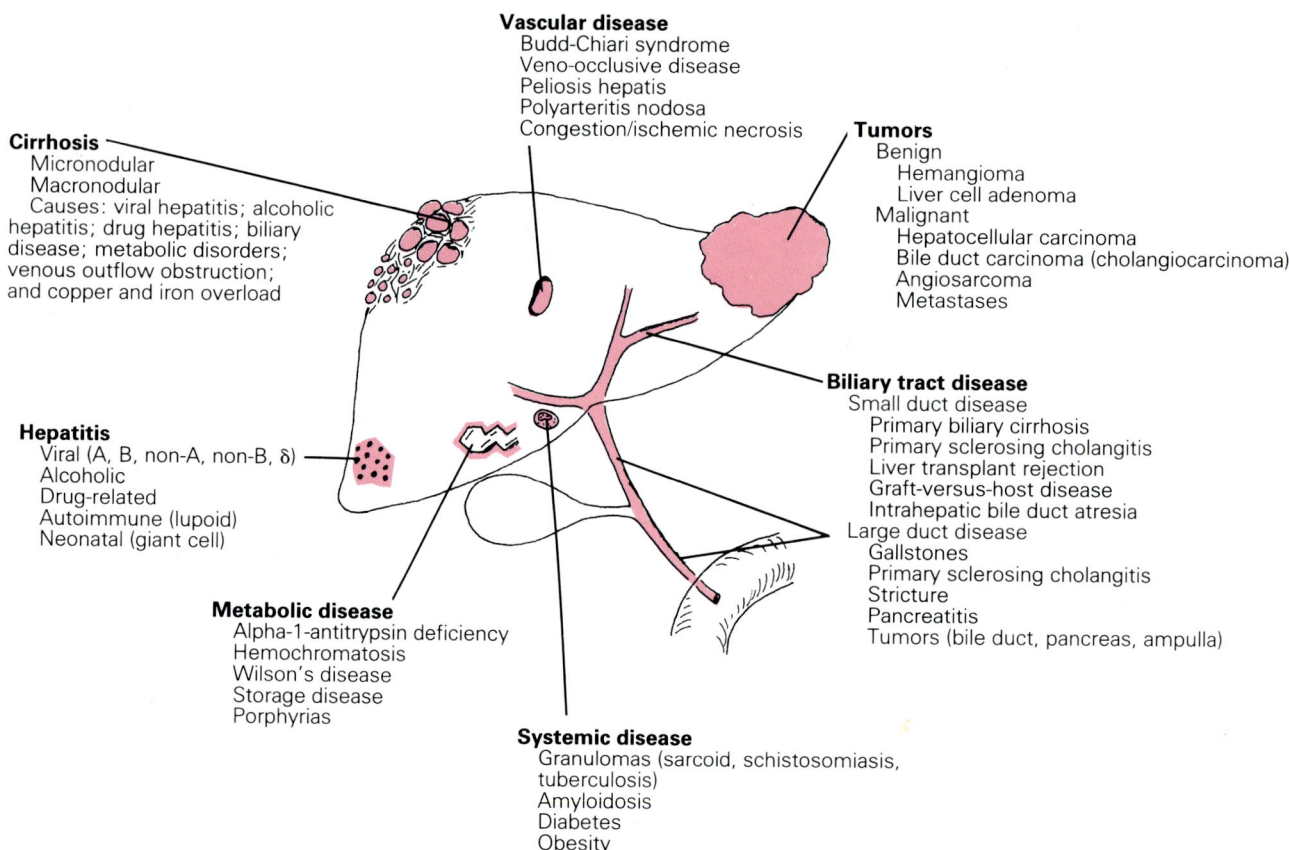

Figure 10.4
Acute hepatitis

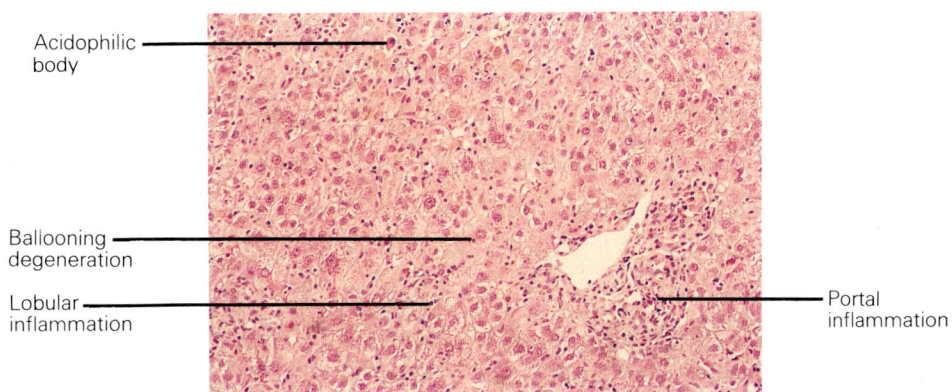

Diffuse inflammation and liver cell degeneration is seen in acute hepatitis due to hepatitis A, B, non-A, non-B, and delta viruses and certain drugs.

Figure 10.5
Acute hepatitis with bridging hepatic necrosis

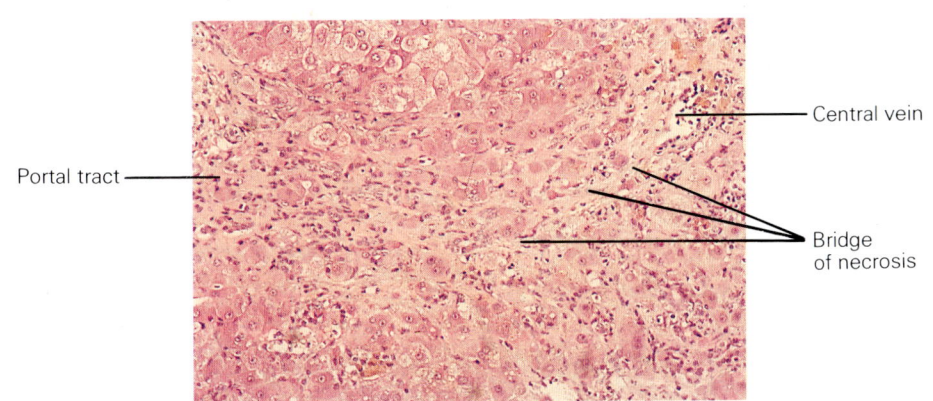

This form of hepatitis is marked by confluent necrosis bridging between central veins and portal tracts. It may presage the development of chronic hepatitis.

Figure 10.6
Massive hepatic necrosis

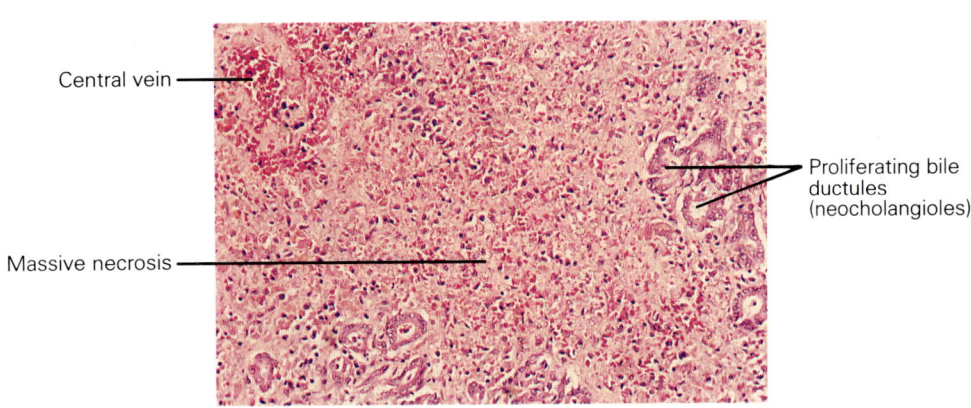

This severe form of hepatitis is associated with a fulminant clinical course and high mortality. Virtually all the parenchyma is necrotic except for islands of proliferating bile ductular structures.

Figure 10.7
Chronic persistent hepatitis (CPH)

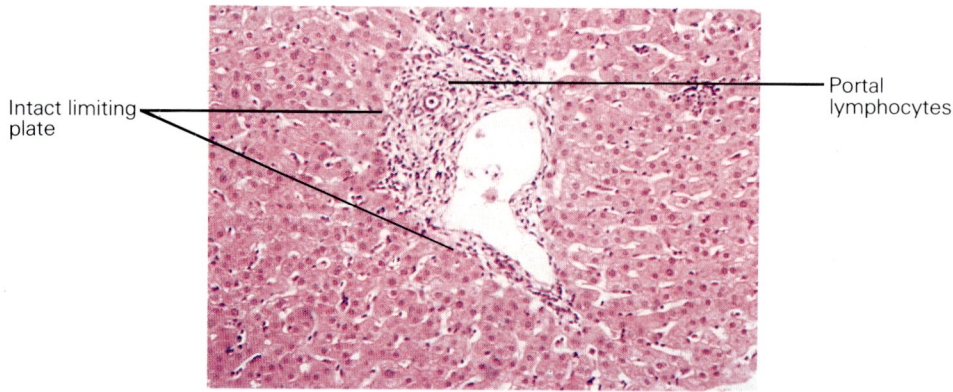

This form of chronic hepatitis shows portal tract lymphocytes with an intact limiting plate. This is considered a "benign" lesion that does not progress to cirrhosis.

Figure 10.8
Chronic lobular hepatitis (CLH)

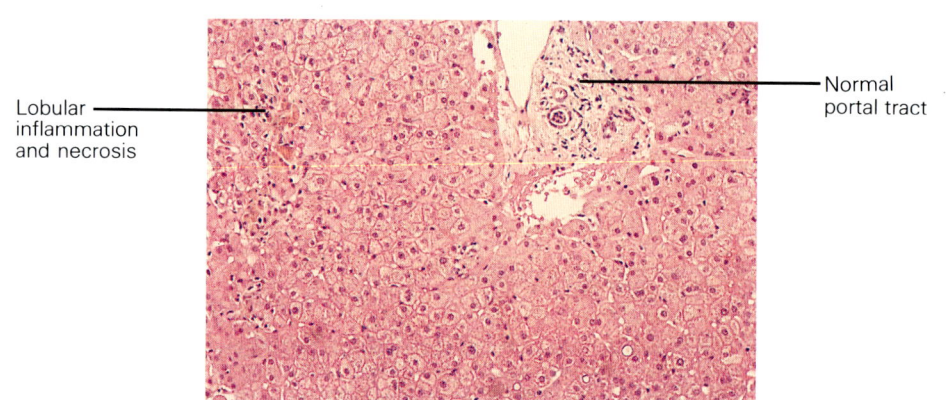

This less common variety of chronic hepatitis shows evidence of lobular inflammation and necrosis only. Cirrhosis does not develop.

Figure 10.9
Chronic active hepatitis (CAH)

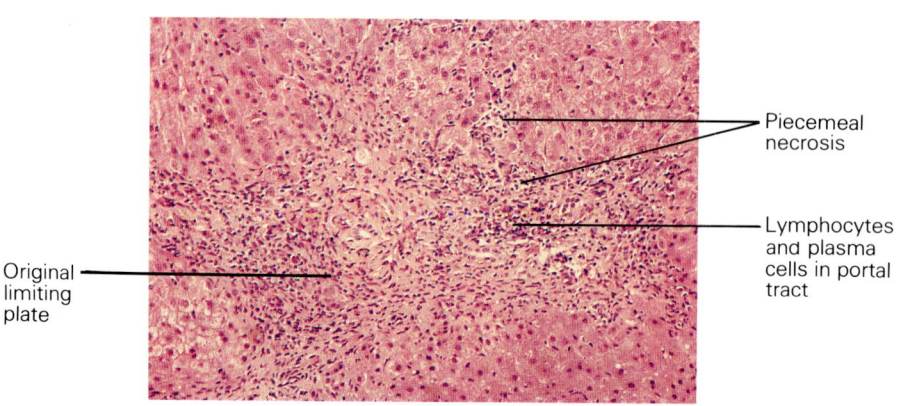

The pathognomonic lesion of CAH is piecemeal necrosis (portal and periportal inflammation and necrosis with erosion of the limiting plate). It may progress to cirrhosis.

Figure 10.10
Piecemeal necrosis in CAH

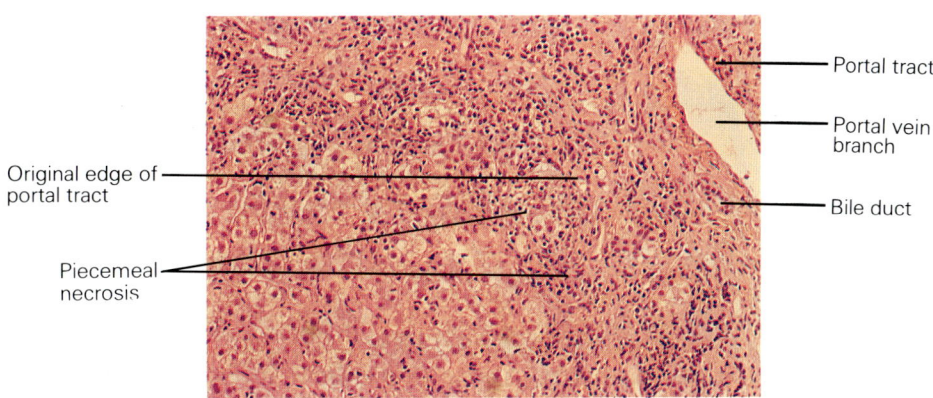

This higher magnification of a portal tract in CAH shows the active lymphocyte-plasma cell infiltrate extending into the periportal region in which liver cells are surrounded and entrapped. Scar tissue is deposited in these regions.

Figure 10.11
CAH with developing cirrhosis

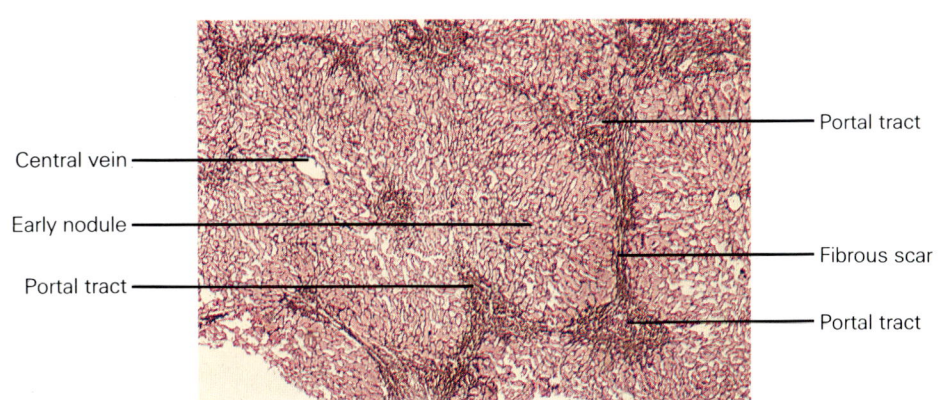

In this reticulin stain, fibrosis of portal tracts is shown, including irregular, scalloped ("arachnoid") edges and bridging between certain portal tracts. Early cirrhotic nodules are developing, but central veins can still be located.

Figure 10.12
Macronodular cirrhosis following CAH

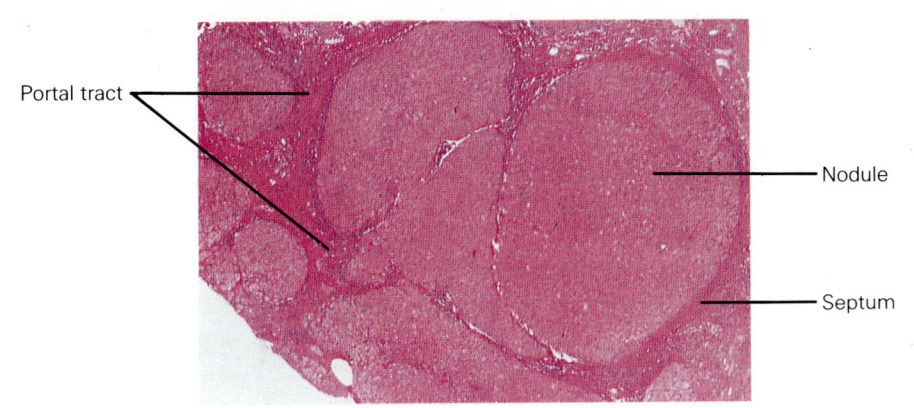

Irregular fibrous septa surround architecturally abnormal nodules in this cirrhotic liver which developed following CAH due to hepatitis B virus infection.

Figure 10.13
"Ground-glass" hepatocytes

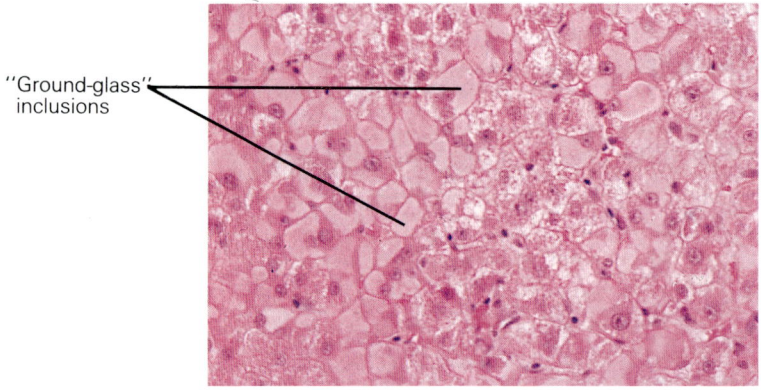

The presence of hepatitis B surface antigen (HBsAg) within chronically infected hepatocytes produces a "ground-glass" cytoplasmic inclusion, often separated from the cell membrane by a clear halo.

Figure 10.14
Orcein stain for HBsAg

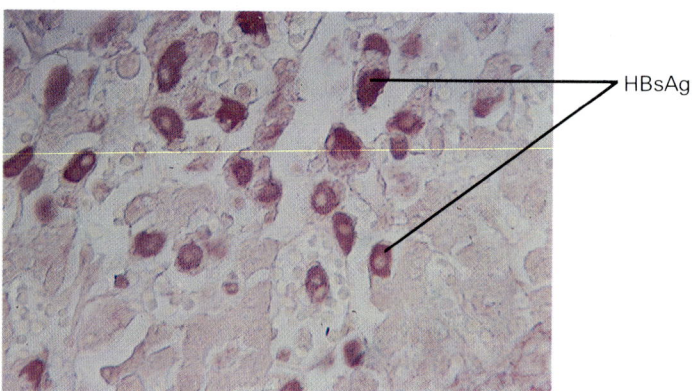

"Ground-glass" hepatocytes containing HBsAg show dark cytoplasmic inclusions with the orcein stain. Note the absence of nuclear staining.

Figure 10.15
Hepatitis B virus particles in carrier serum

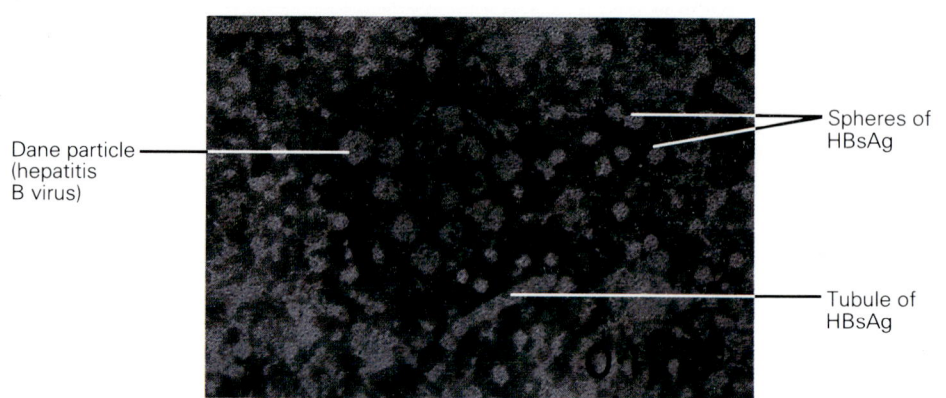

Electron microscopy of serum from individuals with chronic hepatitis B virus infection (carriers) shows spherical and tubular forms of excess HBsAg and rounded hepatitis B virions (Dane particles).

Figure 10.16
Acetaminophen hepatitis

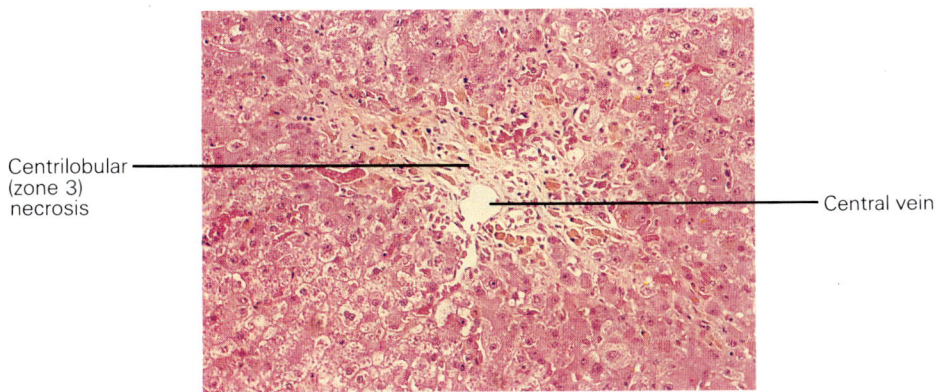

Predictable hepatotoxins such as acetaminophen are metabolized by cytochrome-containing central (Rappaport Zone 3) hepatocytes and result in this pattern of centrilobular necrosis.

Figure 10.17
Giant cell hepatitis

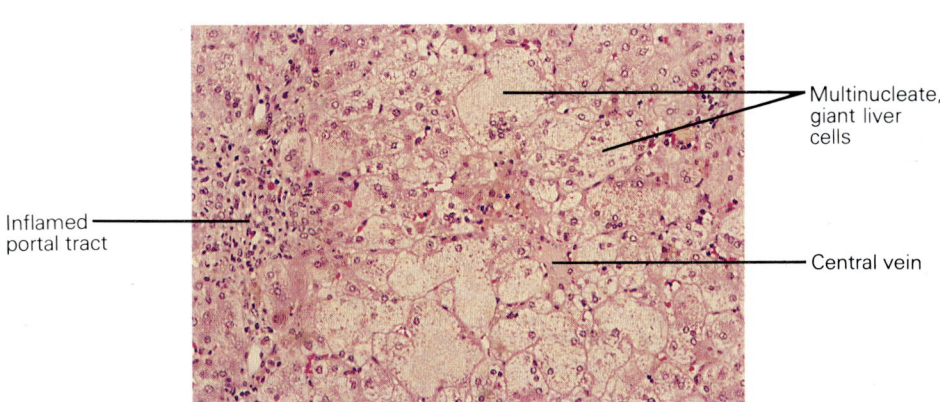

This histologic pattern of hepatitis with prominent "giant cell" hepatocytes is seen in neonatal viral hepatitis, metabolic disorders, and cholestatic diseases.

Figure 10.18
Fatty liver

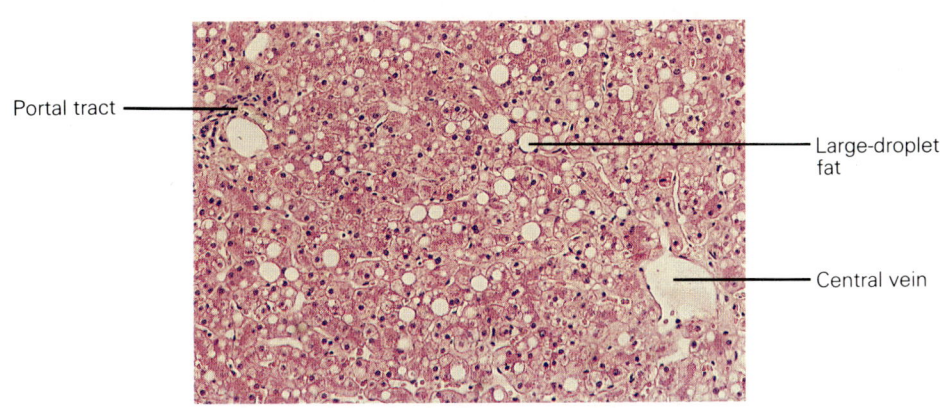

Panlobular fat vacuoles within hepatocytes are seen in this biopsy from an alcoholic. Other causes of fat include obesity, diabetes, and corticosteroid administration.

Figure 10.19
Alcoholic hepatitis

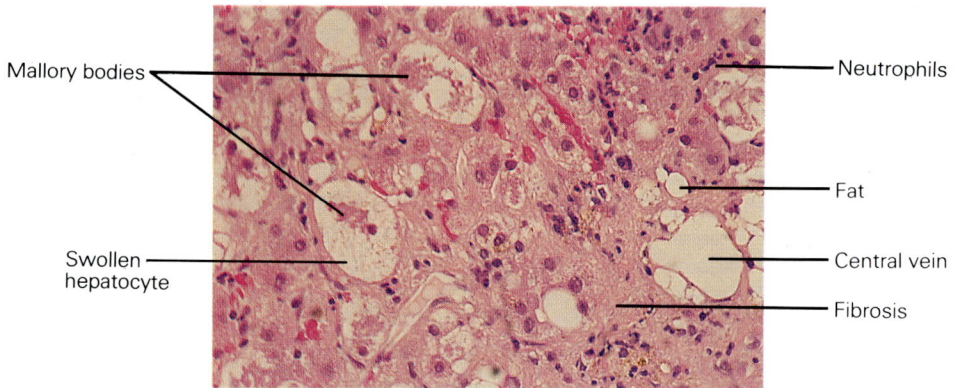

Continual ingestion of large amounts of alcohol produces hepatocyte swelling, Mallory bodies (clumped intermediate filaments), neutrophil infiltrates, and pericentral fibrosis in alcoholic hepatitis.

Figure 10.20
Alcoholic hepatitis and cirrhosis

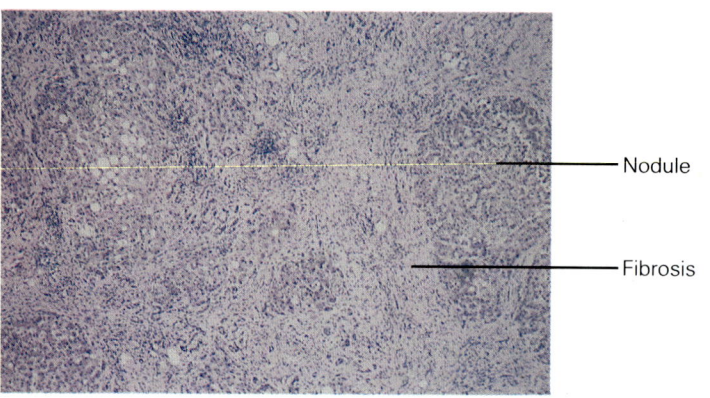

The parenchyma has been dissected by fibrosis, and nodules have developed in this late stage of alcoholic liver disease. Fat (at left) and alcoholic hepatitis often persist at this stage.

Figure 10.21
Microvesicular (small-droplet) fatty change

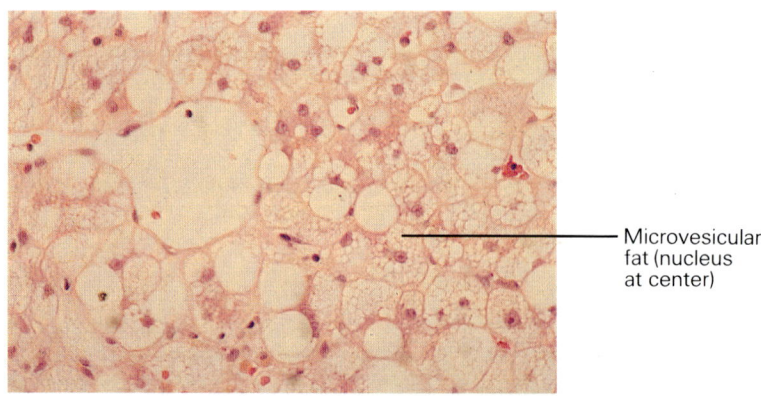

Hepatocytes with microvesicular steatosis (small-droplet fatty change) are a feature of acute fatty liver of pregnancy (third trimester), Reye's syndrome, and tetracycline or valproic acid hepatotoxicity.

Figure 10.22
Alpha-1-antitrypsin deficiency

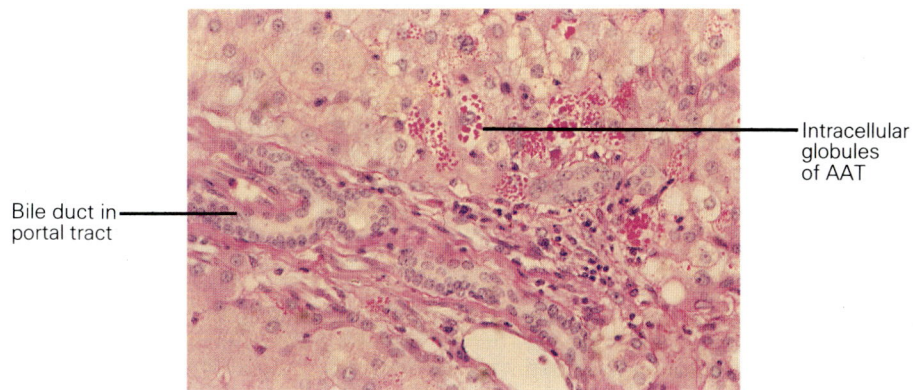

Serum deficiency of the circulating anti-protease, alpha-1-antitrypsin (AAT), is related to structural changes in the enzyme which is retained in globular form in hepatocytes. The globules are demonstrated in periportal hepatocytes by PAS stain with diastase digestion.

Figure 10.23
Type I glycogen storage disease

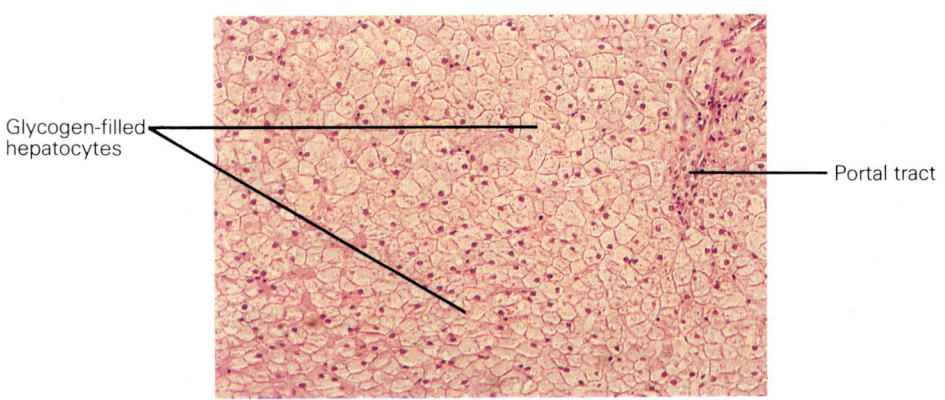

Hepatocytes show pale cytoplasm filled with glycogen in this storage disorder.

Figure 10.24
Niemann-Pick disease

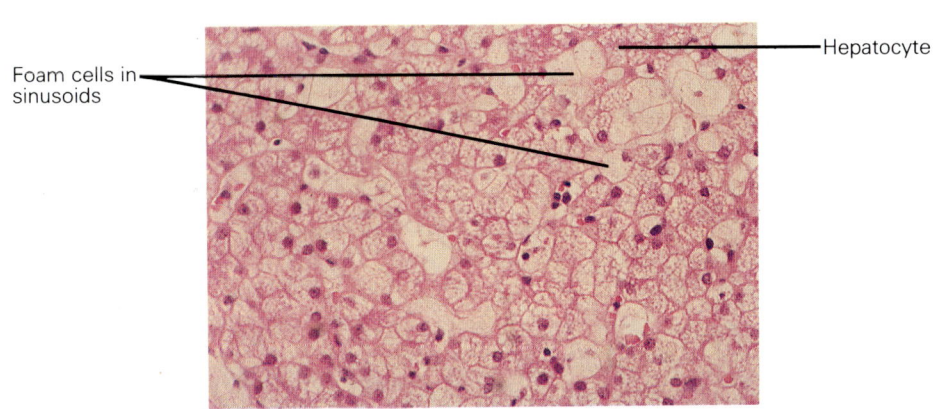

Macrophages containing sphingomyelin (foam cells) are present within sinusoids.

Liver Pathology

Figure 10.25
Hepatic amyloid

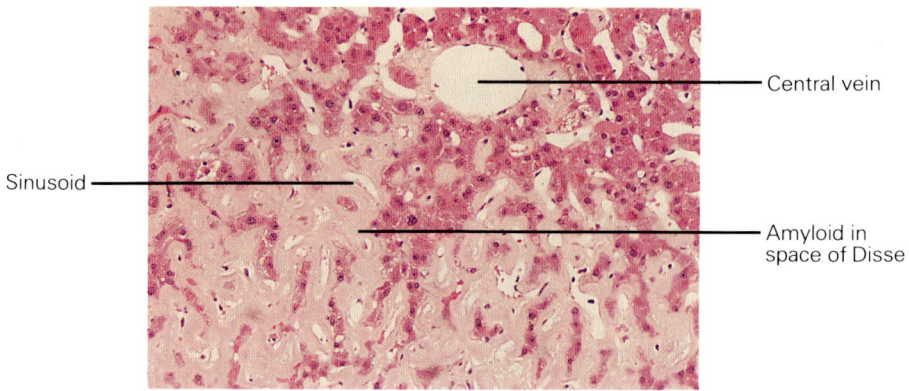

Pink-staining amyloid in the liver characteristically accumulates in the space of Disse and/or in the walls of blood vessels.

Figure 10.26
Hemosiderosis in Kupffer cells

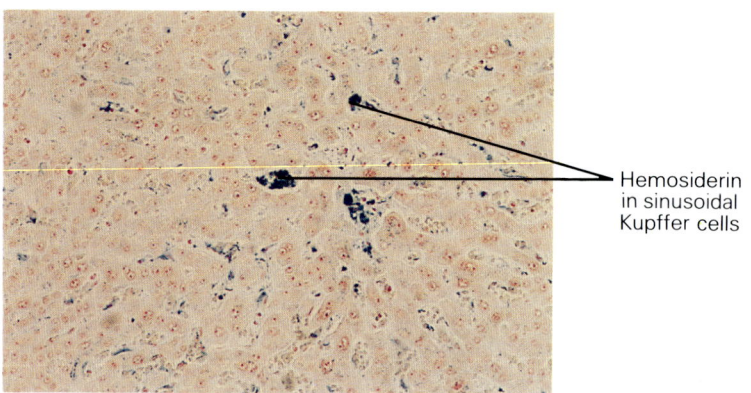

The presence of stainable iron in the liver is known as hemosiderosis. Hemosiderin (blue on Prussian blue iron stain) is most often found in Kupffer cells and may be due to hemolysis or transfusion.

Figure 10.27
Hemochromatosis

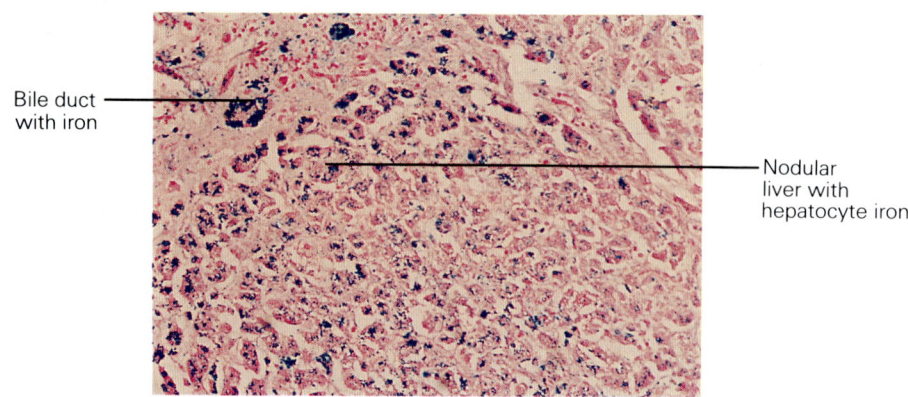

Massive parenchymal iron overload associated with tissue damage is known as hemochromatosis. Marked hemosiderin deposits (blue stain) are present in portal tract bile ducts and macrophages and in hepatocytes.

Figure 10.28
Wilson's disease

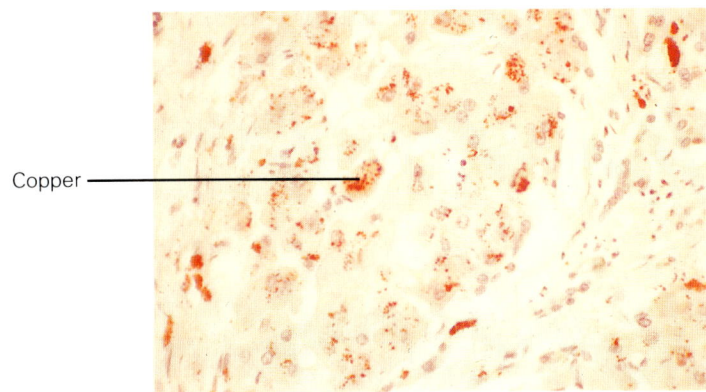

Rhodanine stain for copper (orange granules) shows marked copper deposition in hepatocytes. Routine histology shows chronic active hepatitis and/or cirrhosis in advanced Wilson's disease.

Figure 10.29
Cholestasis

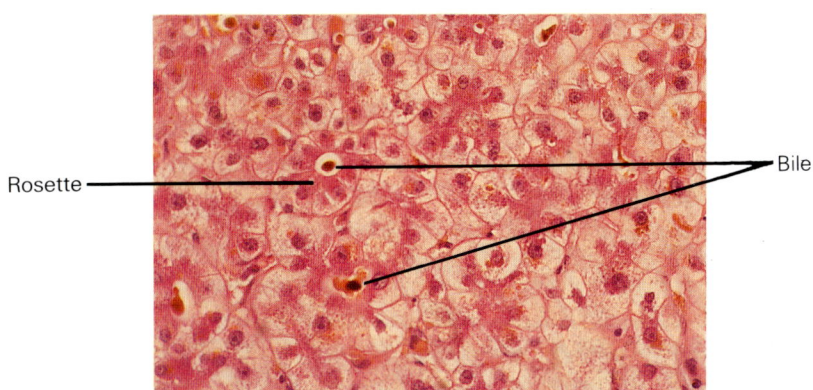

The histologic presence of bile in liver tissue (cholestasis) results from stagnated bile flow. This may be due to drug injury, mechanical bile duct obstruction, and systemic conditions such as *E. coli* sepsis. Hepatocytes may become re-organized into "rosettes" around bile plugs.

Figure 10.30
Large bile duct obstruction

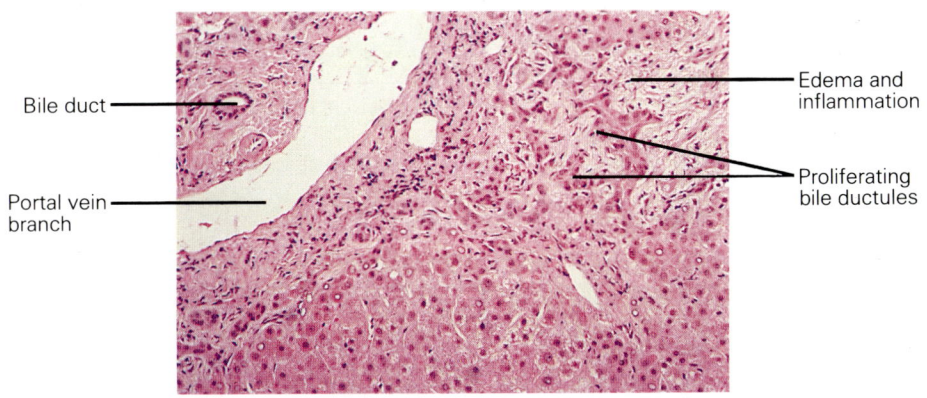

Typical changes in mechanical obstruction of large bile ducts include portal tract edema, bile ductular proliferation, and a neutrophil infiltrate.

Figure 10.31
Cholangitis

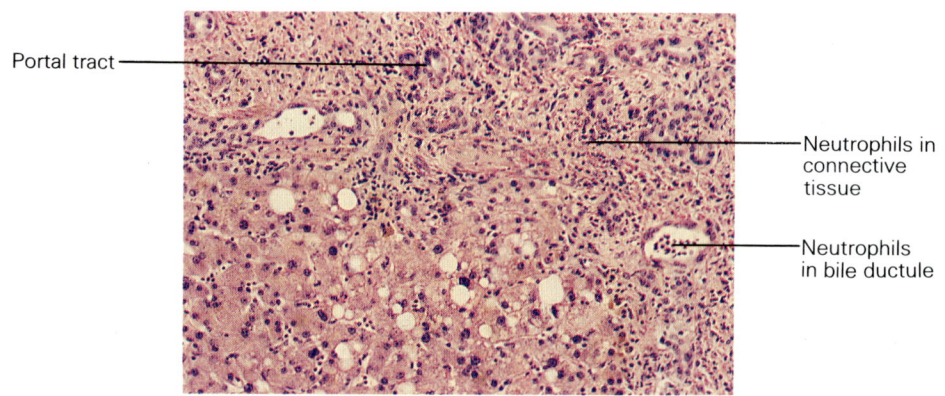

Ascending infection of the biliary tree (cholangitis) results in a heavy neutrophil infiltrate within portal connective tissue, bile ducts, and bile ductules. *E. coli* is the most common etiologic agent.

Figure 10.32
Chronic biliary obstruction and developing biliary cirrhosis

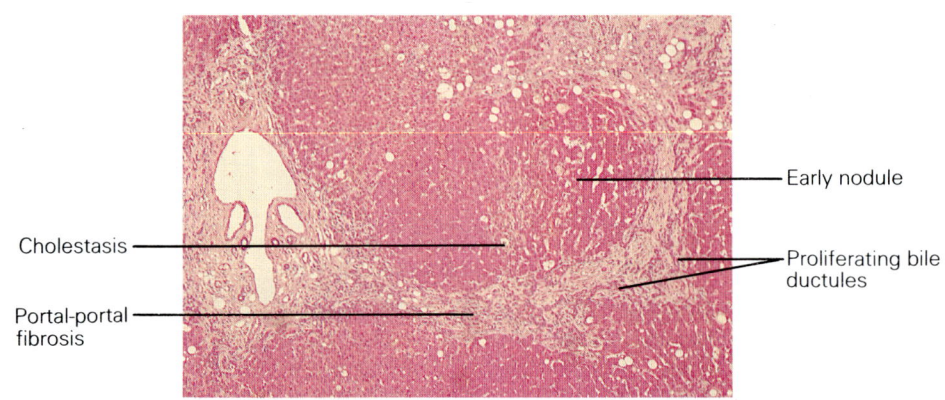

Unrelieved biliary tract obstruction, regardless of etiology, causes portal fibrosis, portal-to-portal fibrous linking, and development of nodules.

Figure 10.33
Biliary cirrhosis

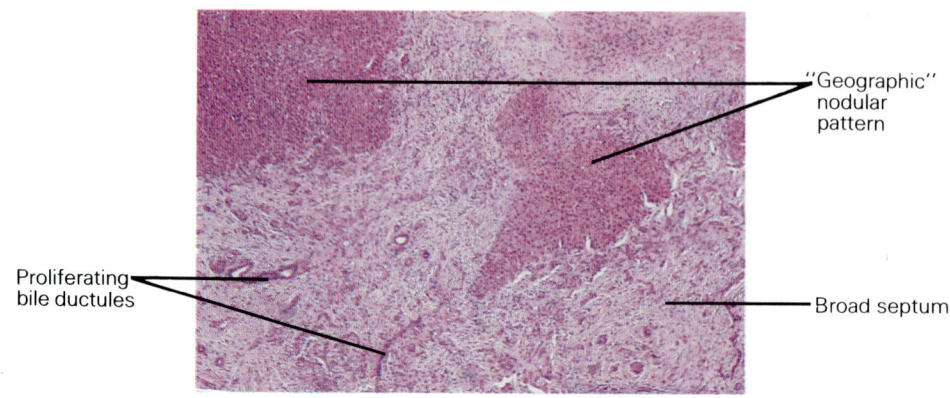

The final architectural stage of many biliary diseases is biliary cirrhosis (so-called secondary biliary cirrhosis). Changes include broad septa and a "geographic" pattern of nodules.

134 *Histopathology of Disease*

Figure 10.34
Primary biliary cirrhosis

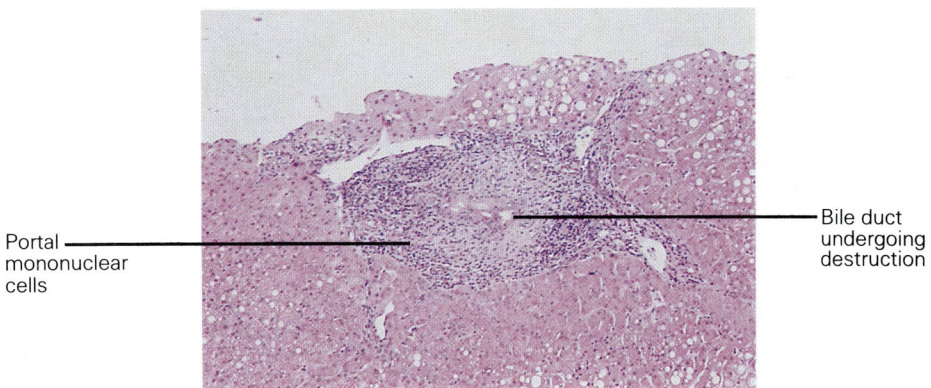

This condition, also called chronic, nonsuppurative, destructive cholangitis, results in destruction of intrahepatic bile ducts by mononuclear inflammatory cells. The disease has four stages: florid bile duct damage (shown above), bile ductular proliferation, portal scarring, and cirrhosis. Affected patients have positive serum anti-mitochondrial antibodies.

Figure 10.35
Primary sclerosing cholangitis

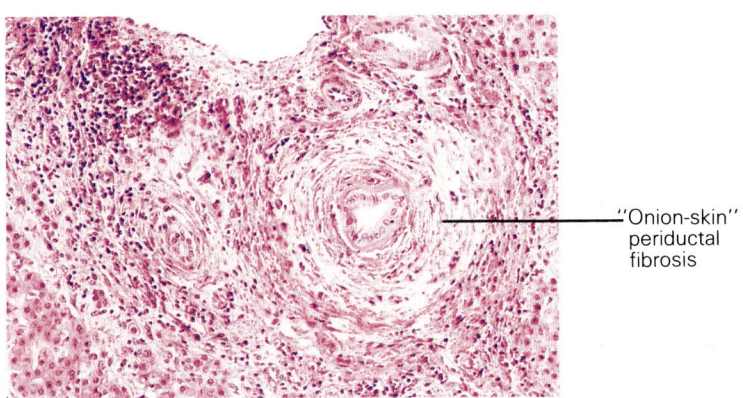

This is a chronic, idiopathic fibrosing disorder involving both intrahepatic and extrahepatic bile ducts, often in patients with ulcerative colitis.

Figure 10.36
Bile duct malformation (microhamartoma)

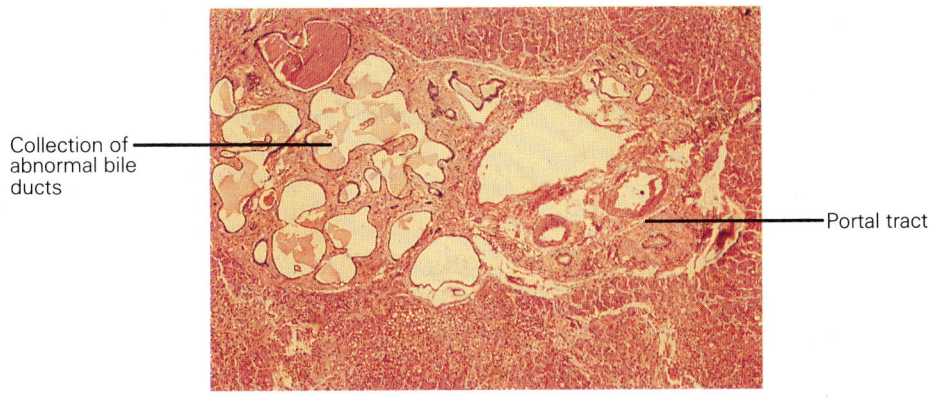

These arise because of embryologic malformation of the bile duct plate. Solitary microhamartomas are incidental histologic findings and are part of the spectrum of fibropolycystic diseases of the liver.

Liver Pathology

Figure 10.37
Congenital hepatic fibrosis

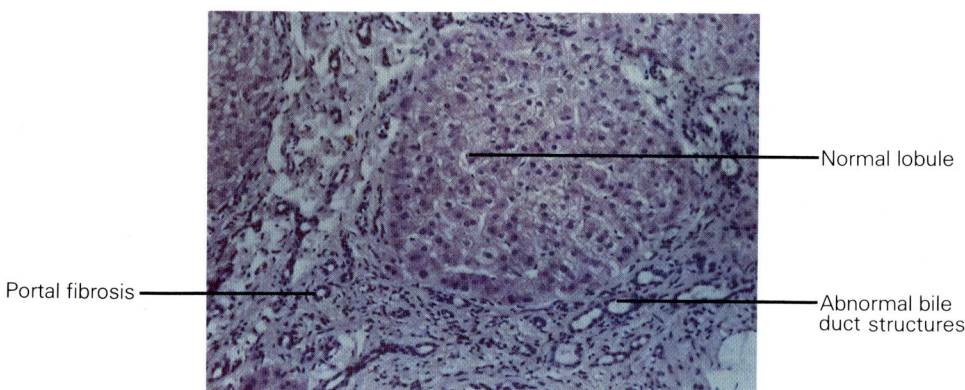

This predominantly childhood condition is associated with portal hypertension. Abnormal biliary structures are embedded in fibrous tissue linking portal areas. Lobular parenchyma is normal.

Figure 10.38
Caroli's disease

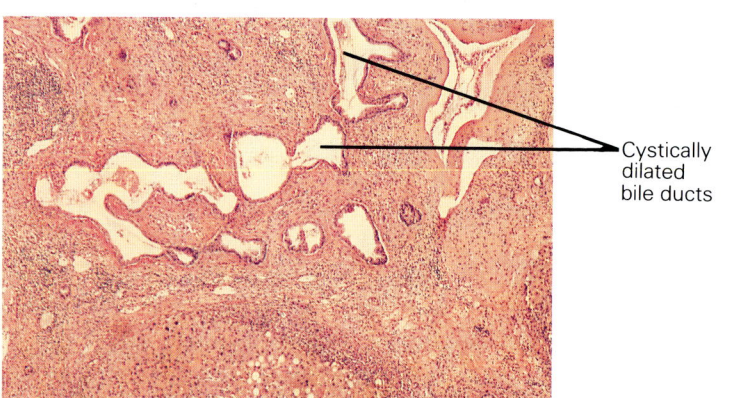

Caroli's disease (congenital dilatation of the intrahepatic bile ducts) is another disease featuring malformed, dilated bile ducts and a predisposition to recurrent cholangitis.

Figure 10.39
Congestion of liver ("nutmeg" liver)

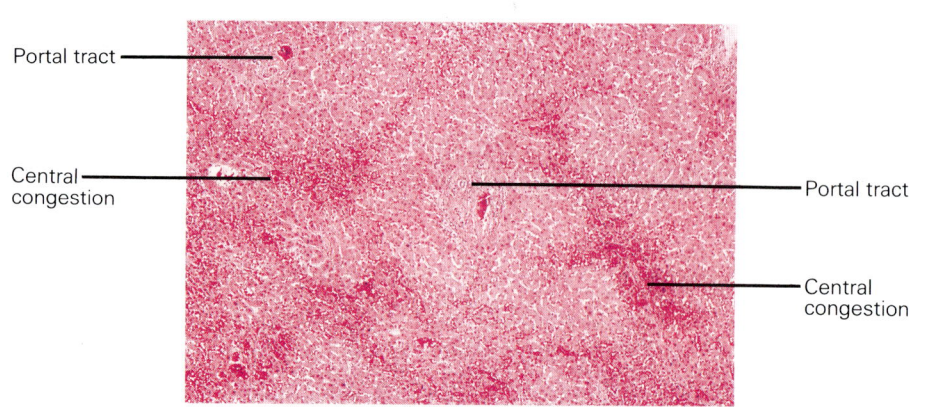

Right heart failure commonly results in congestion of centrilobular veins and sinusoids and a grossly mottled, "nutmeg" appearance. Note the spared periportal regions.

Figure 10.40
Shock liver (ischemic necrosis)

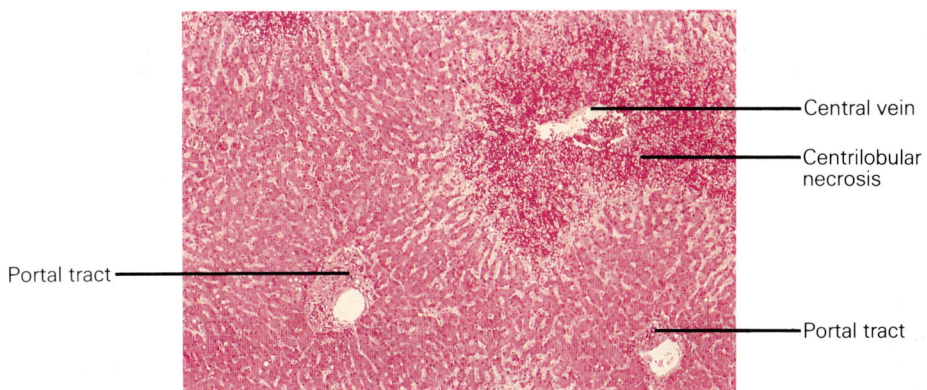

Necrosis of hepatocytes in centrilobular regions (zone 3) often develops following episodes of left ventricular failure and hypotensive shock.

Figure 10.41
Peliosis hepatis

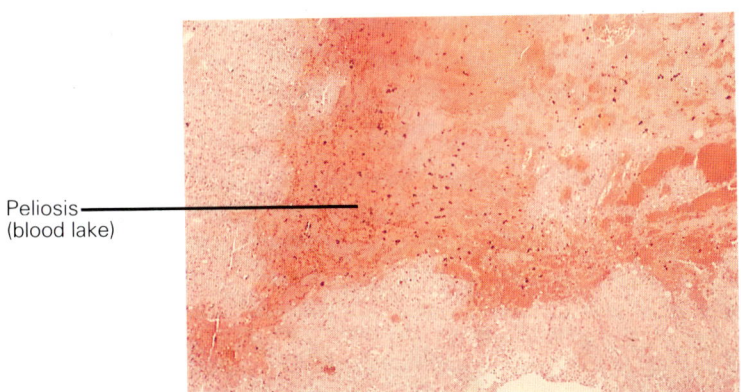

These irregular pools of blood lack a fibrous capsule and are only partly endothelial-lined. This is a rare lesion seen with anabolic steroid use, systemic debilitating diseases, and malignancy.

Figure 10.42
Budd-Chiari syndrome

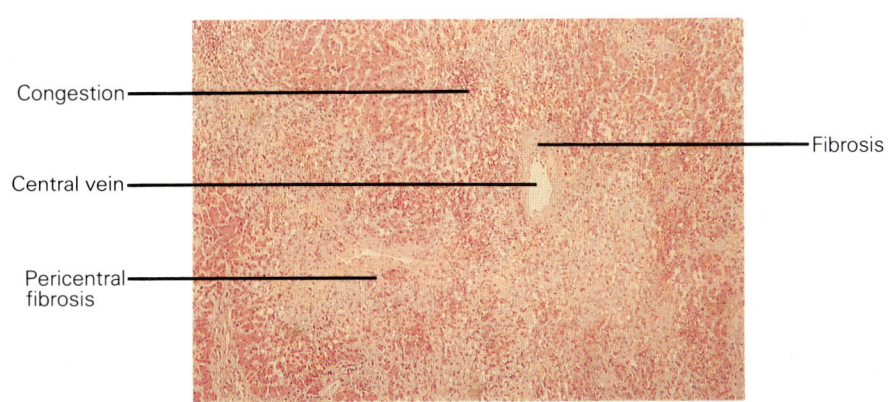

This syndrome of hepatic venous outflow obstruction results in marked centrilobular congestion with fibrosis in the walls of central veins and perisinusoidal regions. Hepatic vein obstruction by thrombi, invasive tumor, or congenital webs are the major causes.

Figure 10.43
Sarcoidosis

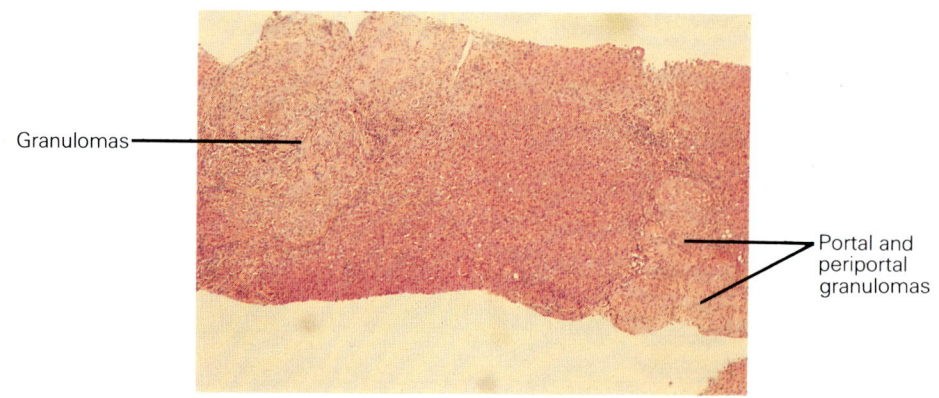

Sarcoid granulomas in the liver often undergo hyalinization and are typically located in the portal and periportal regions.

Figure 10.44
Mycobacterial granulomas in AIDS

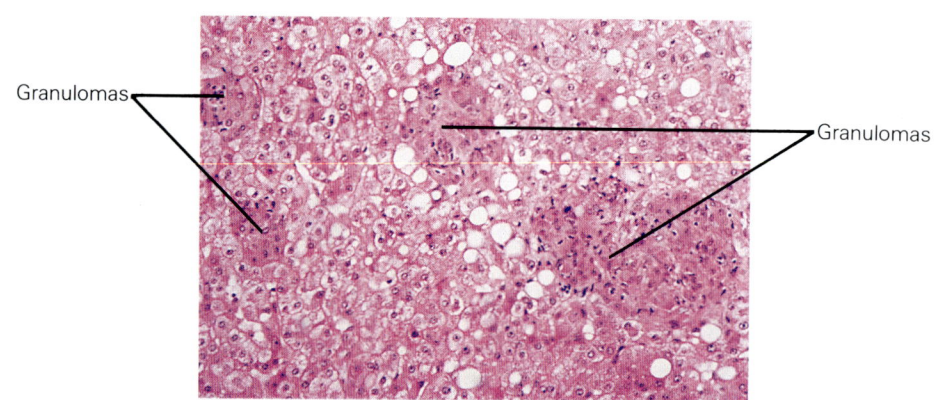

Mycobacterium avium-intracellulare infection often produces noncaseating granulomas composed of plump macrophages in the liver.

Figure 10.45
Acid-fast stain in Mycobacterial granuloma

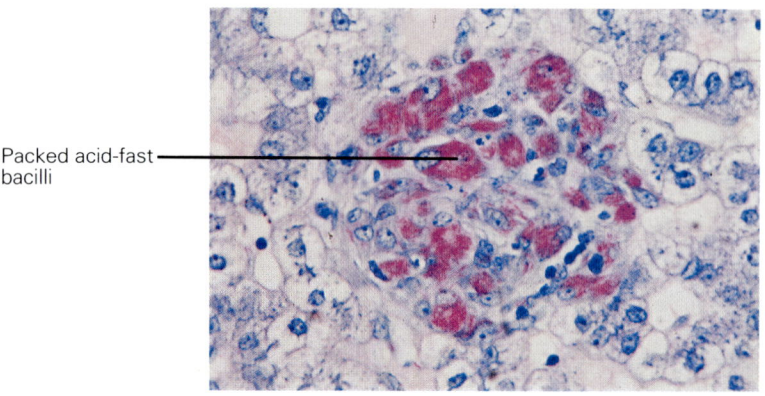

Mycobacterium avium-intracellulare granulomas typically contain abundant acid-fast bacilli packed in macrophages.

Figure 10.46
Cytomegalovirus (CMV) cholangitis and hepatitis in AIDS

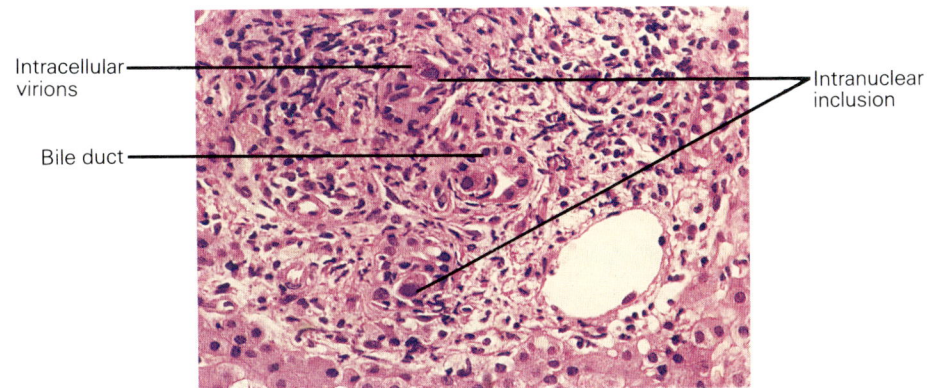

CMV may infect hepatocytes, endothelial cells, Kupffer cells, and bile duct cells (shown above). Several ducts show cells with both intranuclear and intracellular viral inclusions.

Figure 10.47
Cirrhosis

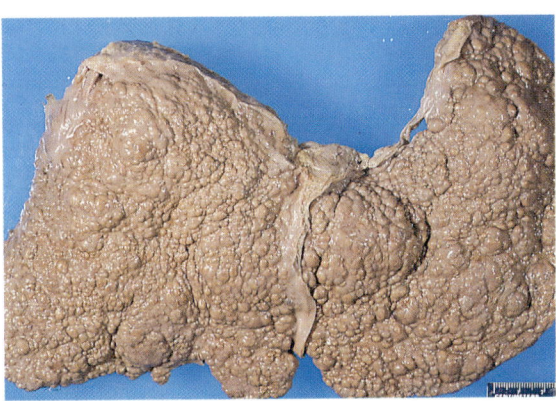

Gross specimen of micronodular cirrhosis. Cirrhosis is defined as diffuse fibrosis associated with architecturally abnormal regenerative nodules.

Figure 10.48
Cirrhosis

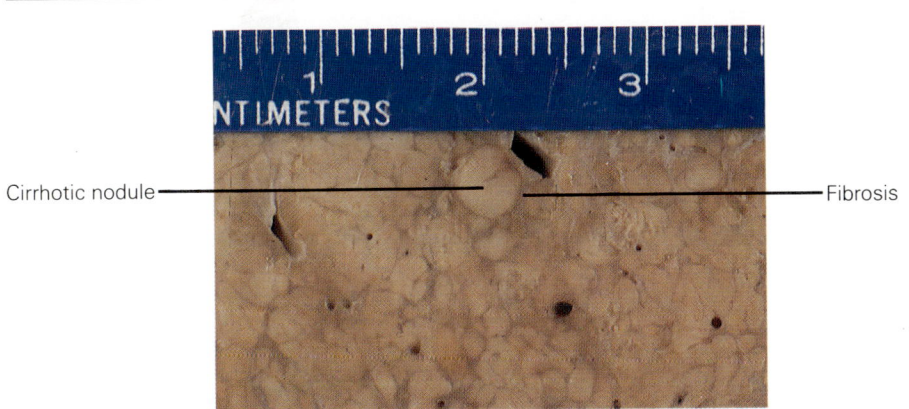

Cut section of cirrhotic liver demonstrating gray areas of fibrosis surrounding pale, cirrhotic nodules.

Figure 10.49
Micronodular cirrhosis

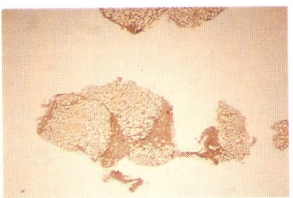

Nodules are 3 mm or less in diameter. Causes include alcoholism, hemochromatosis, and chronic biliary tract disease.

Figure 10.50
Macronodular cirrhosis

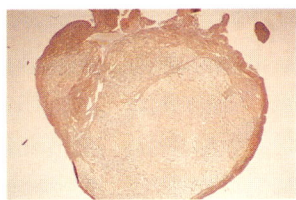

Nodules are 3 mm or more in diameter. Causes include chronic viral hepatitis and autoimmune chronic active hepatitis.

Figure 10.51
Liver cell dysplasia

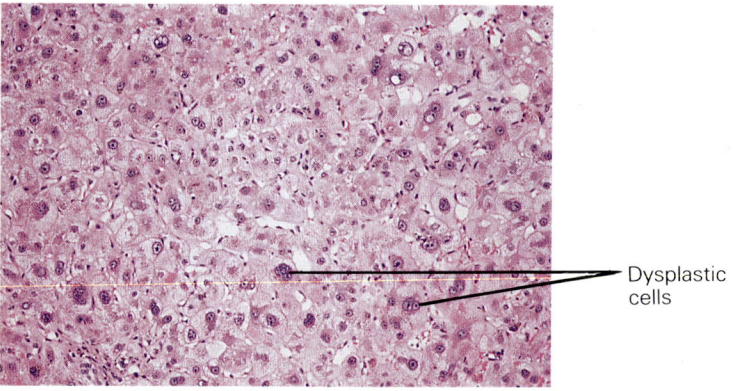

This is considered a premalignant change which is highly associated with cirrhosis, particularly due to hepatitis B virus infection. Dysplastic cells are enlarged and show hyperchromatism, multinucleation, and multiple nucleoli.

Figure 10.52
Liver cell (hepatocellular) carcinoma

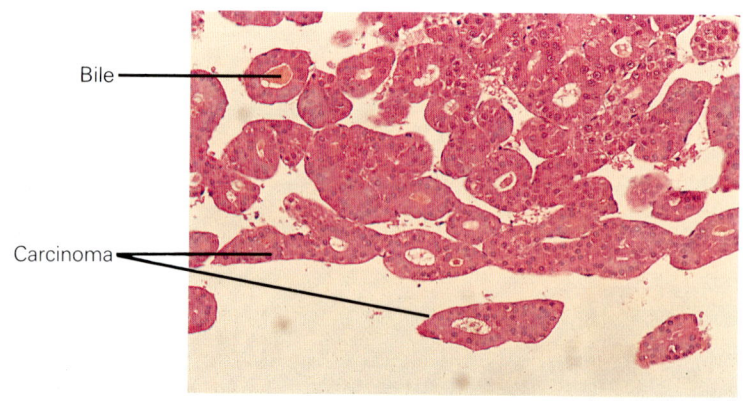

The tumor grows in microtrabeculae and may show histologic bile. Chronic hepatitis B virus infection, hemochromatosis, and alcoholism are major causes.

Figure 10.53
Hemangioma

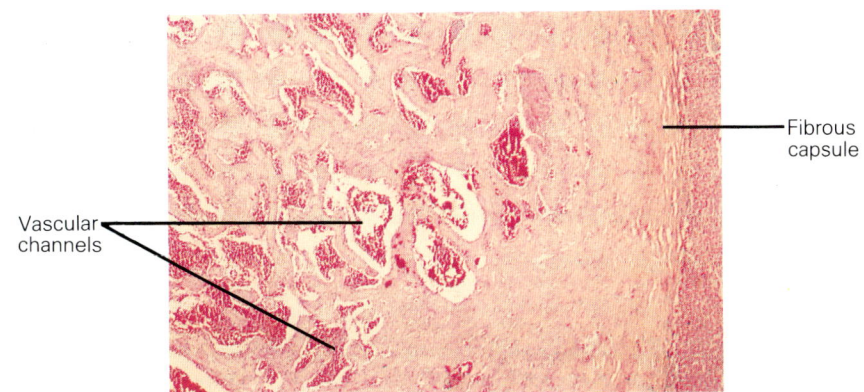

This is a common benign tumor consisting of vascular channels enclosed by dense fibrous stroma.

Figure 10.54
Liver cell adenoma

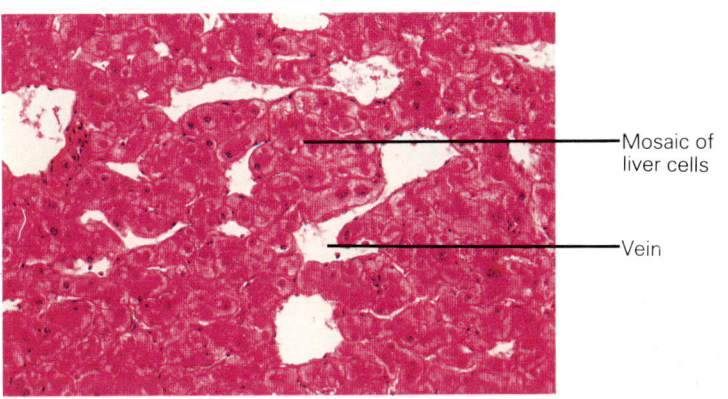

This benign tumor of hepatocytes is related to oral contraceptive use. Hepatocytes grow in thickened plates or a mosaic pattern with interspersed venous and arterial channels. Portal tracts are absent.

Focal Nodular Hyperplasia

Figure 10.55
Focal nodular hyperplasia

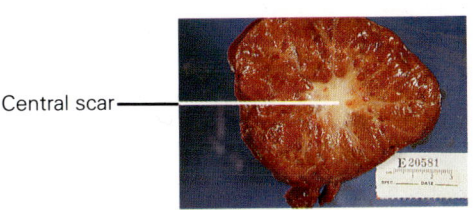

Figure 10.56
Focal nodular hyperplasia

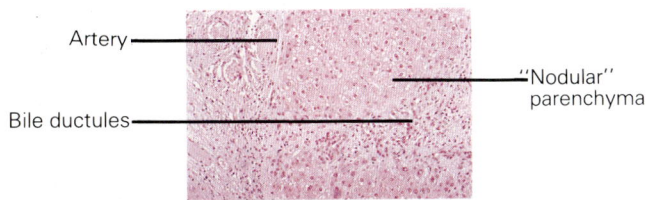

These solitary lesions characteristically show a central, stellate scar that subdivides the liver into cirrhotic-like nodules. The septa contain prominent arteries and bile ductules. The lesion is believed to be a malformation.

Liver Pathology 141

Figure 10.57
Nodular regenerative hyperplasia

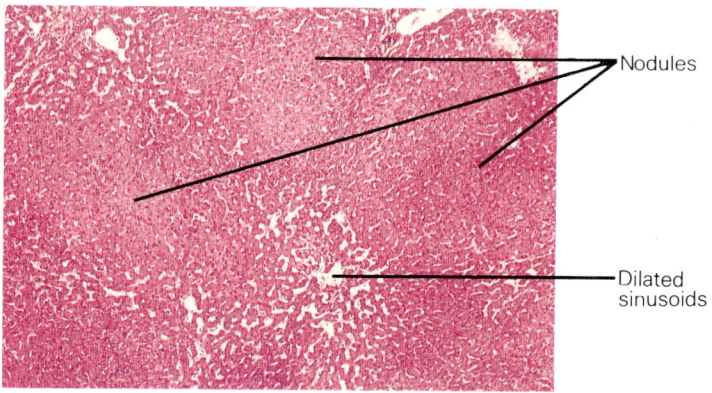

This noncirrhotic nodular condition of the liver causes portal hypertension. Proliferation of hepatocytes produces nodules (without fibrosis) that are separated by dilated sinusoids or compressed hepatocytes.

Figure 10.58
Bile duct carcinoma (cholangiocarcinoma)

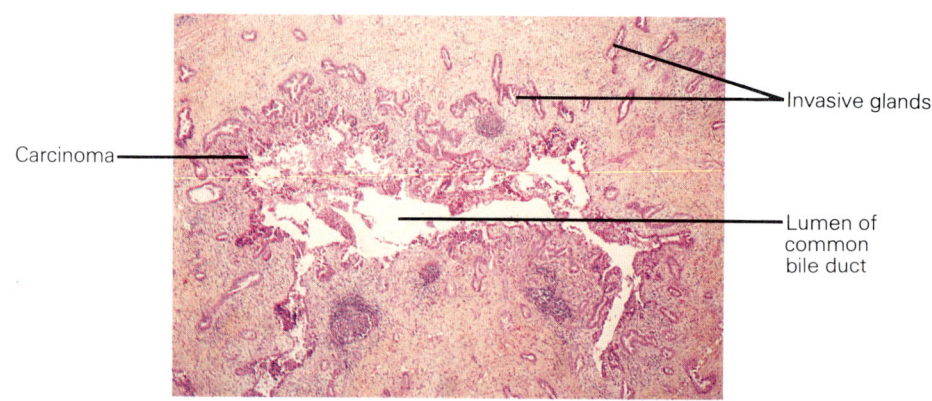

Carcinomas of the common bile duct (shown) or intrahepatic bile ducts are adenocarcinomas which produce glands. Pre-existing sclerosing cholangitis, gallstone disease, or liver fluke infestation are associated factors.

Figure 10.59
Thorotrast

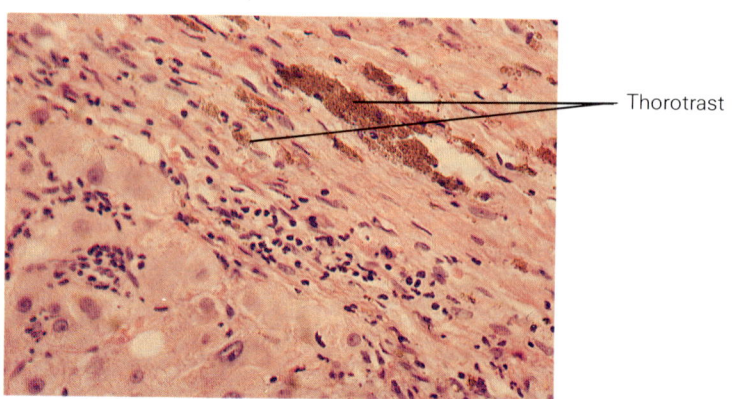

Thorotrast, a colloidal solution of radioactive thorium dioxide, was used for sinus and abdominal films until the 1950s when its association with various malignancies was noted. It is seen here as green-brown refractile granules in portal macrophages.

Figure 10.60
Thorotrast in liver (autoradiography)

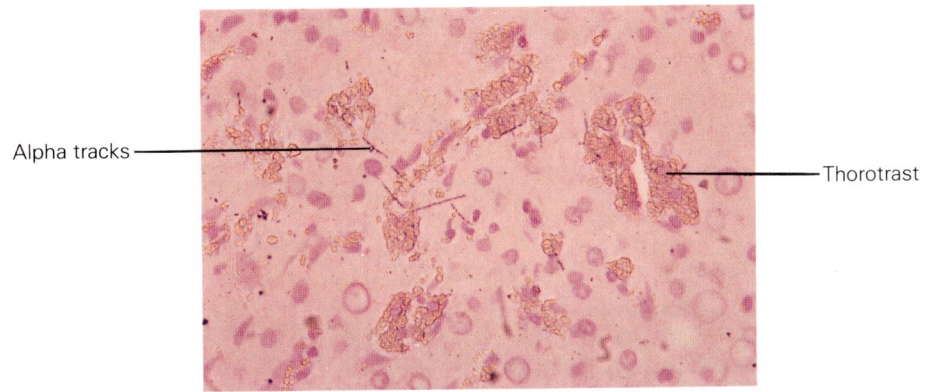

Autoradiography of liver tissue thorotrast shows ongoing emission of alpha particles (tracks) from the green, refractile granules. It is associated with angiosarcoma, cholangiocarcinoma, and liver cell carcinoma.

Figure 10.61
Angiosarcoma

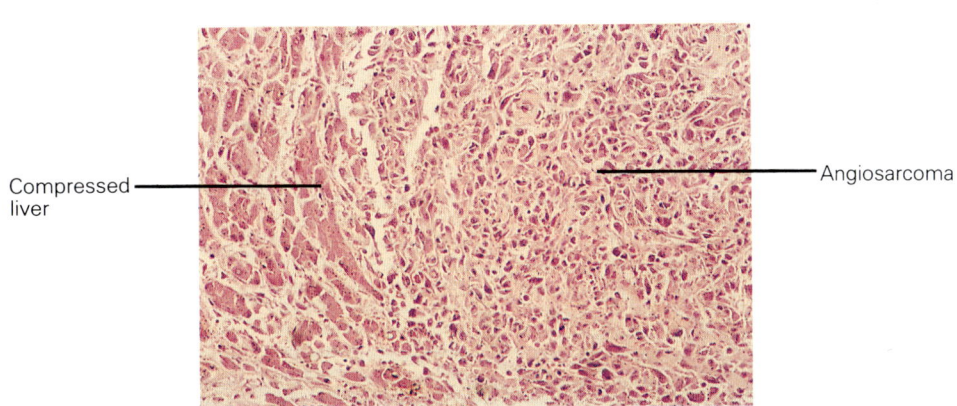

This is a malignant tumor of vascular endothelium, growing as pleomorphic spindle cells with formation of vascular spaces.

Figure 10.62
Liver transplant rejection

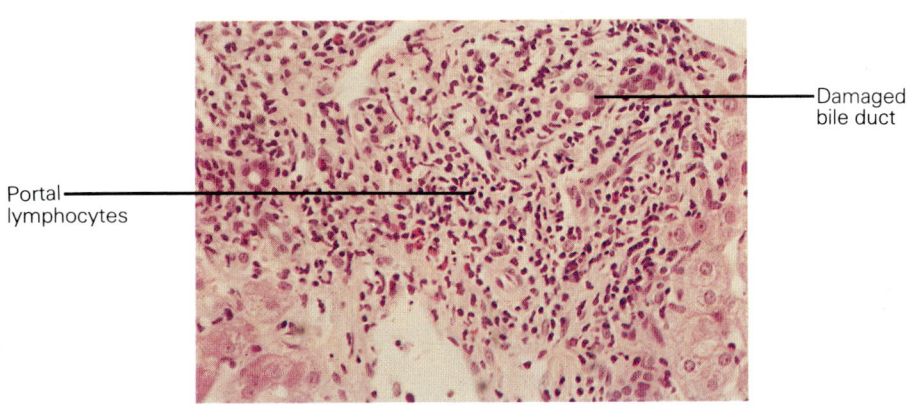

Rejection of liver transplants is commonly manifested by T-lymphocyte infiltration of portal tracts and damage to interlobular bile ducts that express HLA-Dr antigens.

Liver Pathology

CHAPTER 11

GALLBLADDER AND PANCREAS PATHOLOGY

Figure 11.1
Gallbladder and extrahepatic ducts

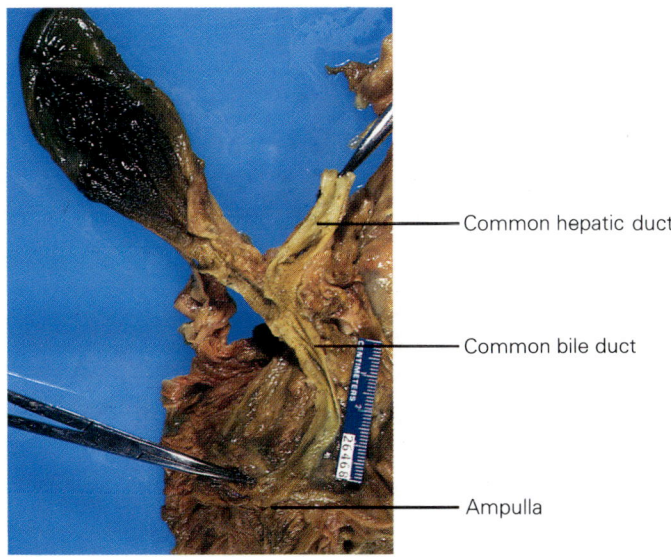

Normal specimen with opened gallbladder, common hepatic duct, and common bile duct.

Figure 11.2
Chronic cholecystitis

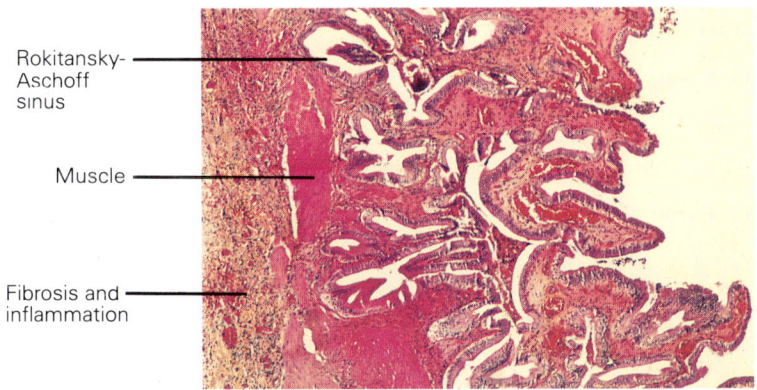

Chronic inflammation of the gallbladder related to the presence of gallstones is manifested by herniations of mucosa through the muscle layer (Rokitansky-Aschoff sinuses) and fibrosis with inflammation of the gallbladder wall.

Figure 11.3
Cholesterolosis (gross)

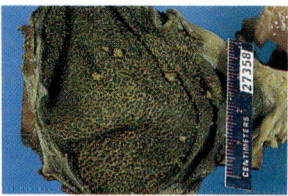

Figure 11.4
Cholesterolosis

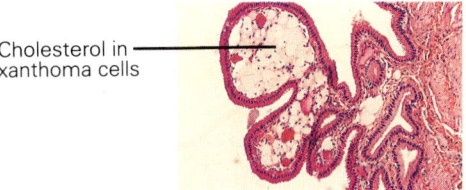

The gallbladder grossly shows a lacy yellow mucosal stippling ("strawberry gallbladder") due to the presence of cholesterol in macrophages (xanthoma cells) within mucosal papillae.

Gallbladder and Pancreas Pathology 147

Figure 11.5
Gallbladder and pancreas: major pathologic lesions

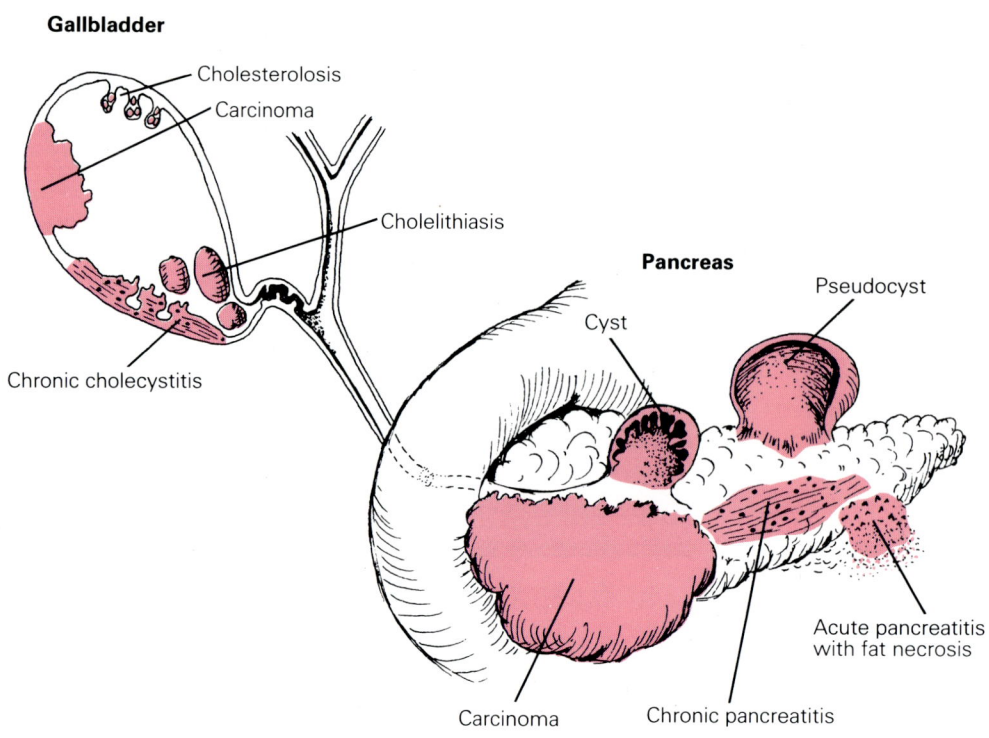

Figure 11.6
Adenocarcinoma of gallbladder

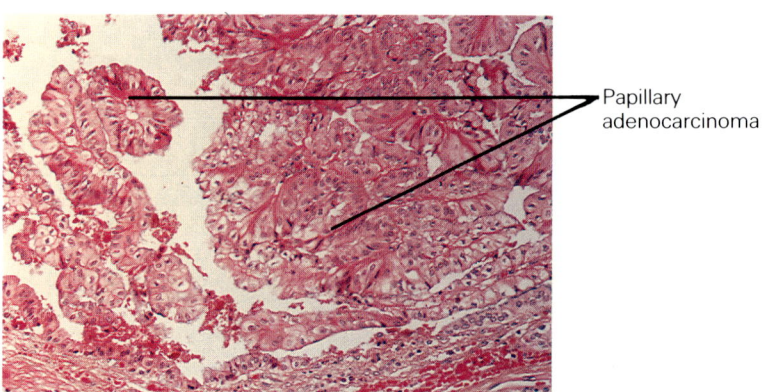

Adenocarcinomas of the gallbladder often present as occult, invasive tumors in the elderly. They are commonly associated with chronic cholecystitis and cholelithiasis.

Figure 11.7
Pancreatic fat necrosis (acute pancreatitis)

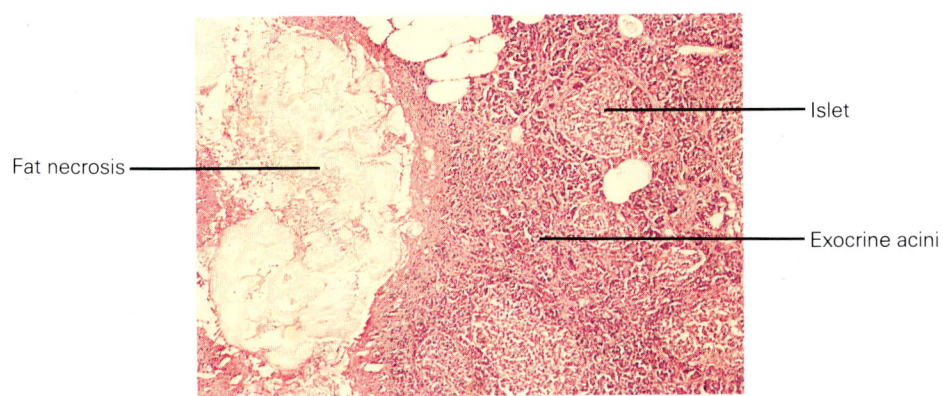

Release of pancreatic enzymes into peripancreatic fat in acute pancreatitis results in necrosis and a ghostlike appearance.

Figure 11.8
Chronic pancreatitis

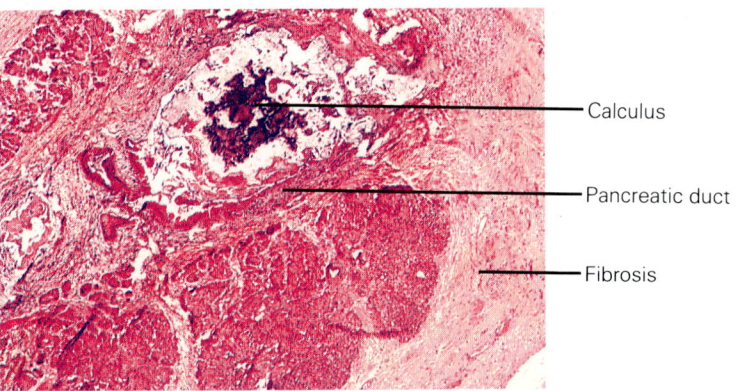

Chronic inflammation of the pancreas causes parenchymal fibrosis with eventual atrophy of exocrine acinar tissue. Inspissated secretions and calculi develop within ducts.

Figure 11.9
Adenocarcinoma of pancreas

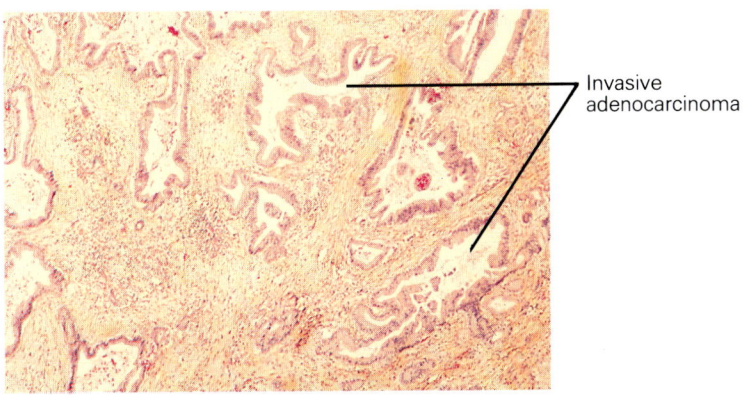

Pancreatic adenocarcinomas arise predominantly from duct epithelium. The well differentiated tumor shown consists of complicated glands invading pancreatic stroma.

CHAPTER 12

REPRODUCTIVE ORGAN PATHOLOGY

Figure 12.1
Uterine leiomyoma

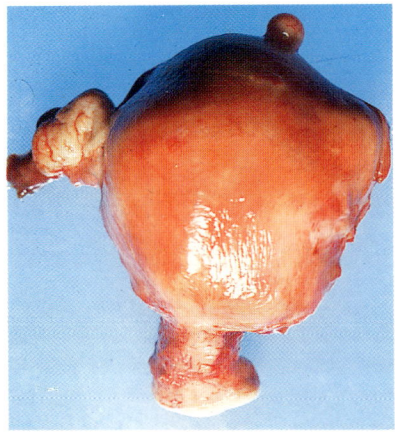

A subserosal leiomyoma ("fibroid") is present on the dome of the uterus in this specimen of right salpingo-oophorectomy and hysterectomy. Normal weights: ovary, 7 g each; testis, 25 g each; and prostate, 20 g (age 51–60), 40 g (age 71–80).

Figure 12.2
Proliferative endometrium

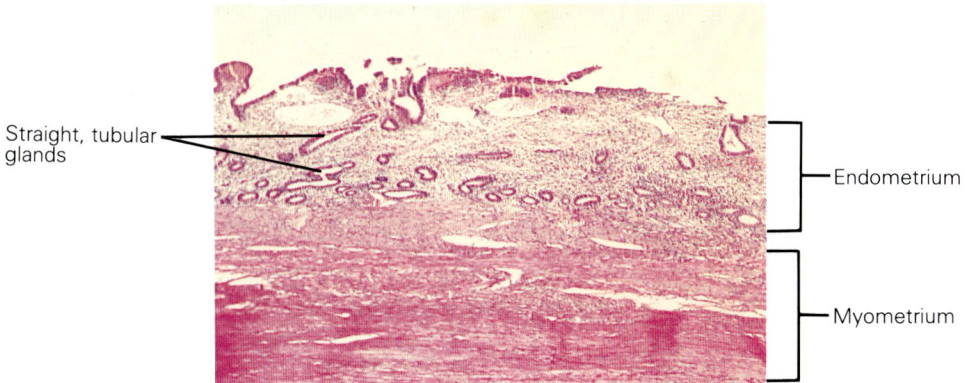

Endometrial glands are straight and tubular. Stroma and glands display mitotic activity.

Figure 12.3
Seventeen-day secretory endometrium

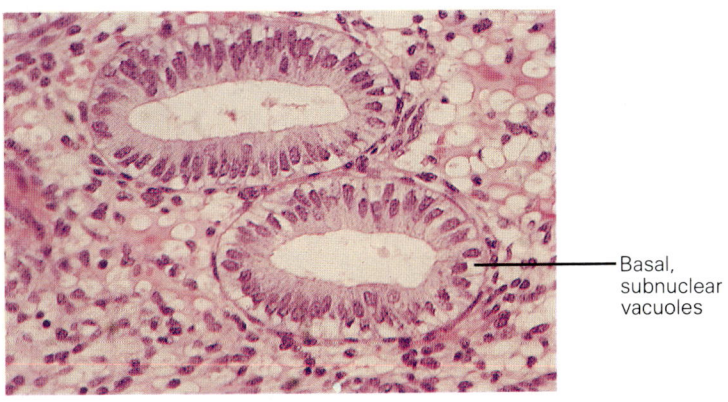

Increased secretory activity in the third week of the menstrual cycle results in the appearance of subnuclear vacuoles.

Reproductive Organ Pathology

Figure 12.4
Secretory endometrium

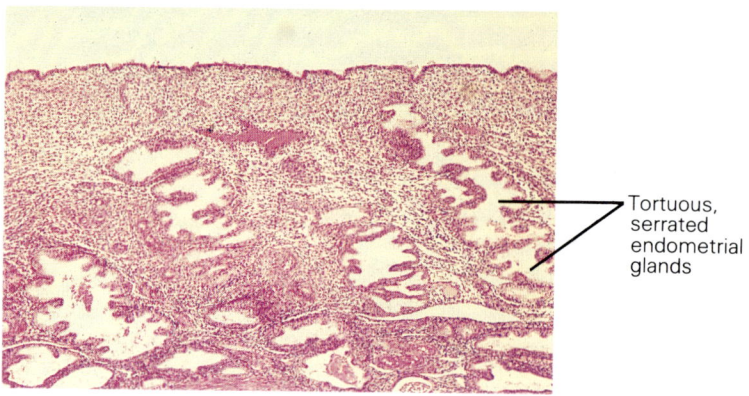

Highly developed, tortuous endometrial glands are present by the fourth week of the menstrual cycle.

Figure 12.5
Menstrual endometrium

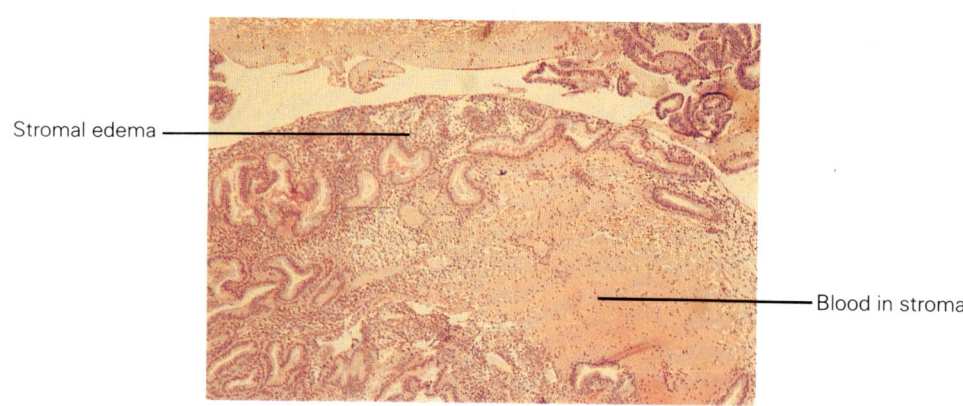

Menstrual shedding is signalled by the appearance of stromal blood. Large, pink stromal cells (predecidual change) and stromal edema accompany prominent sawtooth glands and prominent spiral arterioles.

Figure 12.6
Female reproductive system: major pathologic lesions

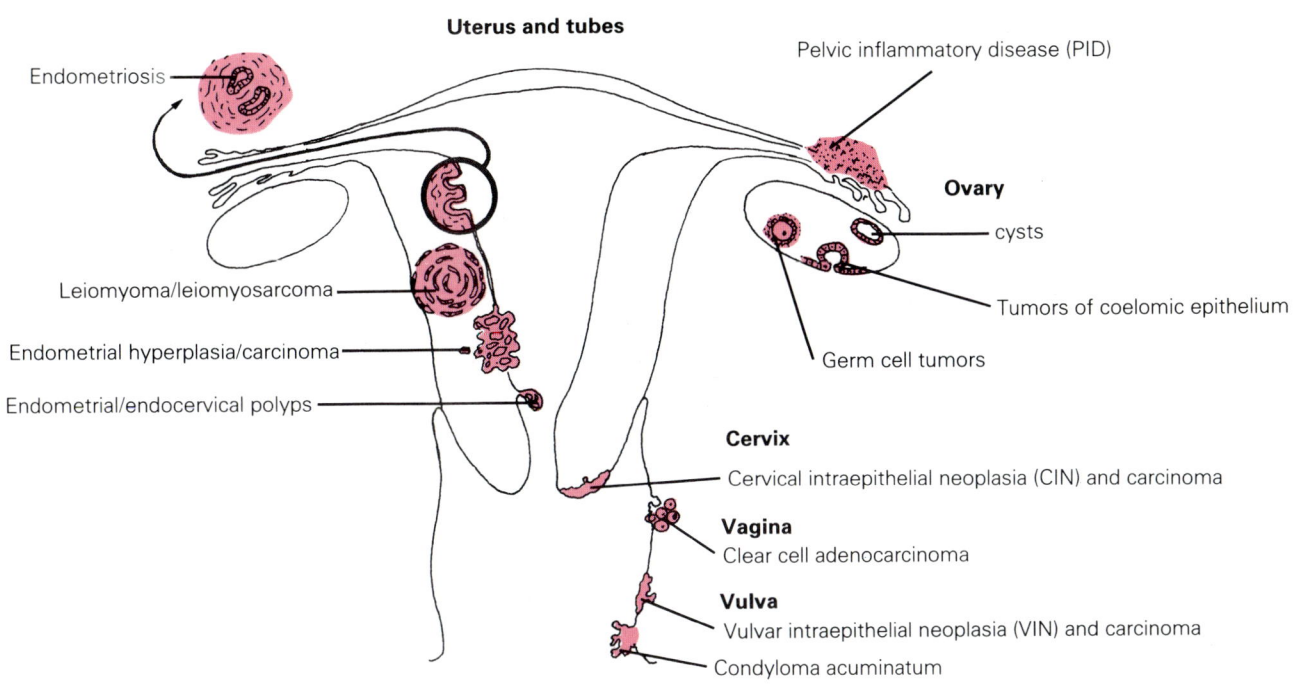

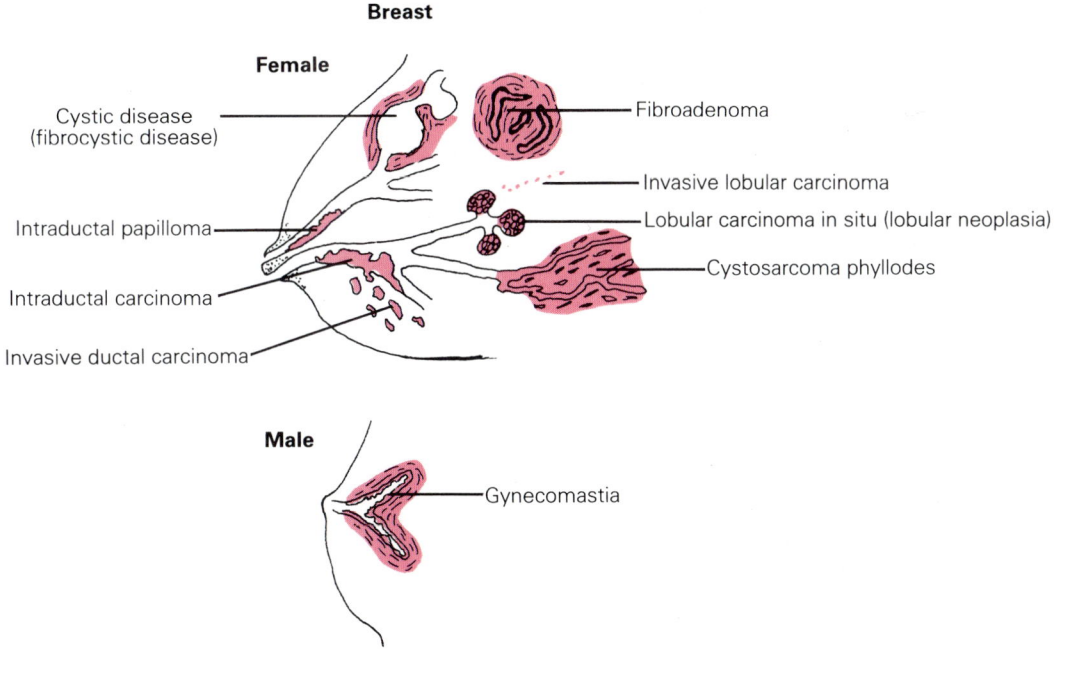

Reproductive Organ Pathology 155

Figure 12.7
Male reproductive system: major pathologic lesions

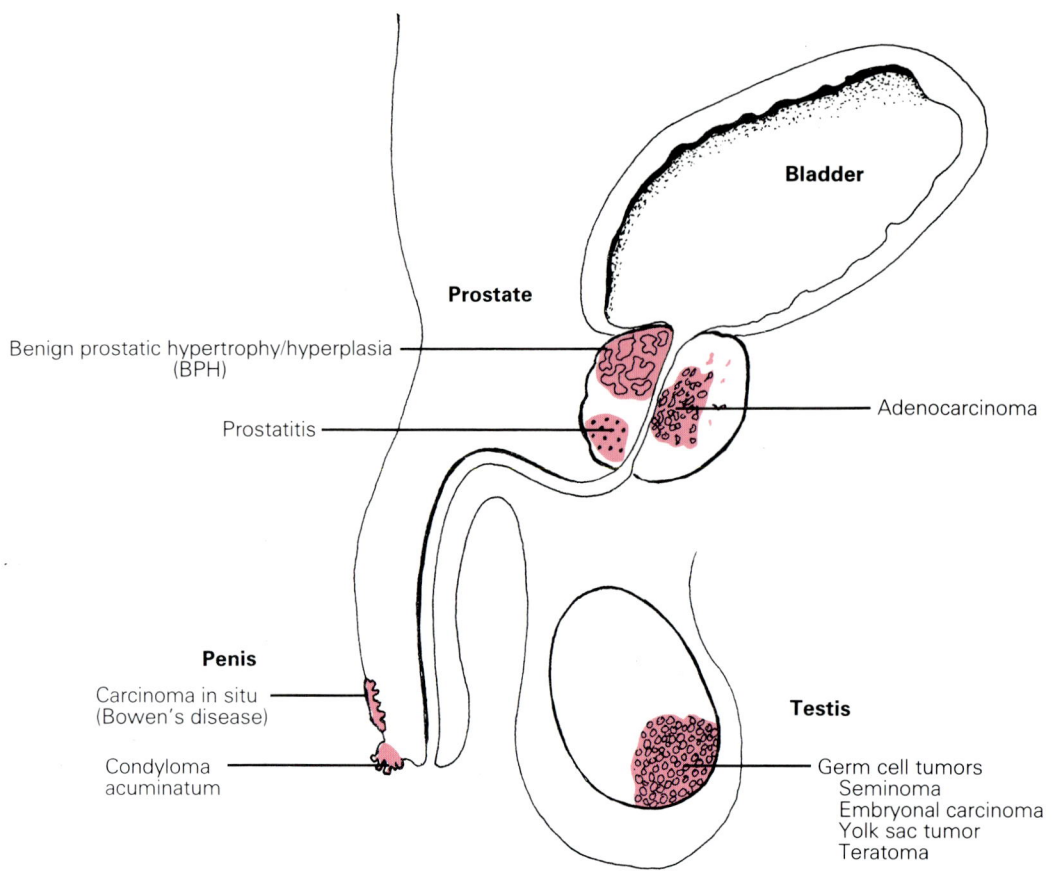

Figure 12.8
Endometrial hyperplasia

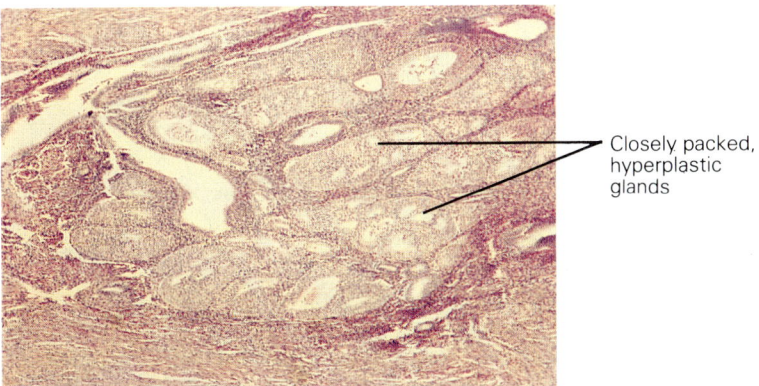

Moderate or severe forms of endometrial gland hyperplasia occur in the menopausal or postmenopausal period under the influence of estrogen stimulation. These are considered precancerous lesions.

Figure 12.9
Endometrial adenocarcinoma

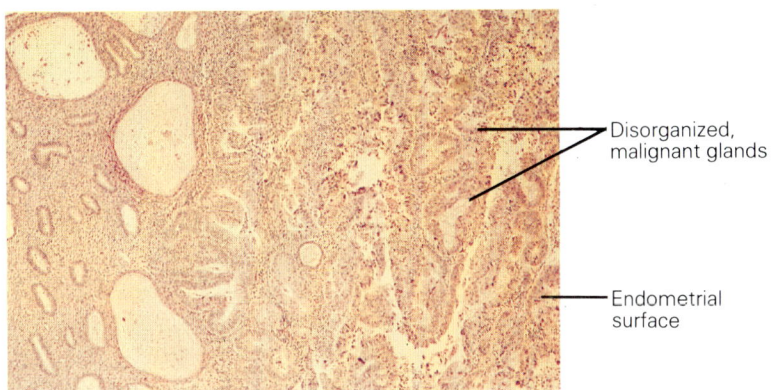

The well differentiated adenocarcinoma shown here is composed of closely packed, disorganized glands with atypical nuclei and mitotic activity.

Figure 12.10
Endometriosis

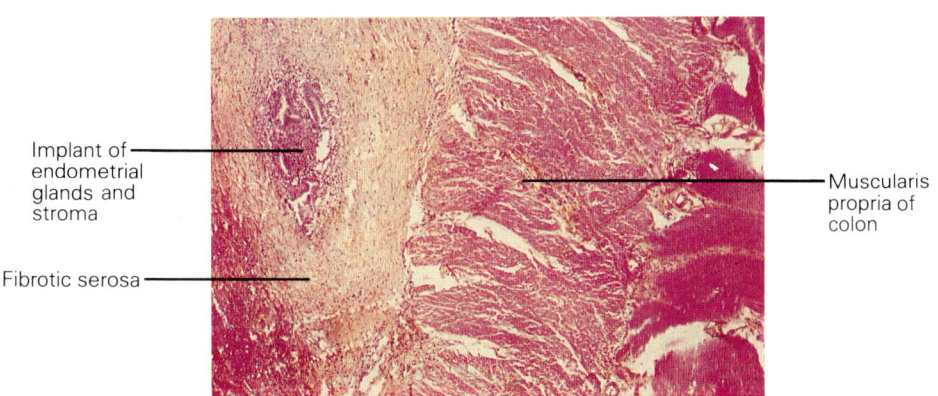

Endometrial glands and stroma at sites outside the uterus (endometriosis) such as ovary, peritoneum, and serosa of bowel are likely to result from regurgitation through the fallopian tubes at menses.

Figure 12.11
Uterine leiomyoma

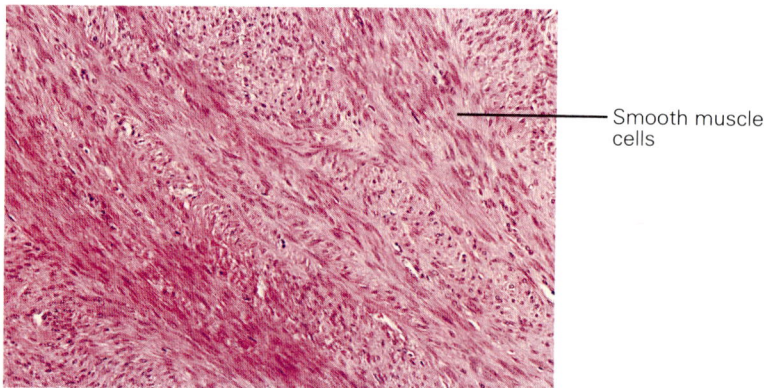

These smooth muscle tumors ("fibroids") are located in the myometrium, submucosal, or subserosal regions. The diagnosis of malignant leiomyosarcoma is based on observing cellular atypia and/or increased mitotic activity.

Figure 12.12
Carcinoma in situ of vulva

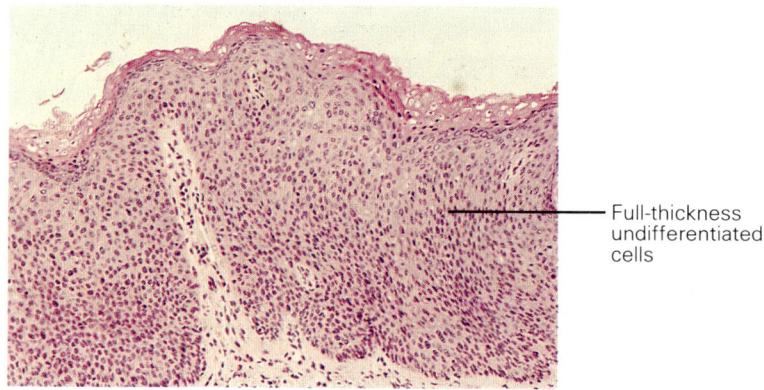

This intraepithelial squamous cell carcinoma (Bowen's disease or vulvar intraepithelial neoplasia—VIN—type III) is related to herpes simplex virus II infection.

Figure 12.13
Clear cell adenocarcinoma of vagina

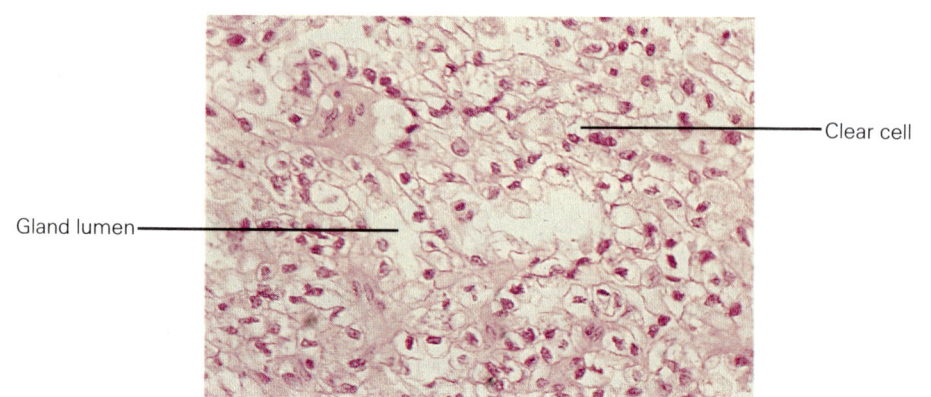

This malignancy may develop in young women who received diethylstilbesterol (DES) during pregnancy. The malignant glands are composed of clear (glycogen-containing) cells.

Figure 12.14
Condyloma acuminatum (wart) of vulva

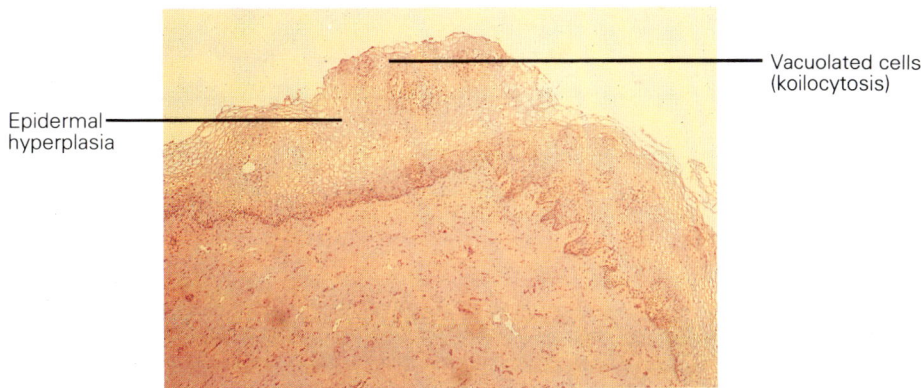

Warty, cauliflower-like epidermal hyperplasia with distinct vacuolization of the epithelium (koilocytosis) is associated with human papilloma virus (HPV) infection.

Figure 12.15
Cervical intraepithelial neoplasia (CIN) I

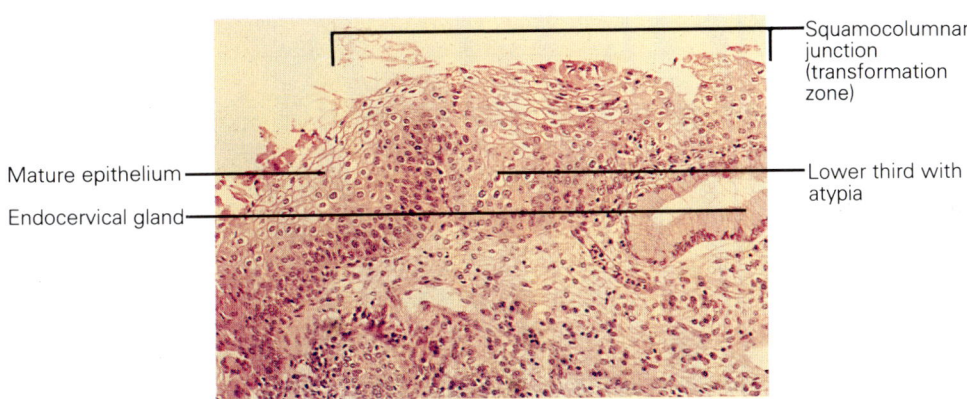

Cervical dysplasias (or cervical intraepithelial neoplasia, CIN) begins at the squamocolumnar junction. In this example of mild dysplasia (CIN I), less than one-third of the epithelium is involved by atypical cells.

Figure 12.16
CIN II (moderate dysplasia)

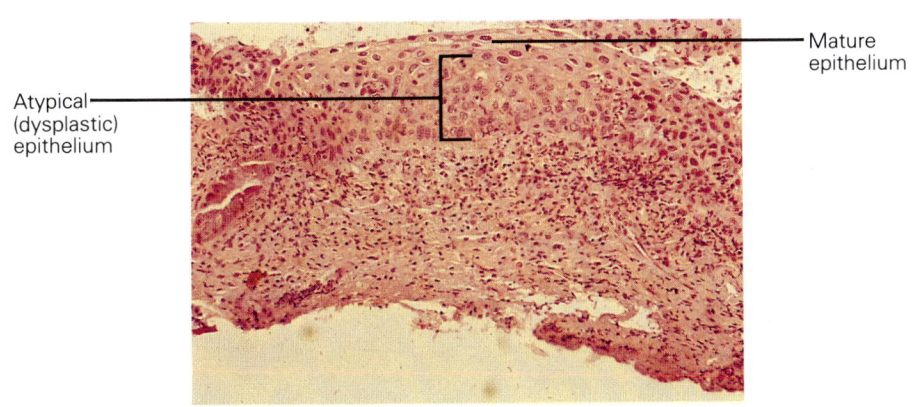

In CIN II, one- to two-thirds of the epithelium is dysplastic. Note the nuclear hyperchromatism and pleomorphism of the dysplastic cells. The subjacent stroma in this field is inflamed.

Figure 12.17
CIN III (severe dysplasia, carcinoma in situ)

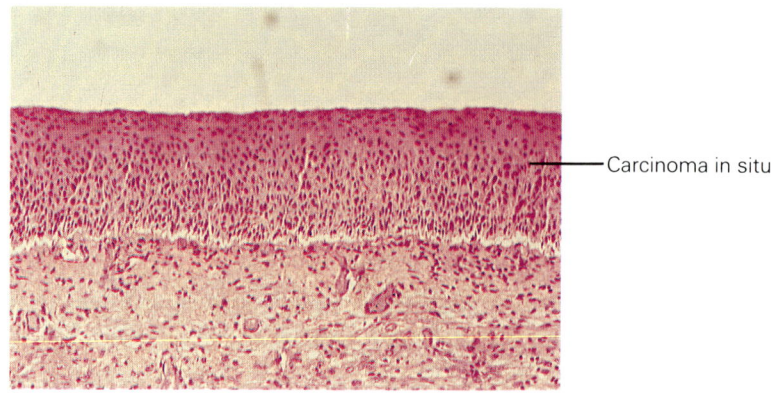

In CIN III, there is two-thirds to full thickness involvement by atypical cells. Note the undifferentiated cells from the base to the superficial region of the epithelium.

Figure 12.18
Invasive squamous cell carcinoma of cervix

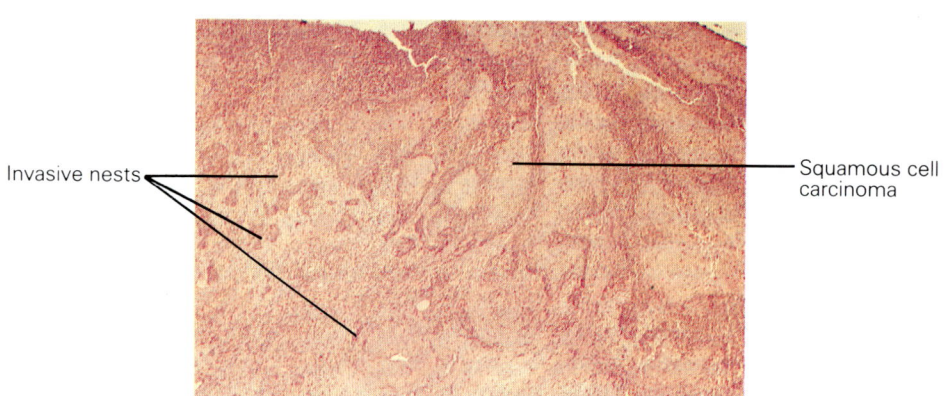

The entire cervical epithelium is replaced by squamous cell carcinoma which invades below. The moderate to well differentiated tumor illustrated here shows obvious squamous differentiation.

Figure 12.19
Ovarian atrophy

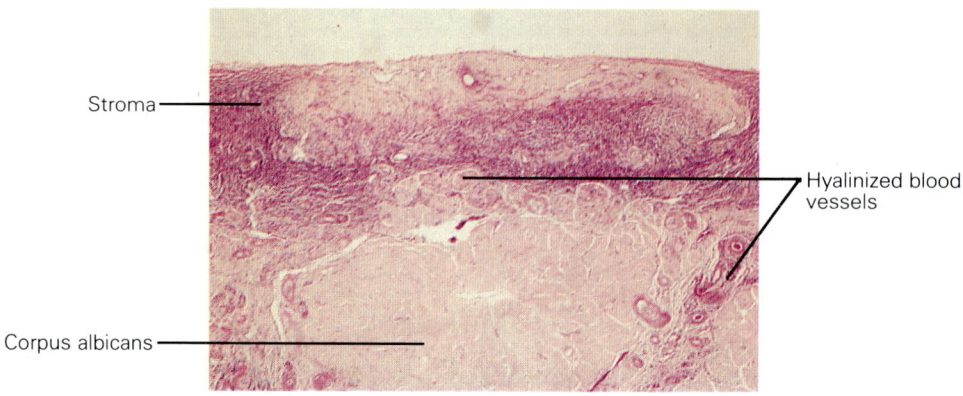

With aging, there is progressive hyalinization of ovarian vessels and increasing numbers of atretic, old corpora lutea (corpora albicantia).

OVARIAN TUMORS
Surface Epithelial (Coelomic) Tumors

Figure 12.20
Serous cystadenoma

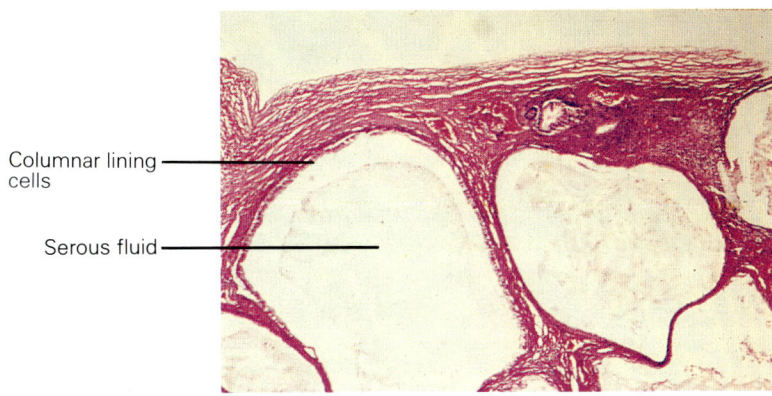

This tumor is of coelomic epithelial origin. The benign, multiloculated cysts comprising the tumor are lined by serous type, ciliated epithelium resembling that of the fallopian tubes.

Figure 12.21
Serous cystadenocarcinoma

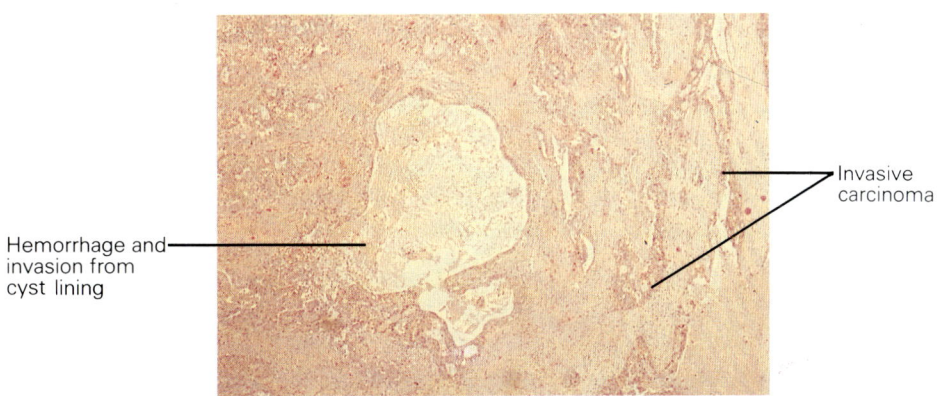

These tumors account for half of ovarian malignancies. In contrast to cystadenomas, the cyst linings are composed of malignant cells which give rise to glands, solid nests, and papillary structures that invade the ovarian stroma. Some contain psammoma bodies.

Figure 12.22
Brenner tumor

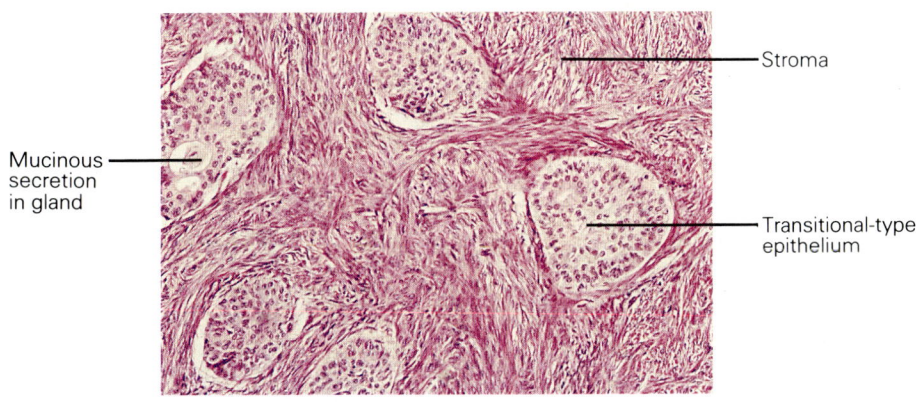

These solid, usually benign tumors, are composed of stroma and epithelial nests resembling transitional urothelium with central mucinous glands.

Germ Cell Tumors

Figure 12.23
Benign cystic teratoma (dermoid cyst)

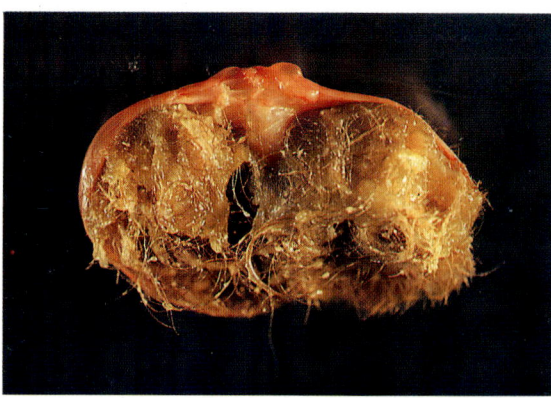

The contents of this ovary include hair and sebaceous material. These skin and adnexal elements are representative of ectodermal tissue present in conjunction with endoderm and mesoderm in this benign tumor of all three germ layers.

Figure 12.24
Benign cystic teratoma (dermoid cyst)

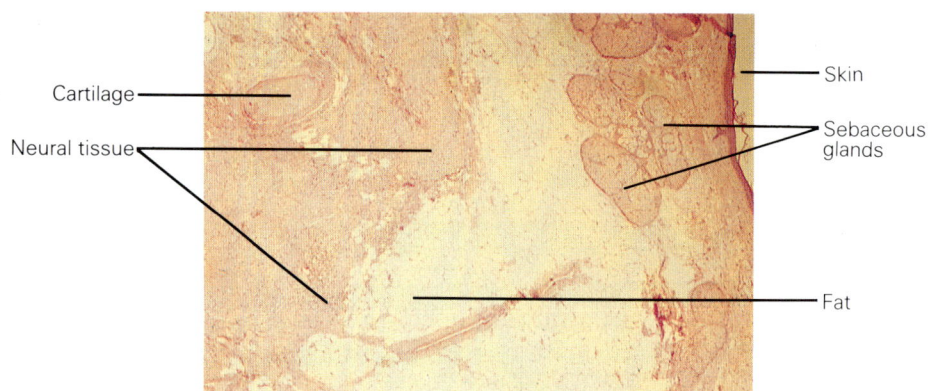

The various histologic structures present in these tumors reflect their origin from all three germ layers (ectoderm, endoderm, mesoderm). Elements as diverse as thyroid and adrenal tissue can be identified in these neoplasms.

Figure 12.25
Dysgerminoma

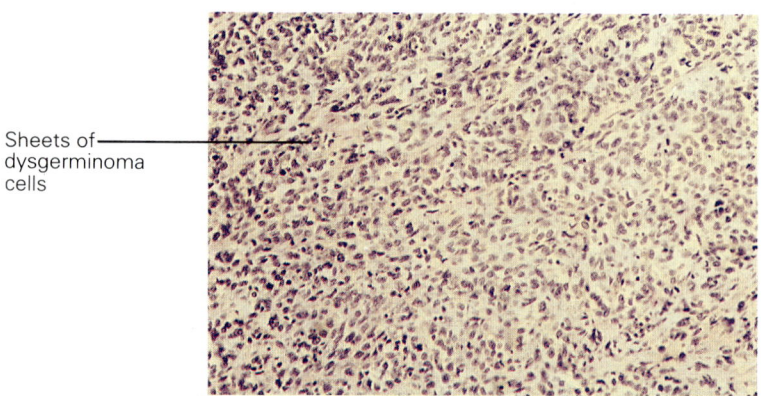

A radiosensitive tumor of varying degrees of malignancy, analogous to the seminoma of the testis. Scattered lymphocytes are seen here throughout the dysgerminoma cells.

Figure 12.26
Endodermal sinus tumor

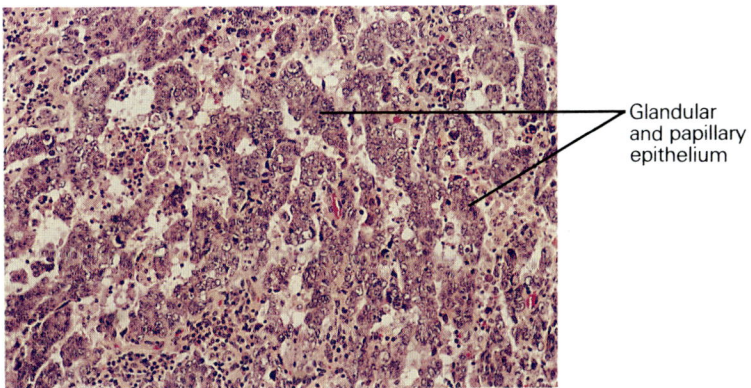

This malignant tumor of yolk sac origin contains alphafetoprotein (AFP) and alpha-1-antitrypsin (AAT).

Figure 12.27
Endodermal sinus tumor (Schiller-Duval body)

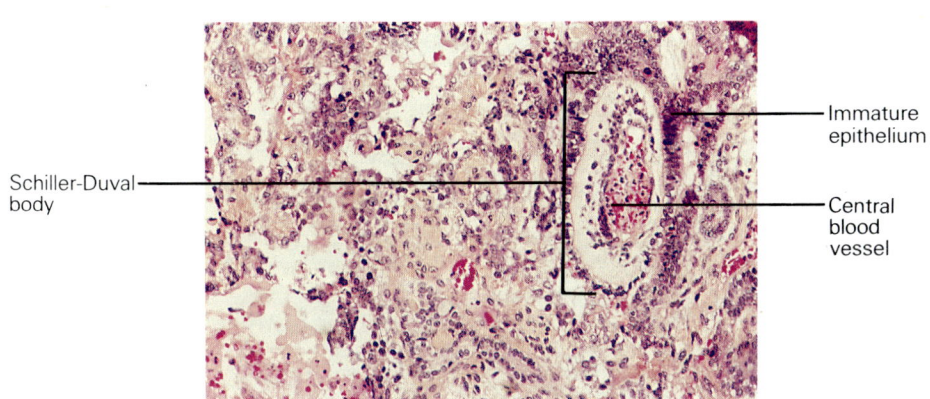

Schiller-Duval bodies, papillary structures containing central blood vessels surrounded by immature epithelium, are characteristic of endodermal sinus tumors.

Figure 12.28
Choriocarcinoma

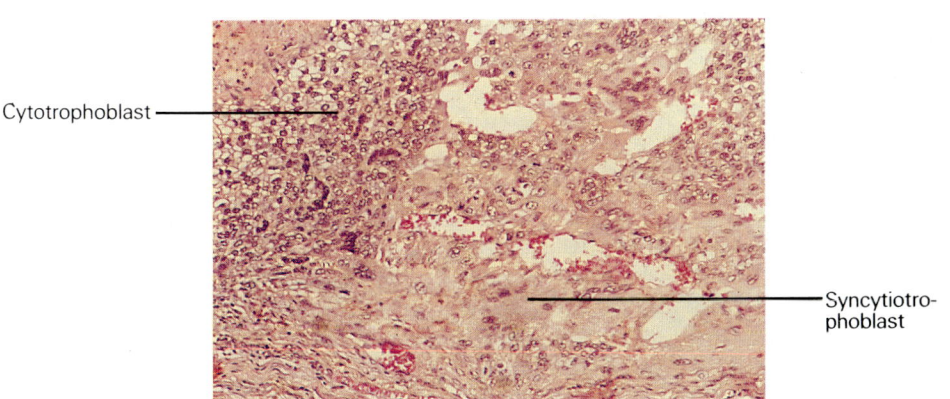

This trophoblast malignancy of ovarian, placental, and testicular origin secretes human chorionic gonadotrophin (HGG). The epithelial cells form cyto- and syncytiotrophoblastic regions.

Sex Cord-Stromal Tumors

Figure 12.29
Granulosa-theca cell tumor

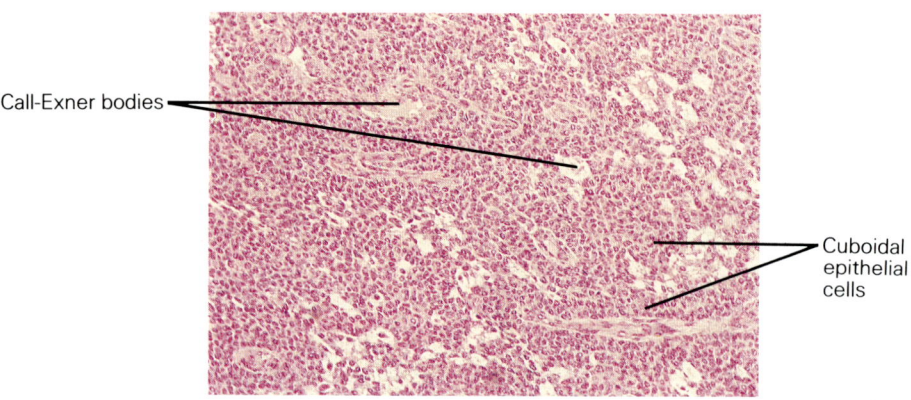

Sheets of cuboidal follicular cells occasionally produce glandular structures containing acidophilic material (Call-Exner bodies).

Figure 12.30
Fibroma

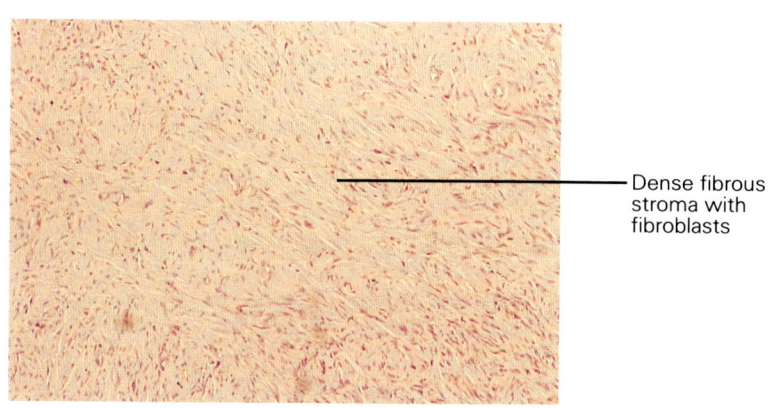

These fairly common benign neoplasms may contain only fibrous tissue (fibroma) or both fibrous tissue and thecal elements (fibrothecomas). The tumor may be associated with ascites and right hydrothorax (Meigs' syndrome).

Figure 12.31
Sertoli-Leydig cell tumor

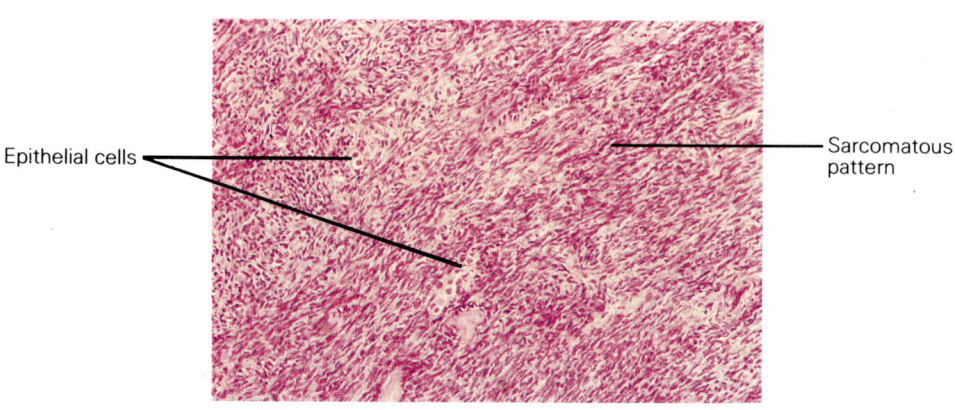

These masculinizing tumors may feature well differentiated tubular structures, Sertoli cells and Leydig cells, or (as shown above) a sarcomatous pattern with few epithelial cells.

Figure 12.32
Pelvic inflammatory disease

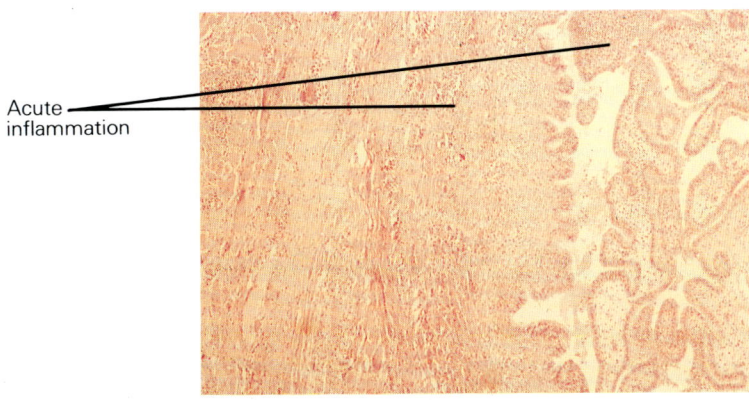

The fallopian tube shown here contains suppurative exudate within its wall and mucosal folds. Involvement of tube and ovary (salpingo-oophoritis) and tubo-ovarian abscesses are complications.

BREAST

Figure 12.33
Cystic disease of the breast

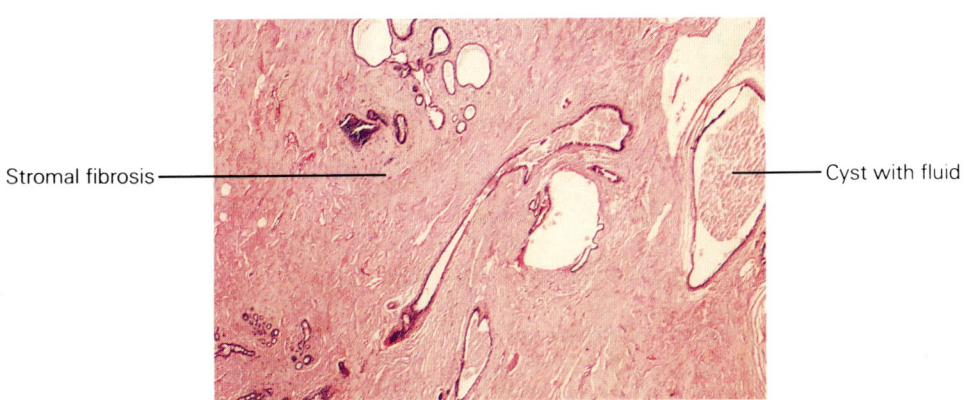

Cystic disease (also known as fibrocystic disease) includes the formation of gross and microscopic cysts, stromal fibrosis, and various forms of epithelial hyperplasia. The condition has been associated with an increased risk of developing breast carcinoma.

Figure 12.34
Fibroadenoma of breast

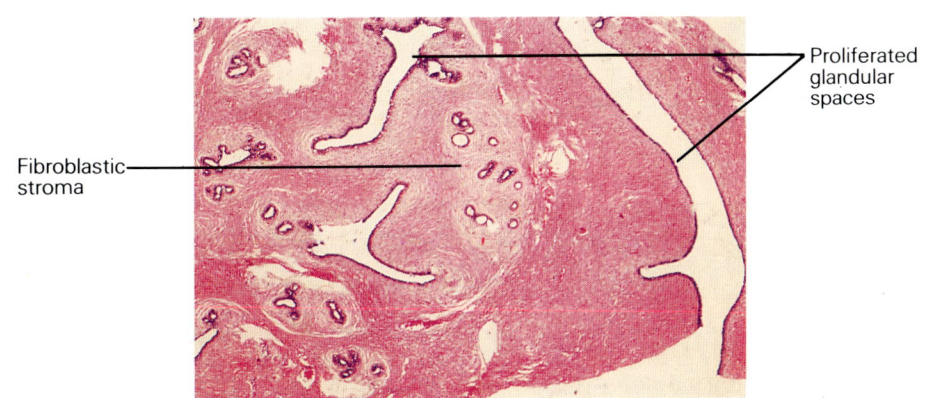

This is the most common benign tumor of the female breast. These well circumscribed lesions show proliferated fibrous tissue stroma and cleft-like or tubular glandular spaces.

Figure 12.35
Gynecomastia of male breast

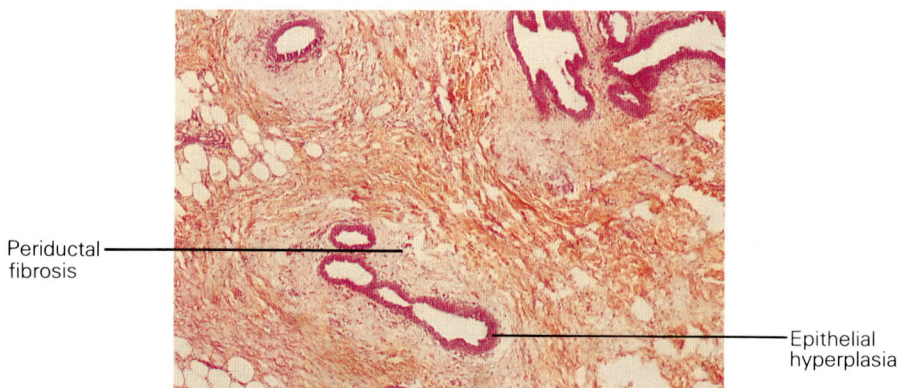

The influence of hyperestrogenism (in cirrhosis or testicular tumors) on the male breast is manifested by periductal fibrosis and hyperplasia of duct epithelium. Note the absence of glandular lobules in the normal male breast.

Figure 12.36
Breast atrophy

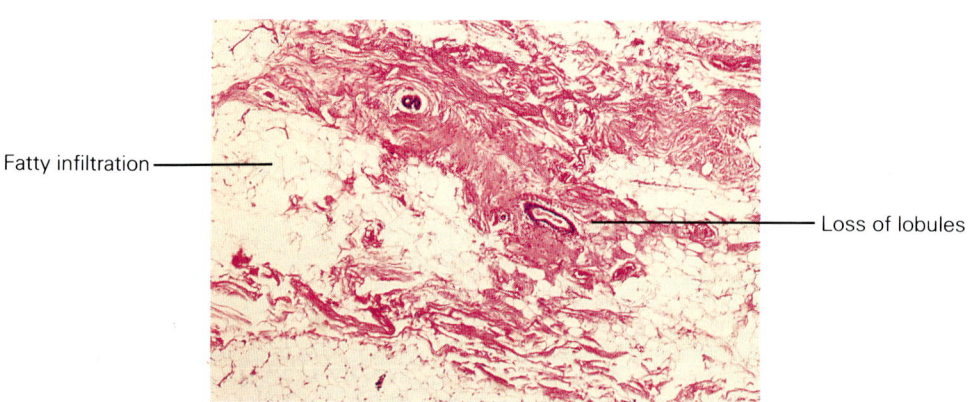

With aging, lobular elements are diminished and the breast tissue is infiltrated by fat.

Figure 12.37
Intraductal papilloma of breast

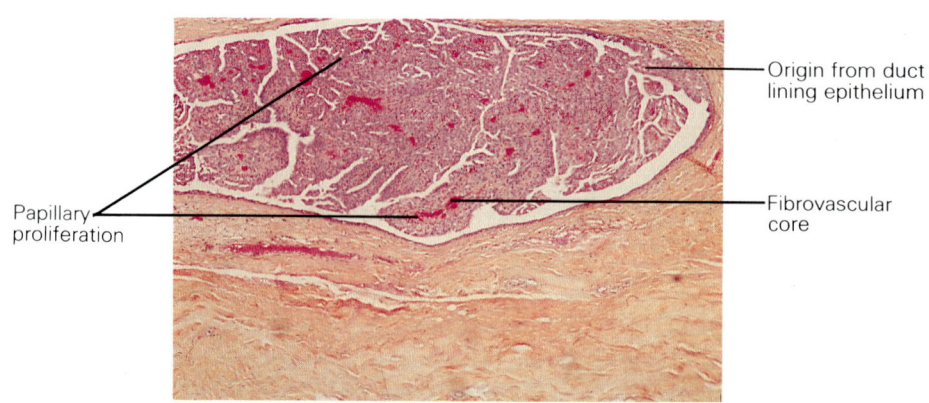

These benign tumors grow within major breast ducts near the nipple and may be a source of bloody discharge. Their internal structure consists of papillary structures lined by cuboidal to columnar epithelium overlying connective tissue cores.

Figure 12.38
Intraductal carcinoma of breast

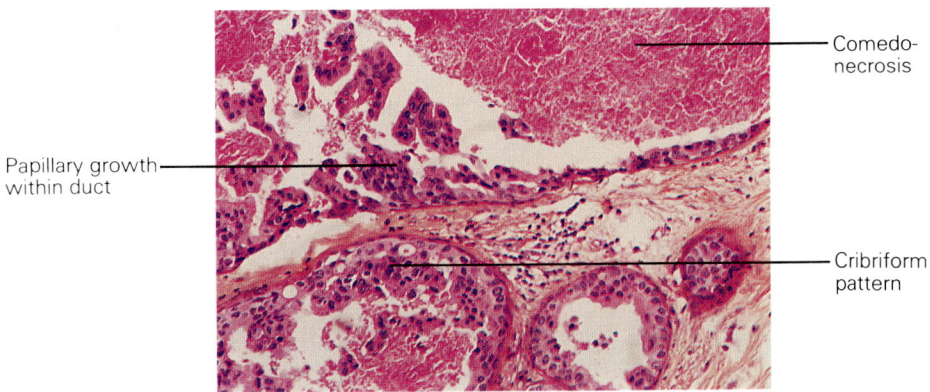

The majority of breast carcinomas originate within ducts. Varied histologic patterns include papillary growth, foci of comedo-necrosis, and complex sieve-like (cribriform) glandular growth. Note the pleomorphism and hyperchromatism of tumor cells seen in this field.

Figure 12.39
Invasive ductal carcinoma of breast

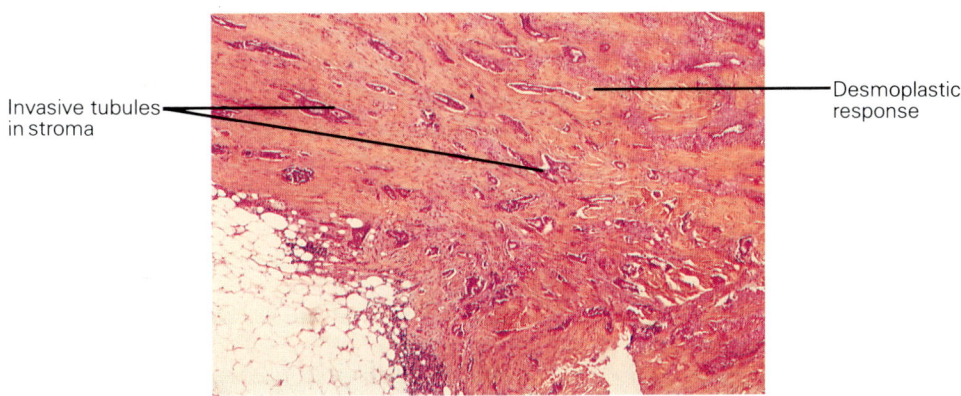

Invasive carcinoma is manifested as nests or tubules growing into breast stroma and fat. Desmoplasia (tumor-related fibrosis) is related to the firm gross consistency of these tumors.

Figure 12.40
Paget's disease of breast

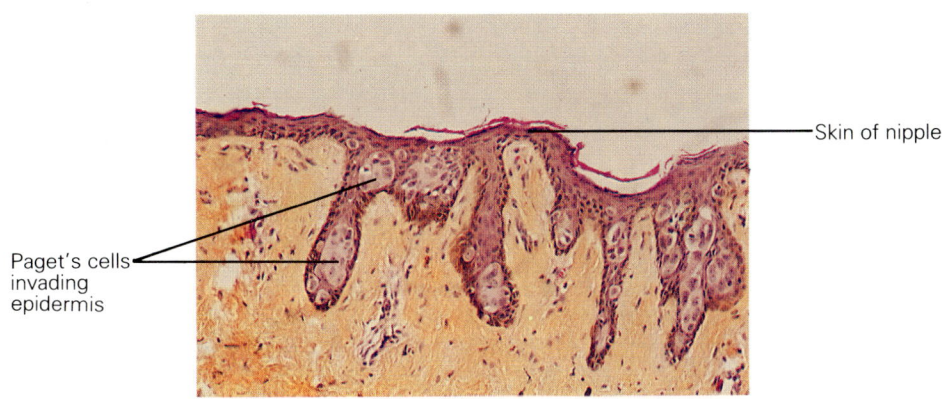

Growth of large, anaplastic carcinoma cells (Paget's cells) from major excretory ducts into the epithelium of overlying nipple and areolae is known as Paget's disease.

Reproductive Organ Pathology

Figure 12.41
Lobular neoplasia (lobular carcinoma in situ)

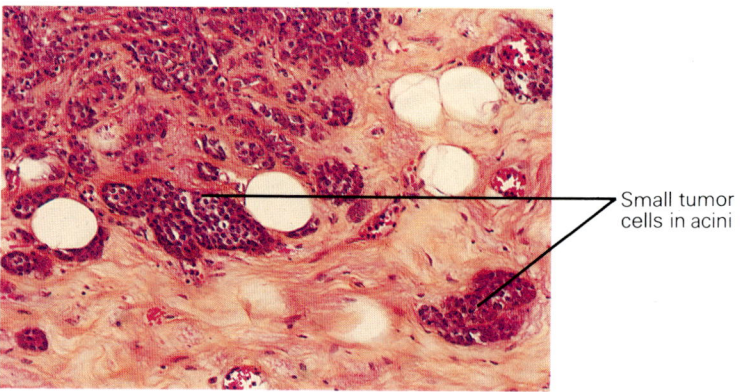

This malignant proliferation of cells of the terminal duct region and acini is associated with an increased incidence of carcinoma in the contralateral breast.

Figure 12.42
Invasive small cell carcinoma of breast

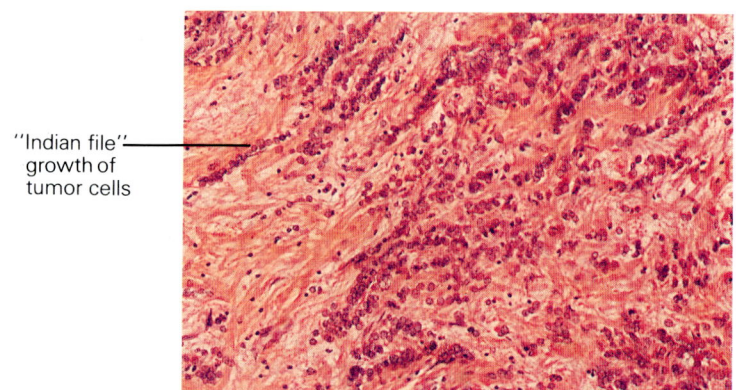

This invasive form of lobular carcinoma is often bilateral and consists of insidious growth of single cells and cells in "Indian file" arrangement within breast stroma.

Figure 12.43
Medullary carcinoma of breast

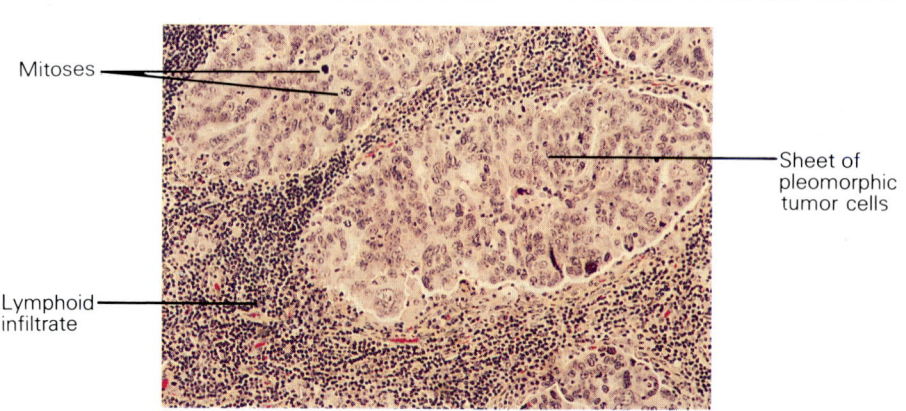

This form of carcinoma is characterized by sheets of pleomorphic tumor cells and prominent lymphoid infiltrates. The latter is believed related to the good prognosis of this tumor.

Figure 12.44
Cystosarcoma phyllodes

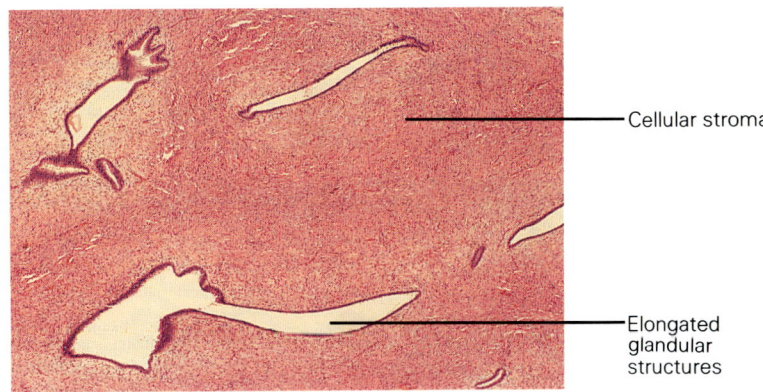

These tumors range from benign to malignant and combine an overly cellular stroma with proliferation of epithelium to form elongated glands. Increasing cellularity of stroma and, particularly, epithelium is associated with malignant behavior.

TESTIS

Figure 12.45
Normal testis

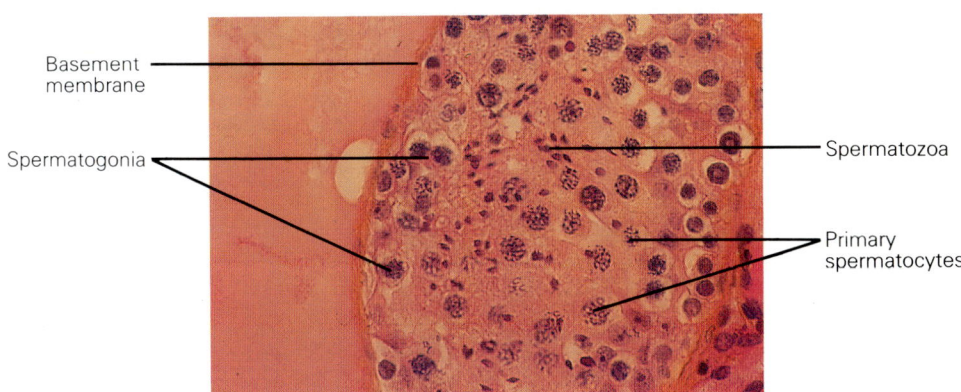

Histologic evaluation of testicular tissue involves assessment of maturation of the spermatogenic series, thickness of basement membrane, and numbers of Sertoli and interstitial (Leydig) cells.

Figure 12.46
Testicular atrophy

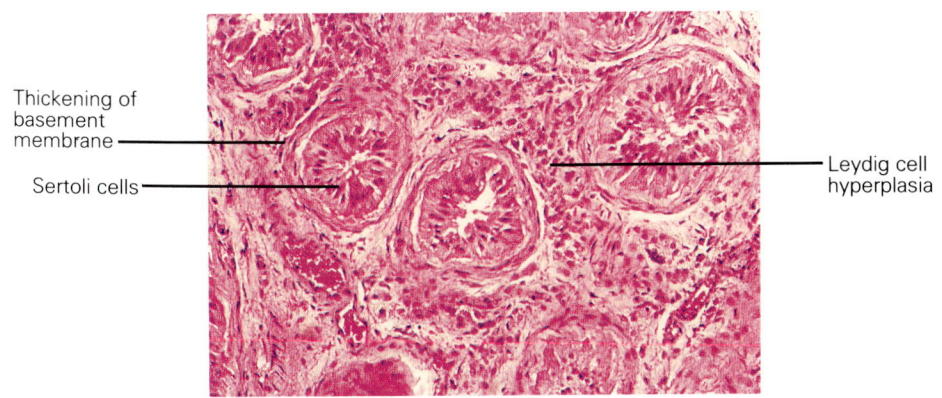

Atrophy results in hyaline thickening of the tubular basement membranes, loss of spermatogenic cells (with persistence of Sertoli cells), and in many cases, hyperplasia of Leydig cells within a fibrotic interstitium.

Figure 12.47
Seminoma of testis

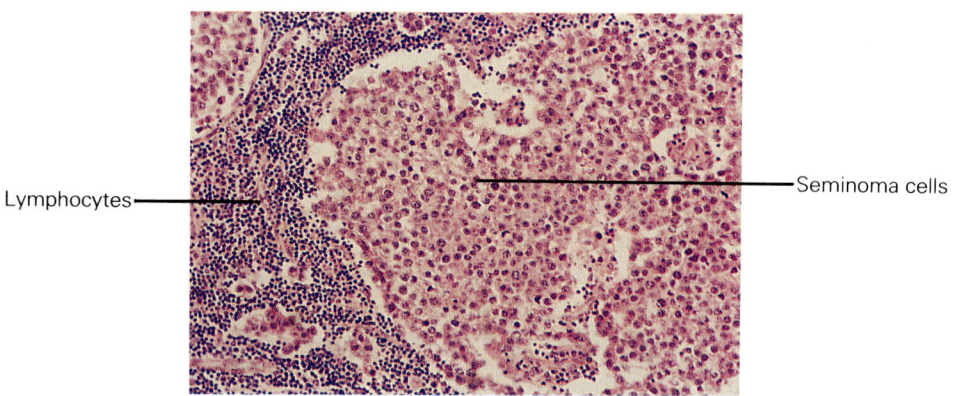

Seminomas are the most common testicular germ cell tumors and consist of lobulated masses of polyhedral seminoma cells with scattered reactive lymphocytes. Their good prognosis is related to its prolonged local growth phase and radiosensitivity.

Figure 12.48
Embryonal carcinoma of testis

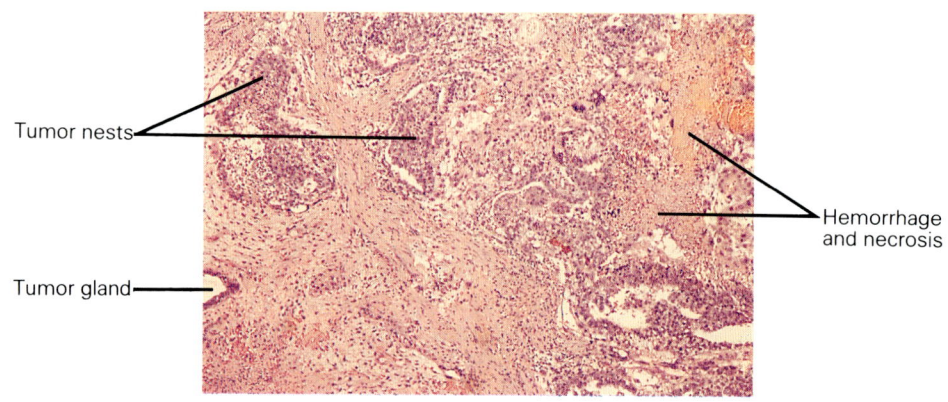

These tumors are more aggressive than seminomas and may produce human chorionic gonadotrophin (HCG) or alphafetoprotein (AFP). Growth is infiltrative, with glandular and nest-like patterns interspersed with zones of necrosis and hemorrhage.

Figure 12.49
Mature teratoma of testis

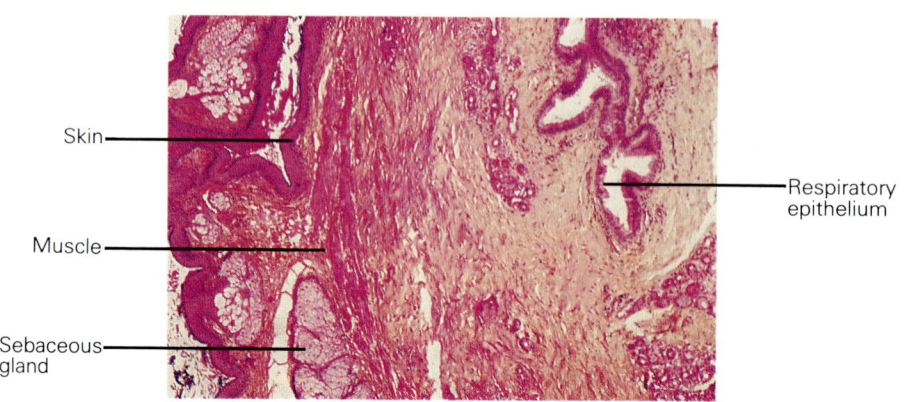

These tumors contain tissues derived from all three germ cell layers. Though most are well differentiated, in adults, foci of malignant transformation may occur.

Figure 12.50
Teratocarcinoma of testis

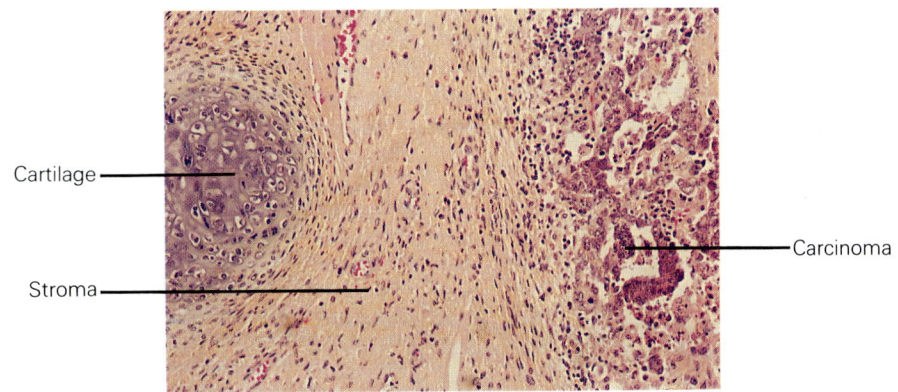

An epithelial malignancy resembling endodermal sinus tumor (at right) has arisen within the mixed tissues in this teratoma. Various types of carcinomas and sarcomas are seen in these malignancies.

PROSTATE

Figure 12.51
Normal prostate

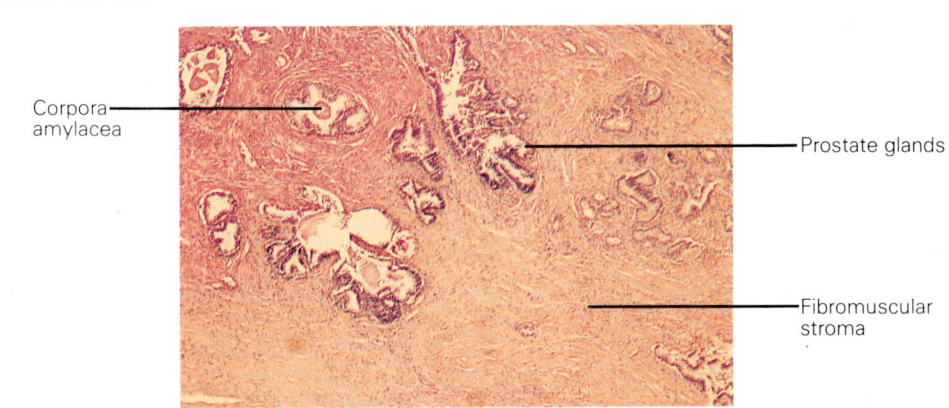

The normal prostate shows lobules of glandular tissue and stroma.

Figure 12.52
Prostatitis

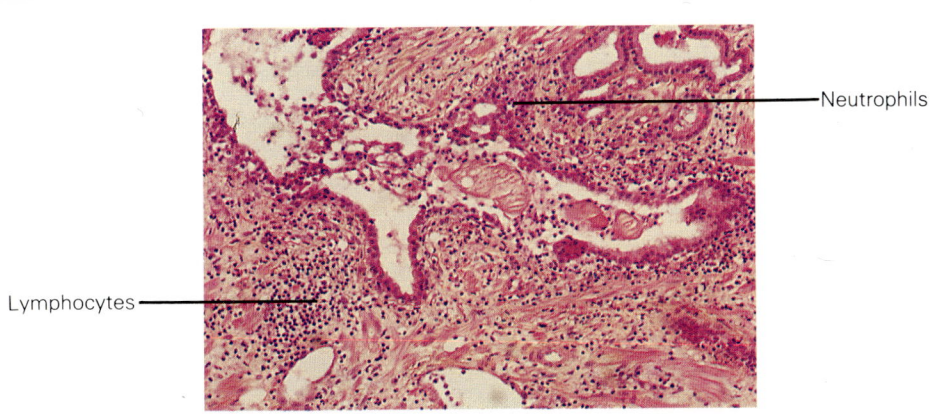

The inflamed prostate tissue shows an admixture of neutrophils and lymphocytes within glands and stroma.

Figure 12.53
Benign prostatic hypertrophy (BPH)

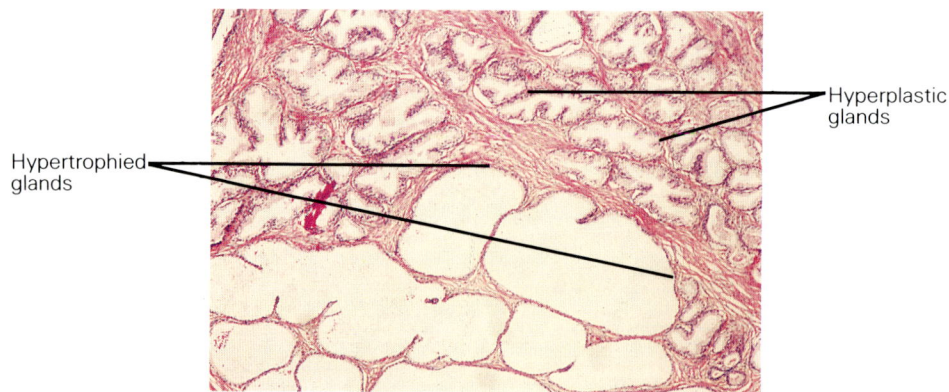

Enlargement of the prostate, though often designated "hypertrophy," consists of both glandular hypertrophy and hyperplasia.

Figure 12.54
Adenocarcinoma of prostate

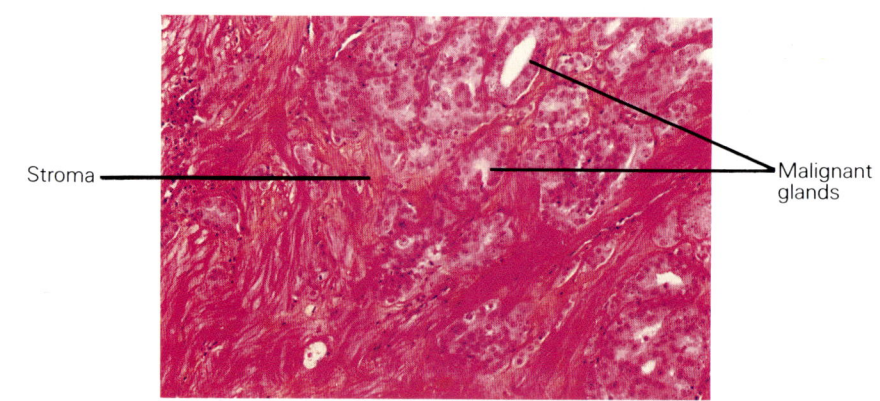

Invasive glandular structures are present within the stroma. Each gland is lined by one-cell only (in contrast to the double-cell layers of normal prostate glands). Note the single prominent nuceolus in the nuclei of these glands, a feature typical of this malignant tumor.

Figure 12.55
Condyloma acuminatum of penis

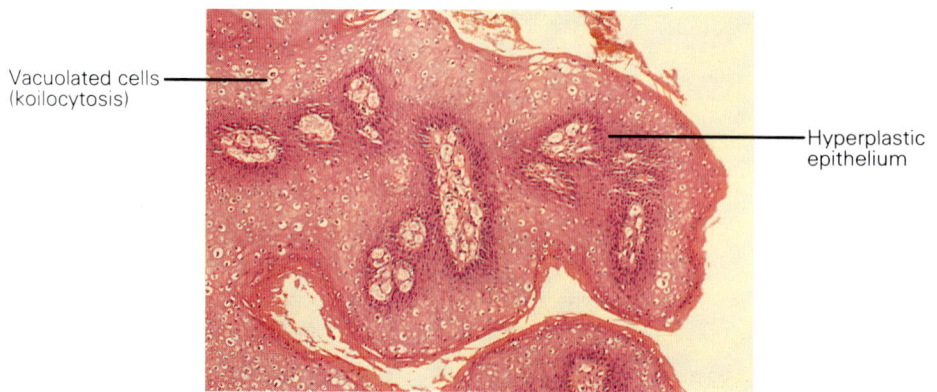

These papillary lesions may develop on the penile or perianal skin and are associated with human papilloma virus (HPV) infection.

CHAPTER 13

ENDOCRINE PATHOLOGY

Figure 13.1
Normal adrenal glands

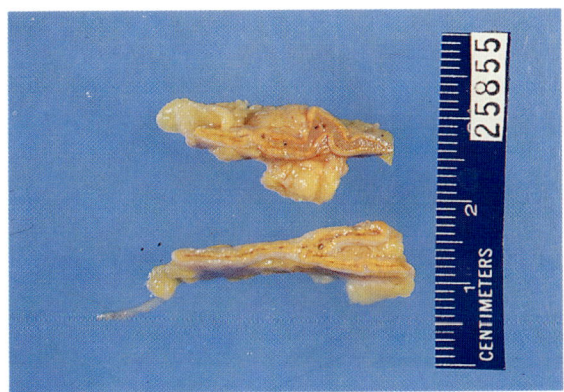

Normal weights: adrenal, 6 g each; parathyroid, 35–45 mg each; pineal, 0.1–0.18 g; pituitary, 0.61 g; and thyroid, 40 g.

Figure 13.2
Normal adrenal

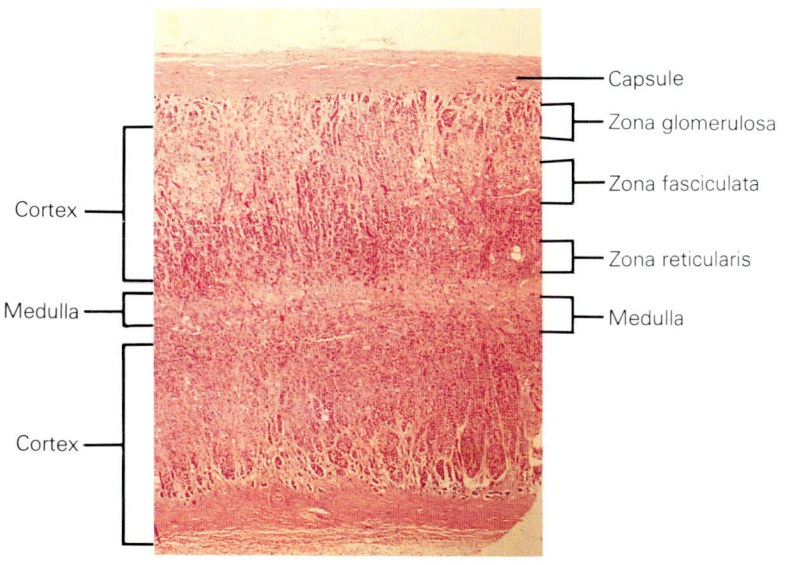

Figure 13.3
Normal thyroid

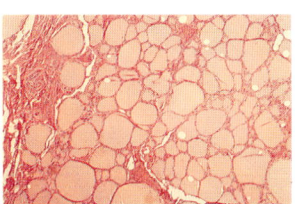

Thyroid follicles containing pink-staining thyroglobulin are lined by low cuboidal cells. The capsule is at left.

Figure 13.4
Normal parathyroid

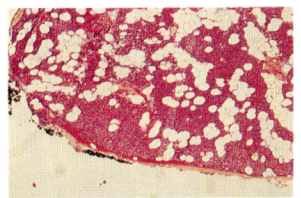

Parathyroid glands consist of approximately 50 percent fat and 50 percent parenchymal cells, including numerous chief cells and scattered plump, pink oxyphils.

Endocrine Pathology 175

Figure 13.5
Endocrine glands: major pathologic lesions

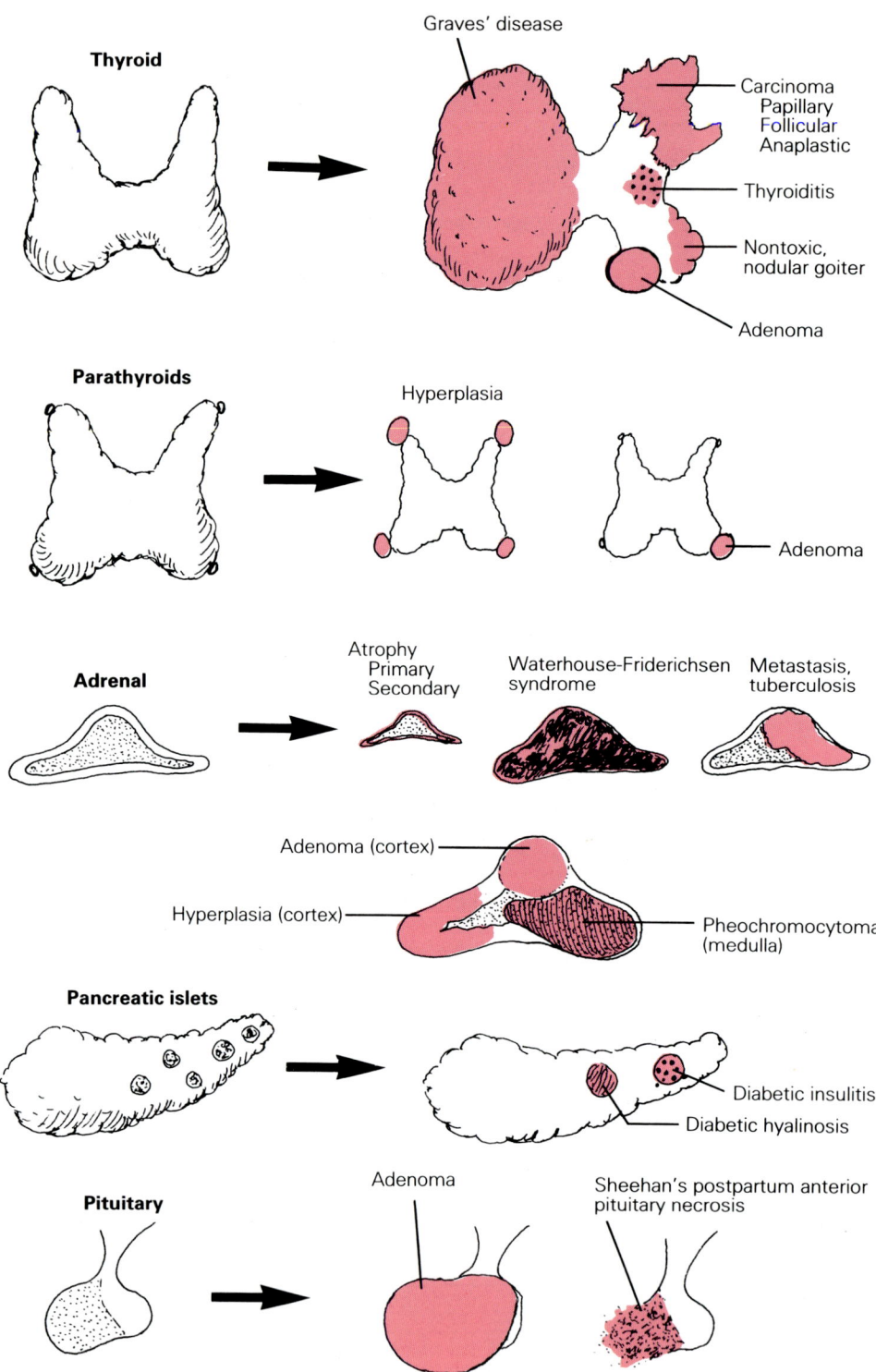

ADRENAL GLAND

Figure 13.6
Adrenocortical atrophy

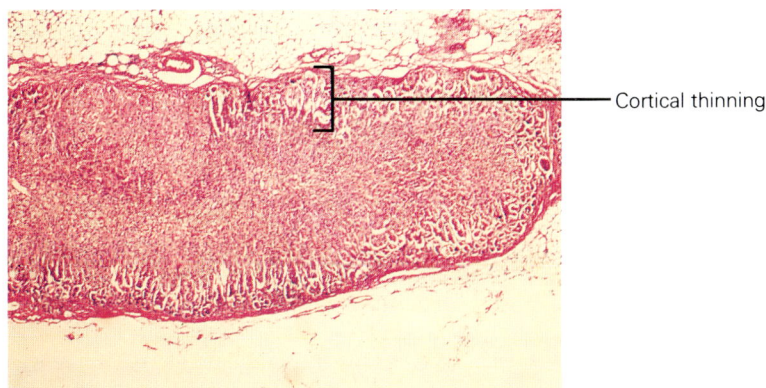

The cortex is atrophic in this section predominantly due to reduction of the thickness of the zona fasciculata. Primary adrenocortical insufficiency (Addison's disease) may be idiopathic, or due to parenchymal replacement by tumor, amyloid, or tuberculosis. Secondary insufficiency results from exogenous steroid administration or interruption of the normal hypophyseal-thalamic axis.

Figure 13.7
Waterhouse-Friderichsen syndrome

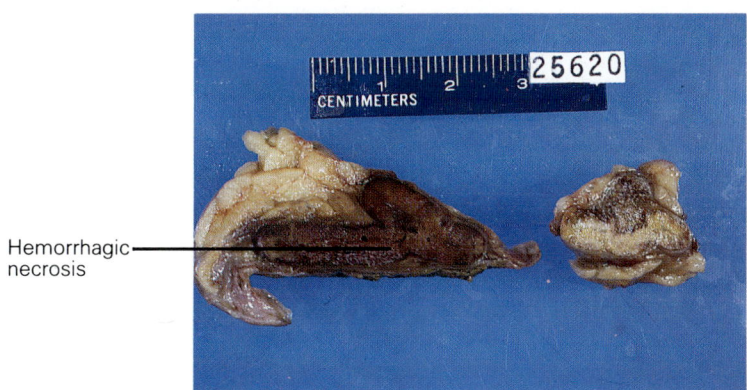

Hemorrhagic necrosis of the adrenals due to meningococcemia resulted in acute adrenocortical insufficiency and cardiovascular collapse in this patient. The left adrenal shows some residual, viable yellow cortical tissue.

Figure 13.8
Waterhouse-Friderichsen syndrome

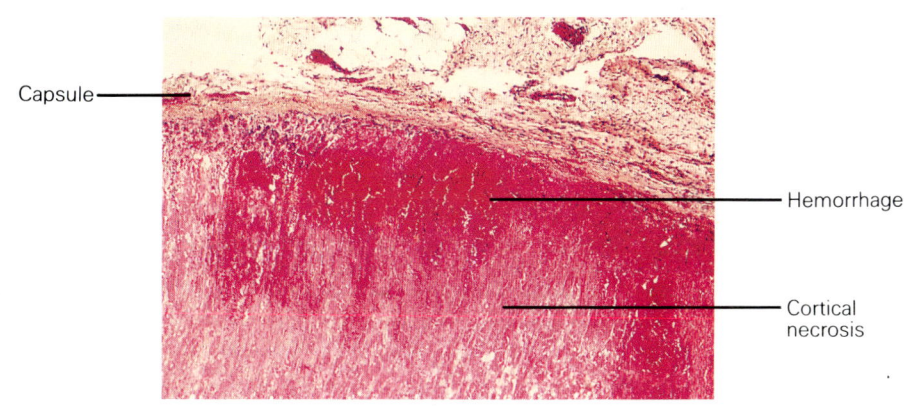

Septicemia with meningococci or, less commonly, pneumococci, staphylococci, or *Hemophilus influenzae* may produce this lesion.

Figure 13.9
Adrenocortical hyperplasia

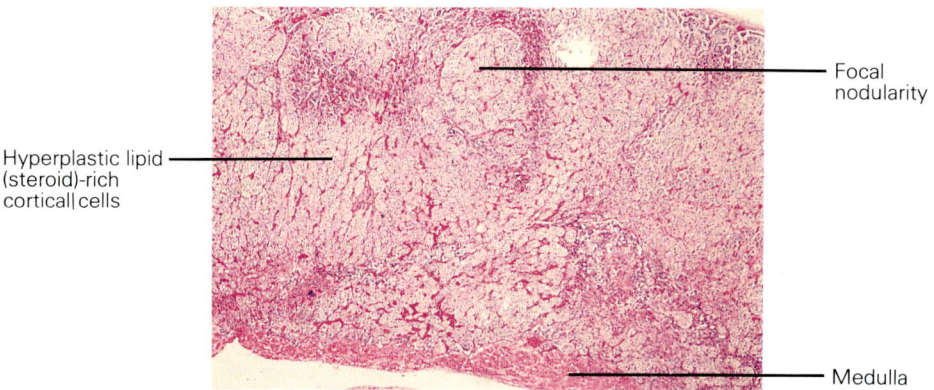

Hyperplasia of the cortex (which may exhibit nodularity) associated with increased cortisol production is one cause of Cushing's syndrome. Pituitary or ectopic adrenocorticotropic hormone (ACTH) is responsible.

Figure 13.10
Adrenocortical adenoma

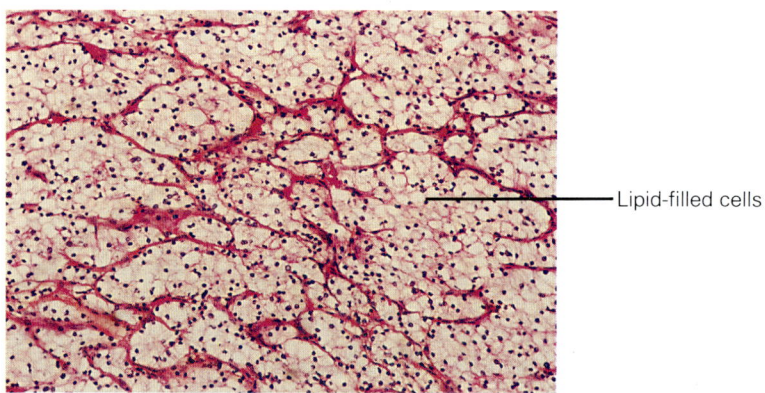

These benign tumors are usually poorly encapsulated and nonfunctional. Their lipid content renders a yellow-orange gross appearance. Histologic growth is in nests and cords, with significant cytologic atypia despite benignity.

Figure 13.11
Adrenal carcinoma

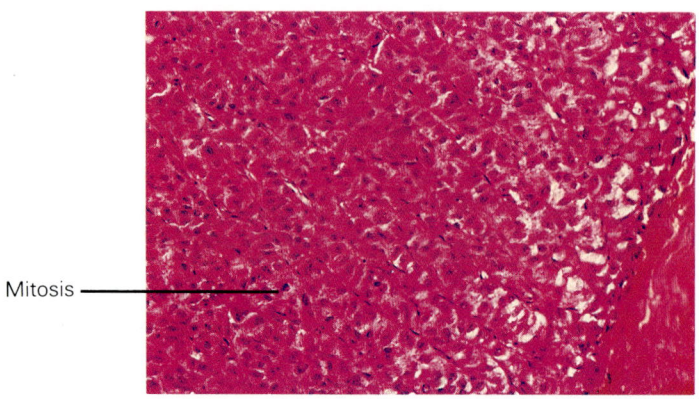

These highly malignant tumors are usually steroid-producing. Mitotic activity, hemorrhage and necrosis, invasion of venous and lymphatic structures, and variable cytologic atypia are characteristic histologic features.

Figure 13.12
Metastatic carcinoma in adrenal cortex

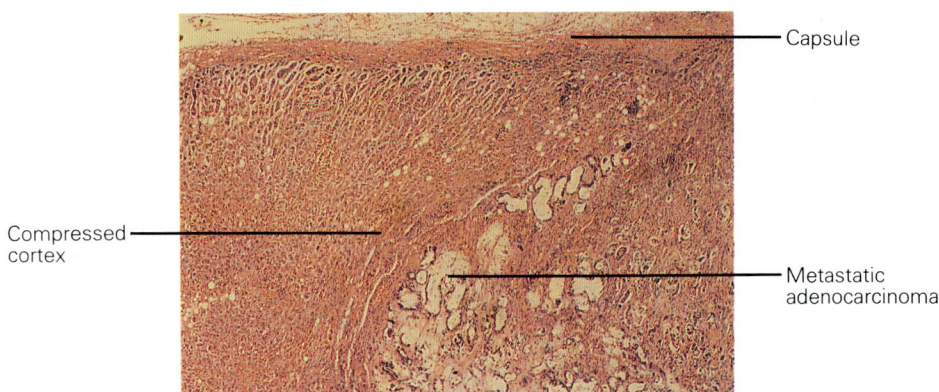

A variety of carcinomas, including squamous cell carcinoma of the lung and adenocarcinomas from several sites, may metastasize to the adrenal gland.

Figure 13.13
Pheochromocytoma

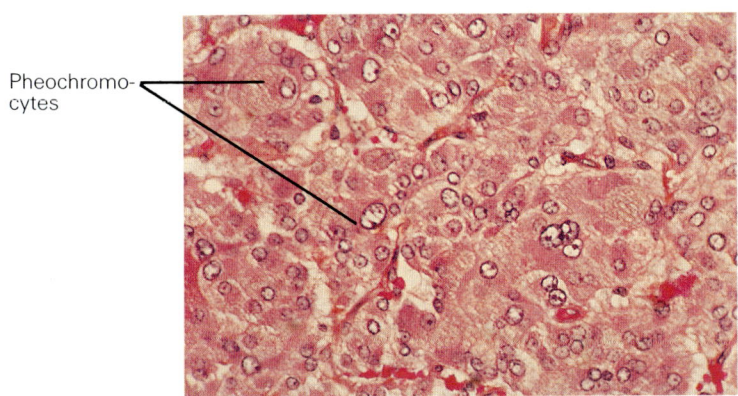

This tumor of the adrenal medulla and occasional other sites produces hypertension through catecholamine secretion. Pheochromocytes, arranged in nests and/or trabeculae, show a granular cytoplasm and nuclear pleomorphism.

THYROID GLAND

Figure 13.14
Nontoxic nodular goiter

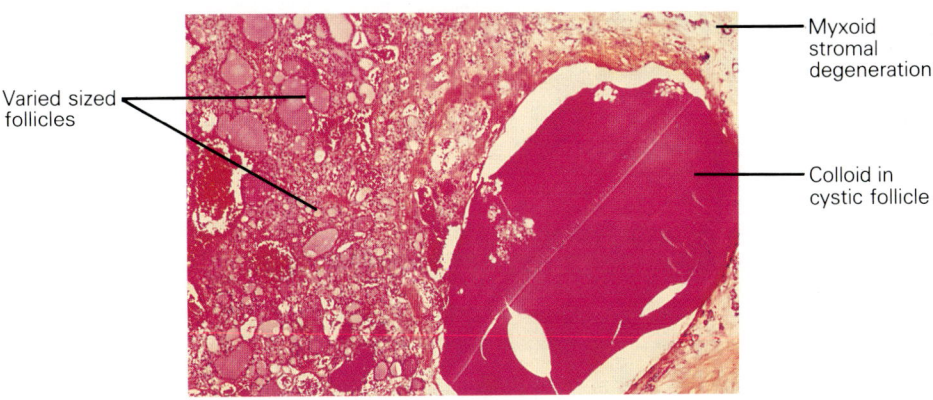

Nodular enlargement of the thyroid in this condition is associated with histologic variations in follicle size, large colloid filled cysts and stromal degeneration, hemorrhage, and calcification.

Figure 13.15
Graves' disease (thyrotoxicosis)

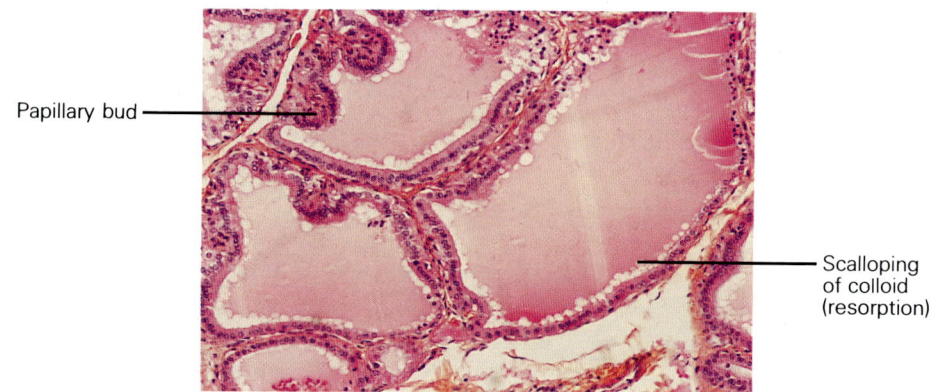

The diffuse thyroid hyperplasia of Graves' disease results in follicular hypercellularity and scattered, simple papillary projections. Active resorption of colloid (scalloping) by plump cuboidal to columnar follicular cells is associated with thyroid hyperfunction and ophthalmopathy.

Figure 13.16
Hashimoto's (autoimmune) thyroiditis

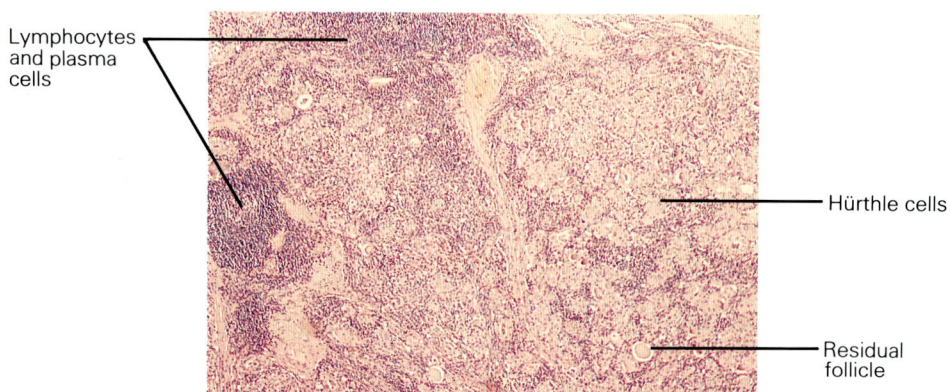

Lymphocytes and plasma cells extensively replace thyroid follicles, and residual thyroid cells are transformed to plump, pink mitochondria-rich Hürthle cells. There is resultant thyroid enlargement and hypothyroidism.

Figure 13.17
Riedel's struma

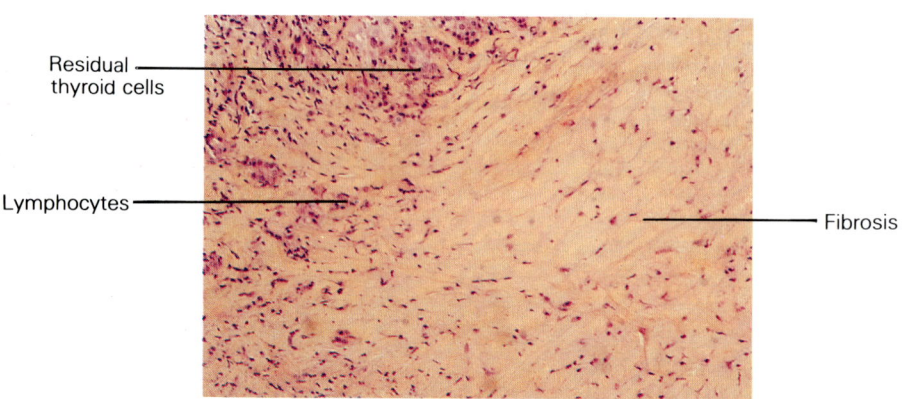

The thyroid parenchyma is diffusely replaced by firm fibrous tissue ("woody thyroiditis") which may extend into adjacent neck structures. It must be clinically distinguished from carcinoma.

Figure 13.18
Thyroid adenoma

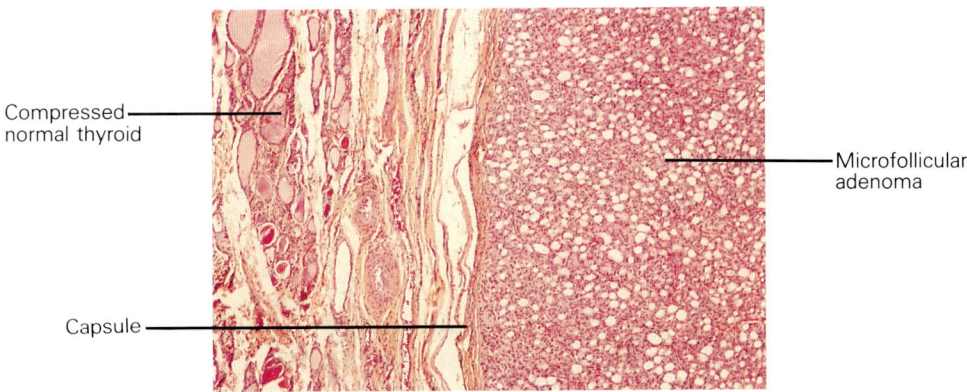

These "cold" nodules are well-encapsulated, compress adjacent normal thyroid, and do not usually cause hyperthyroidism.

Figure 13.19
Papillary adenocarcinoma of the thyroid

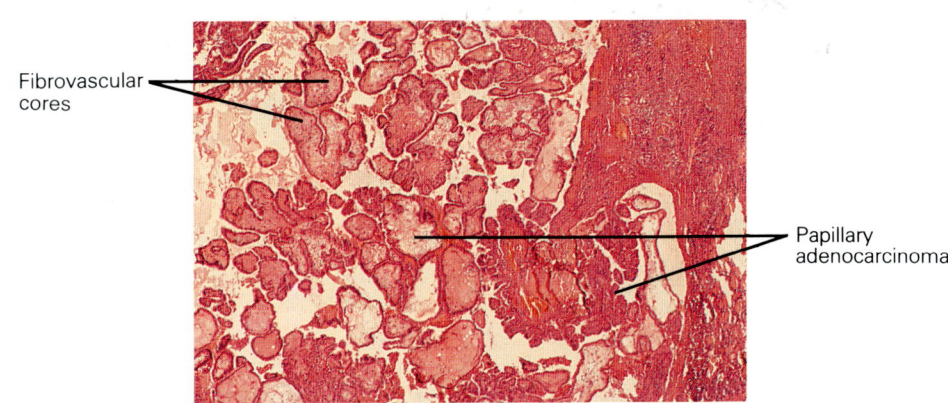

This is the most common type of thyroid carcinoma, growing in papillary structures lined by piled-up cells. Prognosis is good and growth indolent, with metastasis typically to cervical lymph nodes.

Figure 13.20
Psammoma bodies

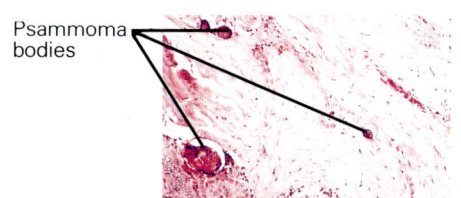

Figure 13.21
Ground-glass nuclei

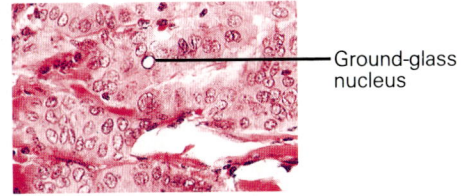

More than 50 percent of papillary thyroid carcinomas contain laminated calcific spheres (psammoma bodies) and "optically clear" ground-glass nuclei.

Figure 13.22
Follicular adenocarcinoma of thyroid

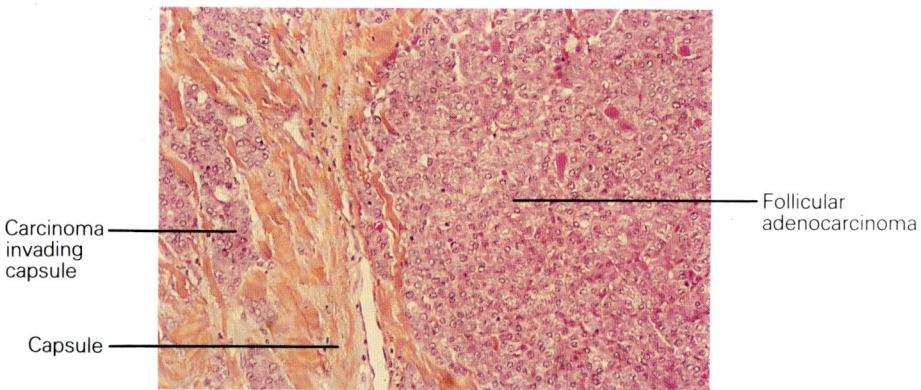

Accounting for approximately 25 percent of thyroid cancers, these tumors grow in follicles and invade the thyroid capsule and blood vessels.

Figure 13.23
Medullary carcinoma of thyroid

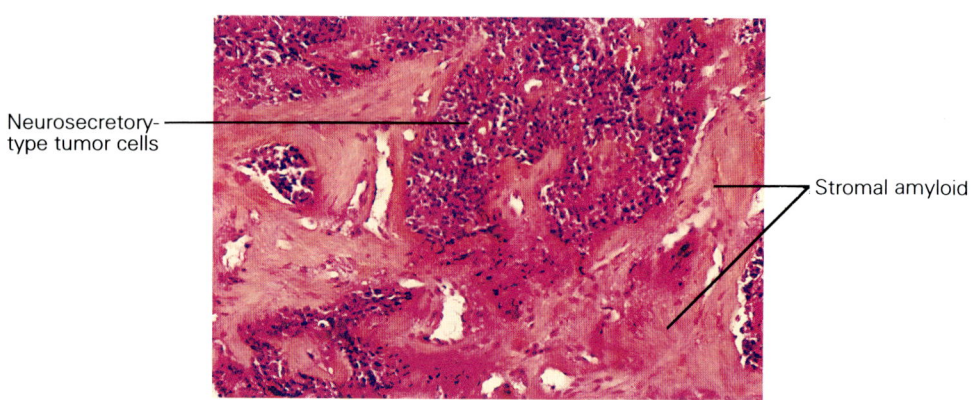

Parafollicular (C) neurosecretory cells comprise this uncommon form of thyroid cancer. Most contain amyloid within their stroma.

PARATHYROID GLAND

Figure 13.24
Parathyroid hyperplasia

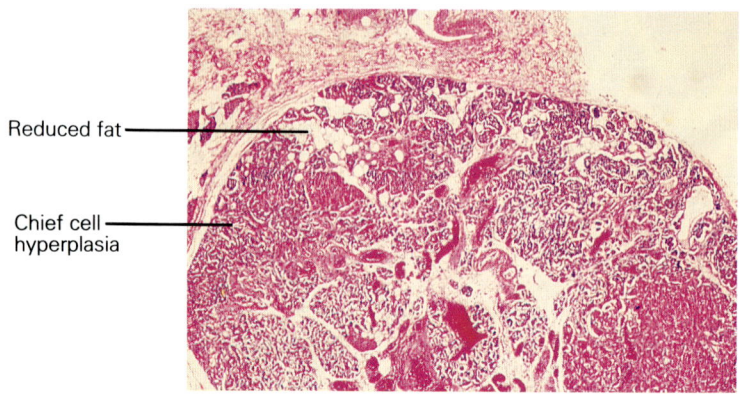

Primary and secondary forms of hyperplasia show sheets, cords, and glands of hyperplastic chief cells in a lobulated pattern replacing normal fat (compare to Figure 13.4).

Figure 13.25
Parathyroid adenoma

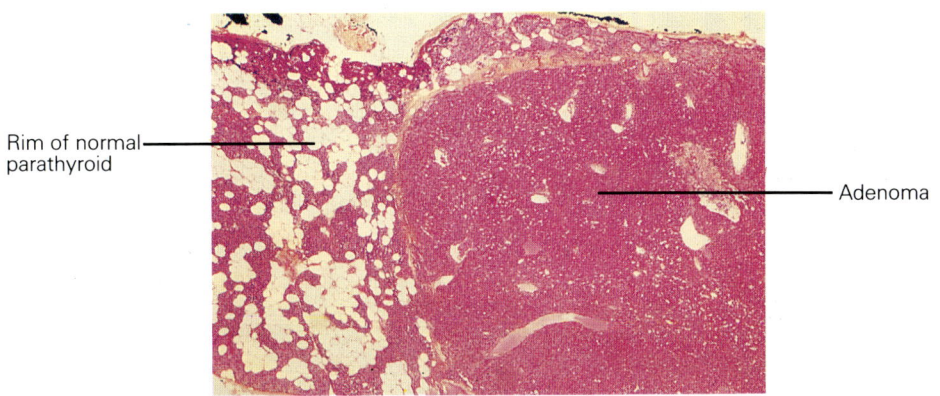

These well-encapsulated lesions are composed of sheets of chief cells, sometimes with admixed oxyphils.

Figure 13.26
Pancreatic islets in diabetes

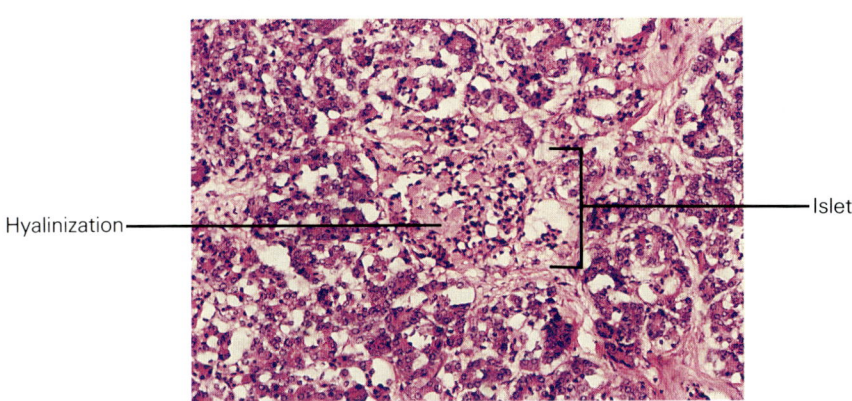

Obliteration of islets by hyalinized connective tissue may be seen in the diabetic pancreas. Another diabetic change (not shown here) is islet infiltration by lymphocytes (insulitis).

CHAPTER 14

BONE AND SOFT TISSUE PATHOLOGY

Figure 14.1
Osteoporosis

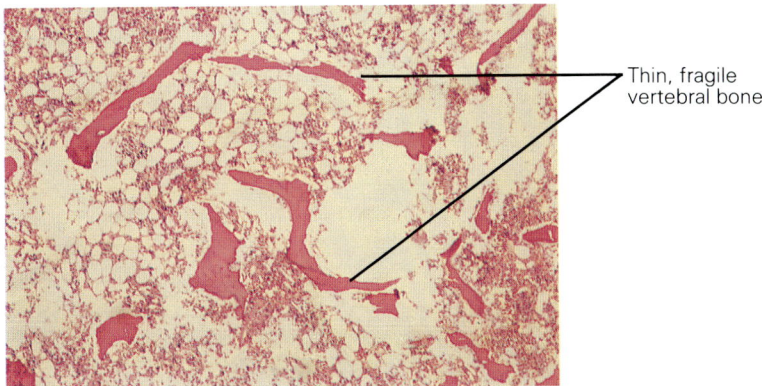

The reduced skeletal mass in osteoporosis results from loss of both bone mineral and matrix.

Figure 14.2
Osteomyelitis

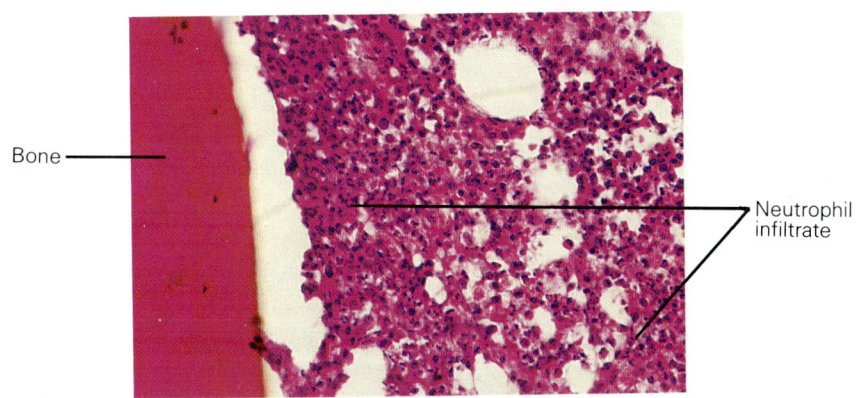

Pyogenic bone infections are due to *Staphylococcus aureus*, group B streptococcus in neonates, and salmonellae in patients with sickle cell disease.

Figure 14.3
Paget's disease of bone (osteitis deformans)

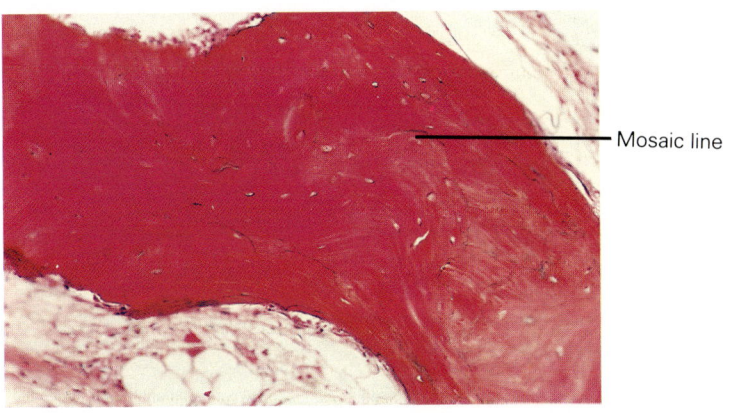

Resorption of bone by osteoclasts, followed by irregular bone formation, leads to thickened cortical and trabecular bone with a mosaic pattern.

Figure 14.4
Bone and soft tissues: major pathologic lesions

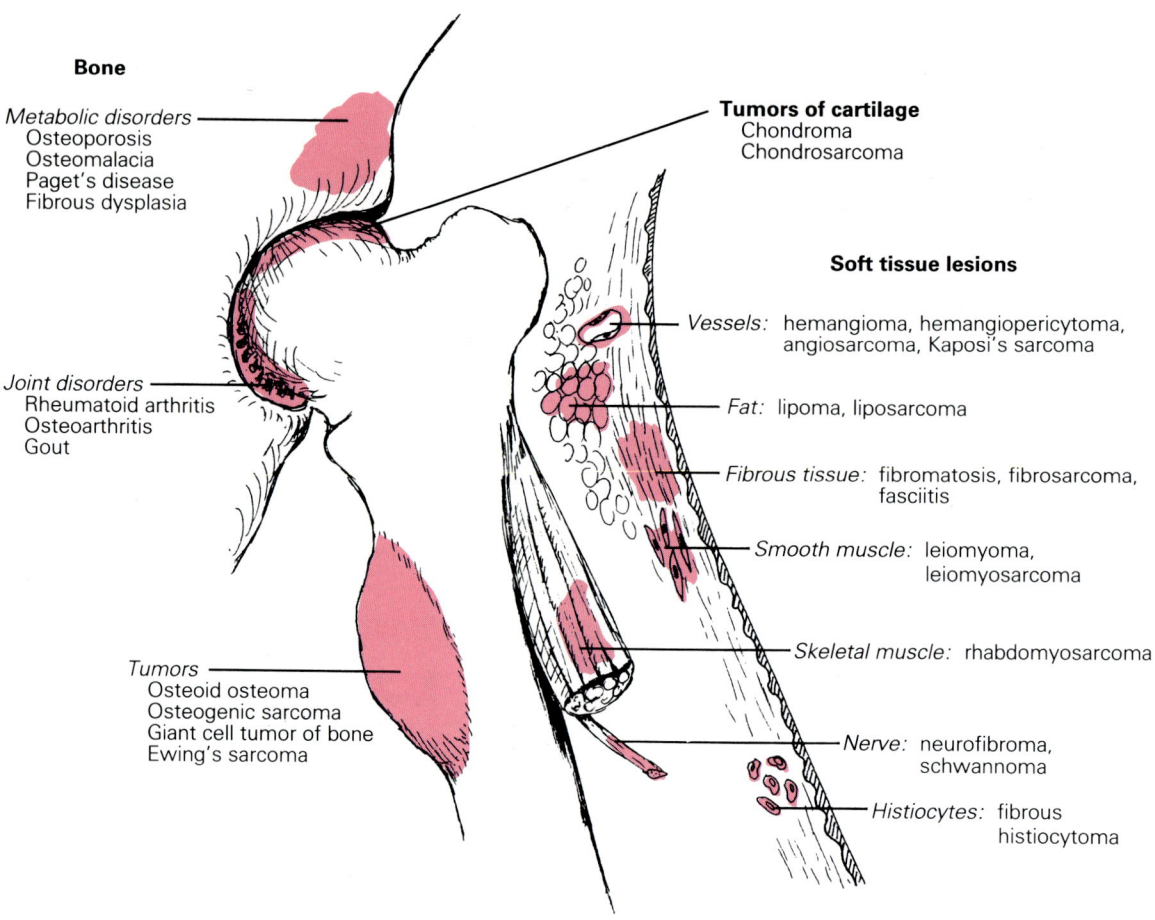

Figure 14.5
Fibrous dysplasia of bone

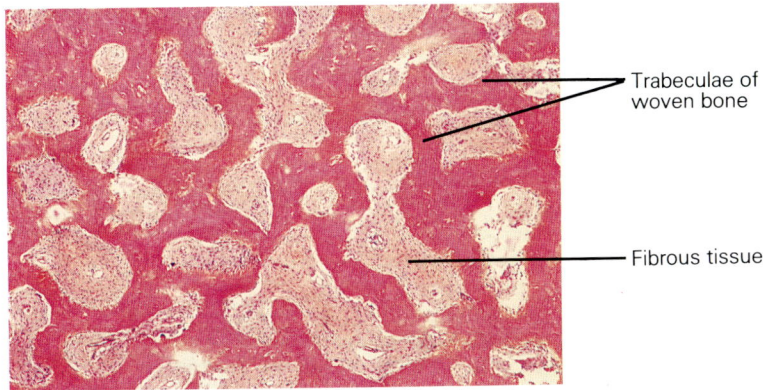

This benign lesion consists of abnormal fibrous tissue deposition and irregular trabeculae of woven bone. The majority of cases involve single bones (monostotic fibrous dysplasia).

Figure 14.6
Osteoid osteoma of bone

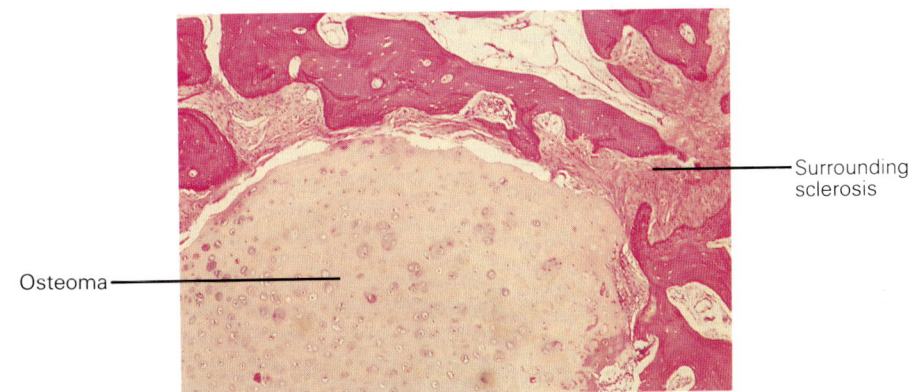

These radiographically radiolucent benign lesions of tibial and femoral diaphyses occur in young individuals and are composed of sheets or anastomosing partly mineralized osteoid trabeculae.

Figure 14.7
Osteogenic sarcoma

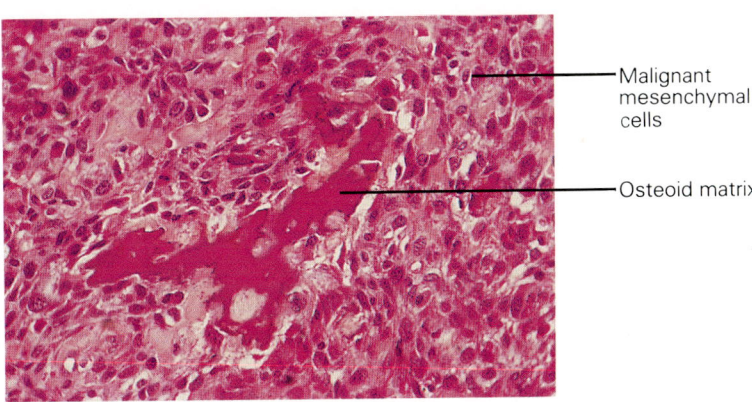

This malignancy of mesenchymal cells produces osteoid or bone in long bones of the extremities.

Bone and Soft Tissue Pathology

Figure 14.8
Chondroma (enchondroma) of bone

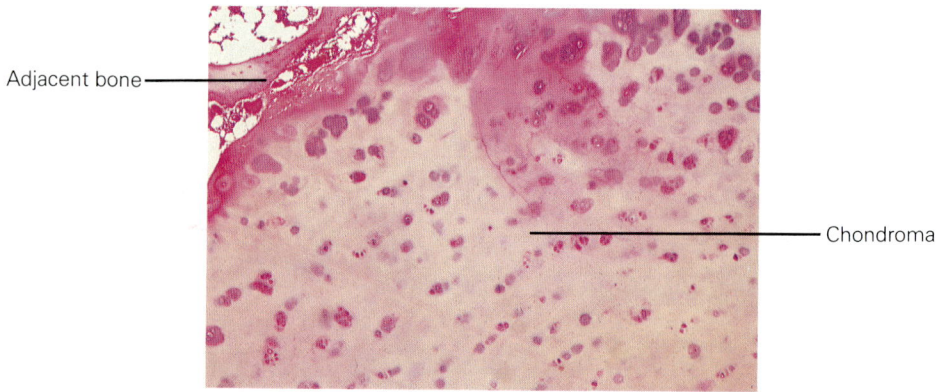

These benign tumors composed of hyaline cartilage develop in small bones of the hands and feet. Compare the small, bland nuclei of the chondrocytes to the malignant nuclei in chondrosarcoma (Figure 14.9).

Figure 14.9
Chondrosarcoma

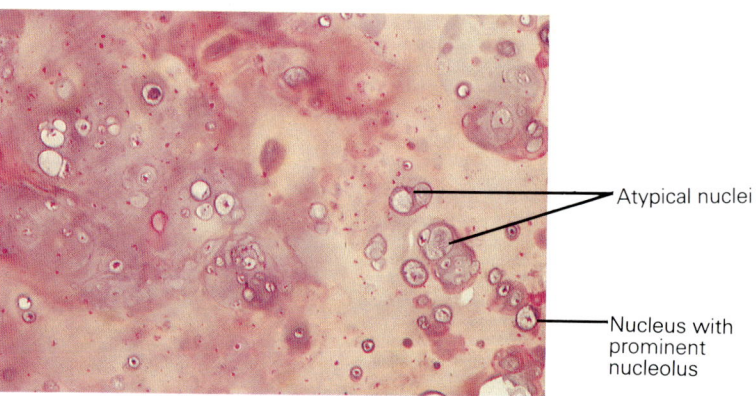

These malignant tumors commonly arise in pelvic bones and show anaplastic nuclei within chondrocytes. Compare the nuclear pleomorphism and atypia to Figure 14.8.

Figure 14.10
Ewing's sarcoma

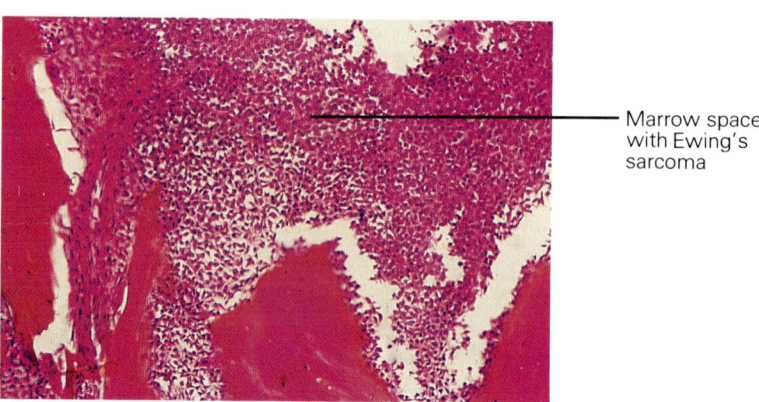

A highly malignant tumor of primitive mesenchymal cells arising in long tubular or innominate bones. Tumor cells are small and rounded and contain PAS-positive cytoplasmic granules.

Figure 14.11
Giant cell tumor of bone

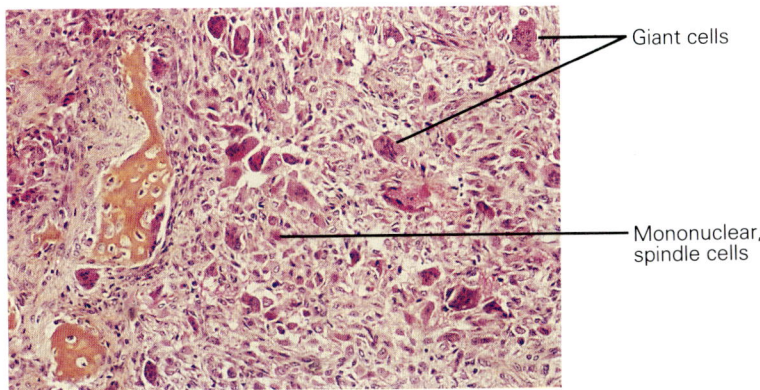

This tumor of epiphyses of the distal femur and proximal tibia or fibula consists of non-neoplastic multinucleate giant cells and neoplastic, plump spindle cells which appear to be osteoclastic in origin.

Figure 14.12
Synovitis in rheumatoid arthritis

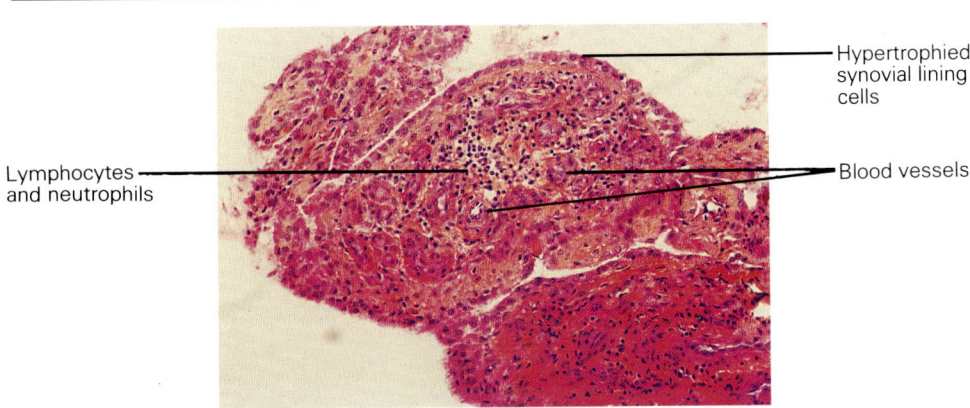

The prominent synovial folds in the synovitis associated with rheumatoid arthritis show hypertrophied synovial lining cells and underlying vascular inflammatory tissue.

Figure 14.13
Pannus in rheumatoid arthritis

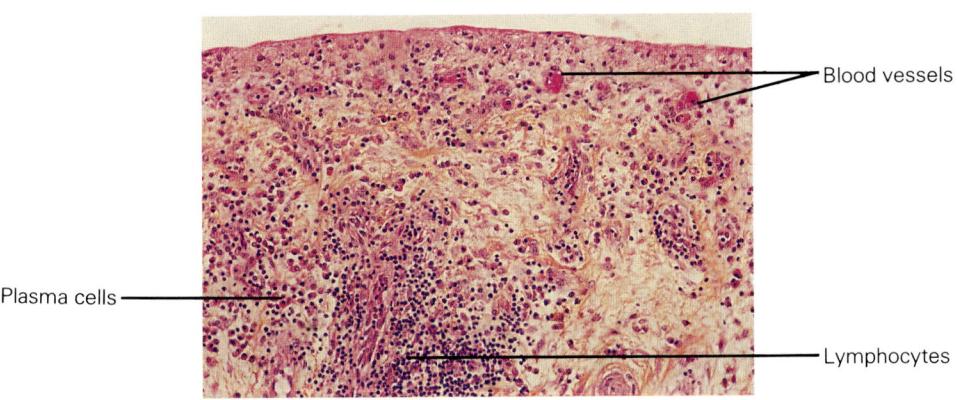

The pannus consists of vascularized connective tissue with plasma cells, lymphocytes, and macrophages replacing the synovial lining. It may erode the underlying articular cartilage and joint capsule.

Bone and Soft Tissue Pathology

Figure 14.14
Pigmented villonodular synovitis

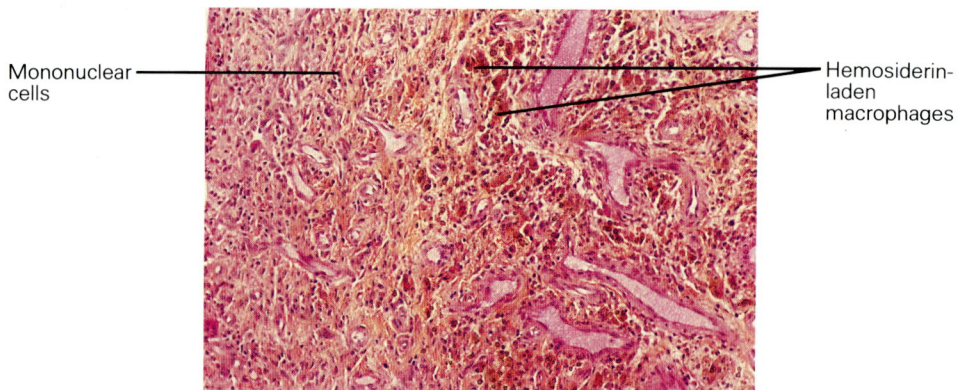

This proliferative lesion consists of polypoid synovial projections containing spindle cells, lymphocytes, and hemosiderin-laden macrophages. This has been considered a reactive lesion to trauma or, alternatively, a neoplastic lesion of synovial cells or histiocytes.

Figure 14.15
Synovial sarcoma

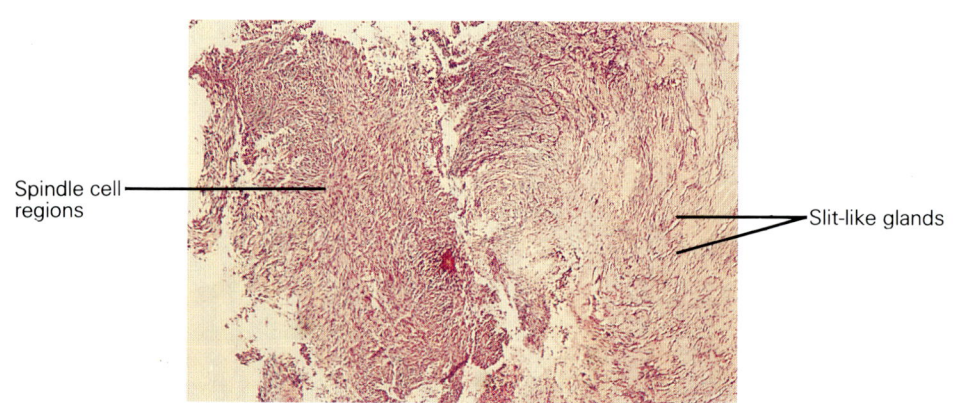

This malignant synovial tumor most often arises in the lower extremities and lower torso. A biphasic glandular and spindle cell pattern is usually present.

Figure 14.16
Ganglion

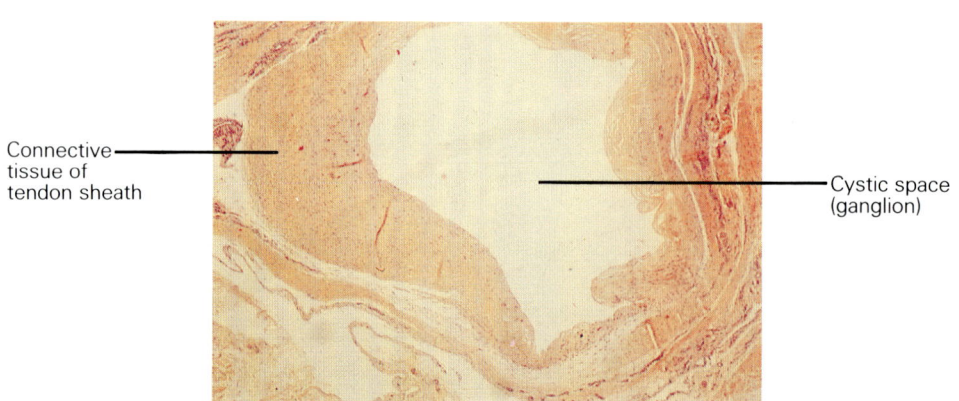

Myxoid degeneration of tendon or joint capsule connective tissue, often in the wrist, leads to an inner cystic space or ganglion.

Figure 14.17
Benign fibrous histiocytoma

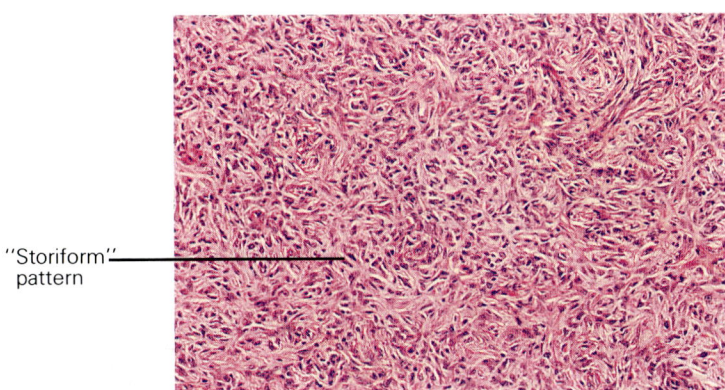

A soft tissue tumor arising within subcutaneous tissue and other sites; these lesions show spindle-shaped histiocytic cells arranged in a whorled ("storiform") pattern with variable facultative collagen production.

Figure 14.18
Fibromatosis

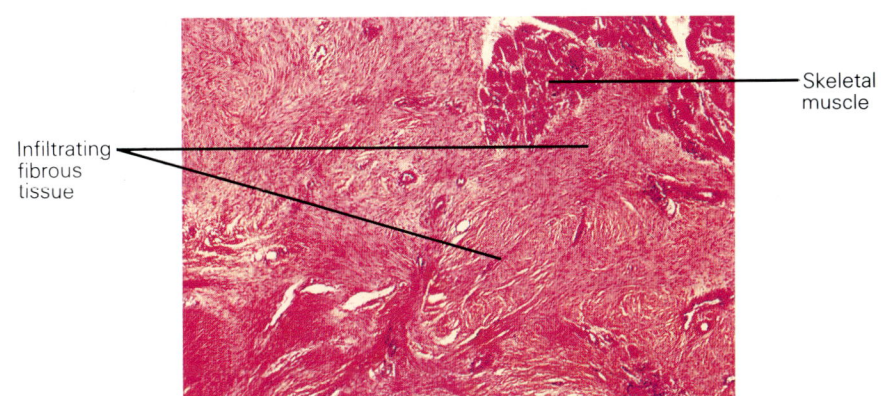

This infiltrative fibroblastic lesion may develop in subcutaneous tissues, fascia, and muscle (desmoid tumor of abdomen).

Figure 14.19
Fasciitis (pseudosarcomatous fasciitis)

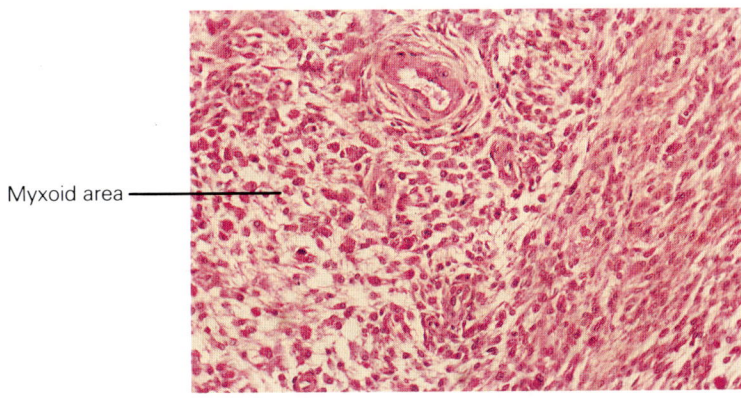

A subcutaneous growth of myxoid fibroblastic tissue admixed with mononuclear inflammatory cells, often in the upper extremity. These lesions resemble reparative tissue.

Figure 14.20
Mesenchymoma (angiomyolipoma)

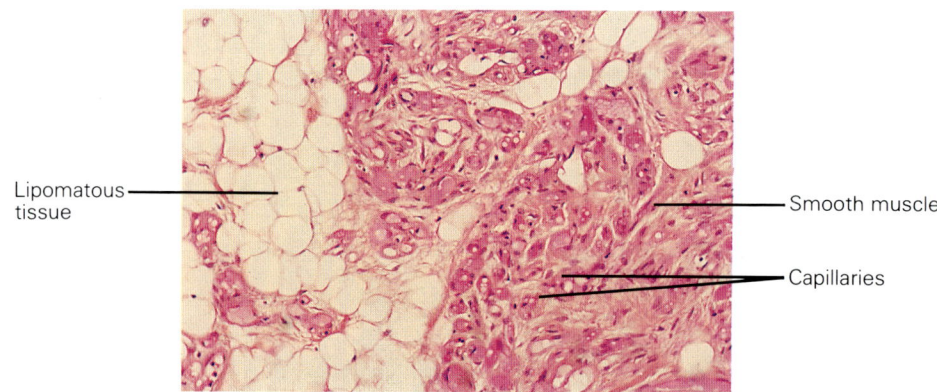

These benign mesenchymal tumors often arise in the kidney and perirenal tissues and are composed of admixed fat, capillary and venous angiomas, and smooth muscle bundles.

Figure 14.21
Lipoma

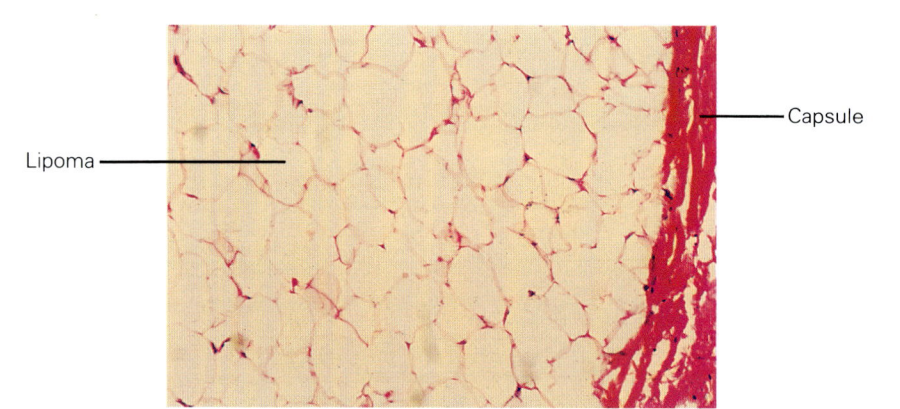

These common benign tumors are collections of adipose tissue which grossly show large size variations.

Figure 14.22
Liposarcoma

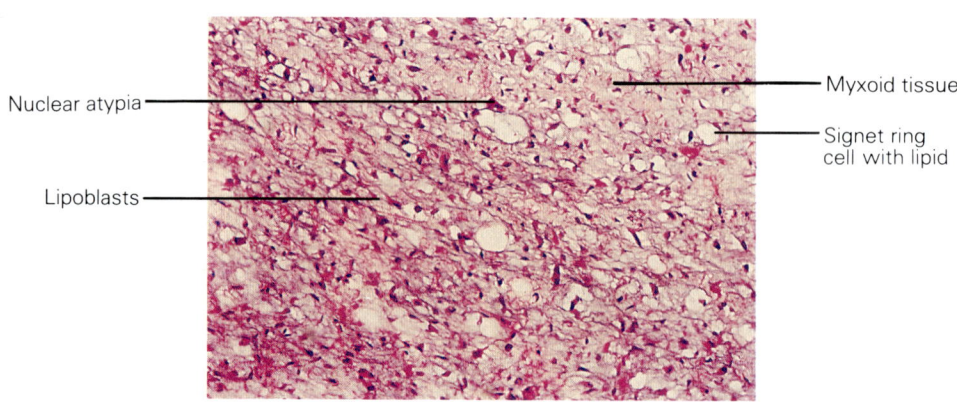

Liposarcomas are malignant tumors of adipose tissue growing in the deep soft tissues in the gluteal region, thigh, retroperitoneum, and other sites. Pleomorphic lipoblasts and adult-appearing adipocytes are admixed with myxoid tissue.

Figure 14.23
Leiomyosarcoma

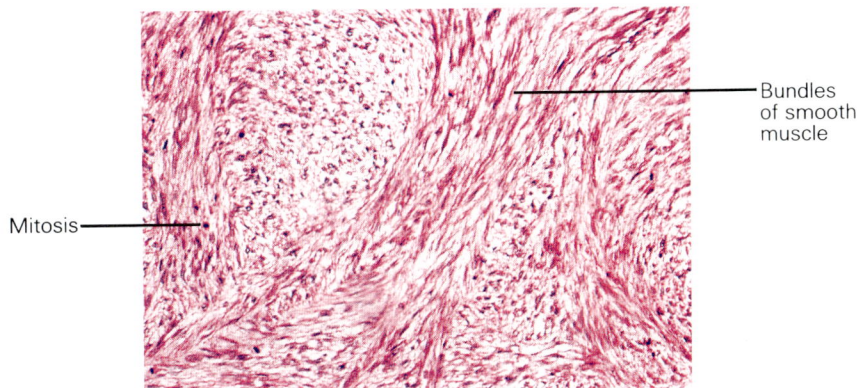

These smooth muscle tumors arise in the uterus, stomach, retroperitoneum, and other sites. Mitotic activity is important in differentiating from benign leiomyomas (see Figures 9.16 and 12.11).

Figure 14.24
Rhabdomyosarcoma

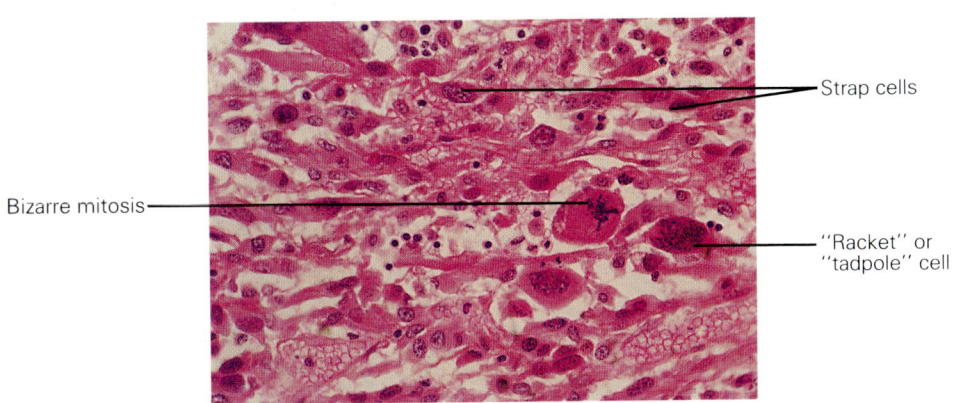

These tumors arise in muscles of children and adults. Tumor cells are strap or racket shaped and may show cross striations or longitudinal myofibrils.

Figure 14.25
Schwannoma (neurilemmoma)

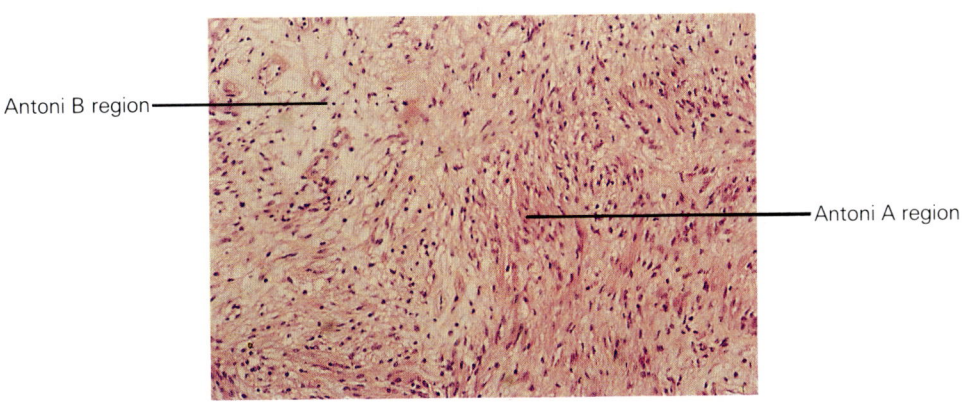

These are benign, encapsulated Schwann cell tumors of proximal nerves or spinal nerve roots. The spindle shaped Schwann cells are organized into cellular (Antoni A) and hypocellular (Antoni B) regions.

Figure 14.26
Neurofibromas

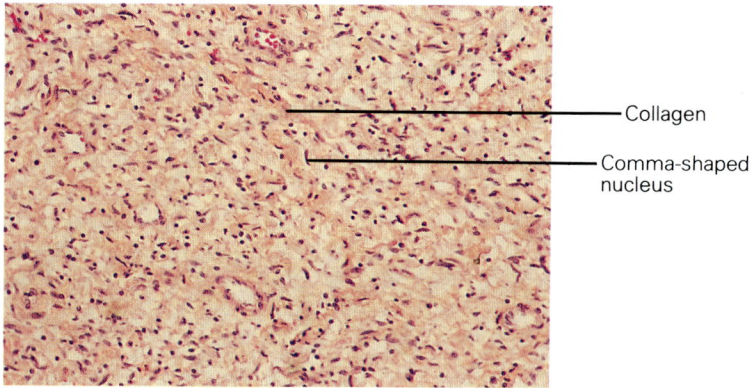

These tumors consist of loosely arranged spindle cells. Nerve fibers may be scattered throughout the tumor. They may be solitary subcutaneous lesions or multiple in the syndrome of neurofibromatosis (von Recklinghausen's disease).

Figure 14.27
Granular cell tumor (esophagus)

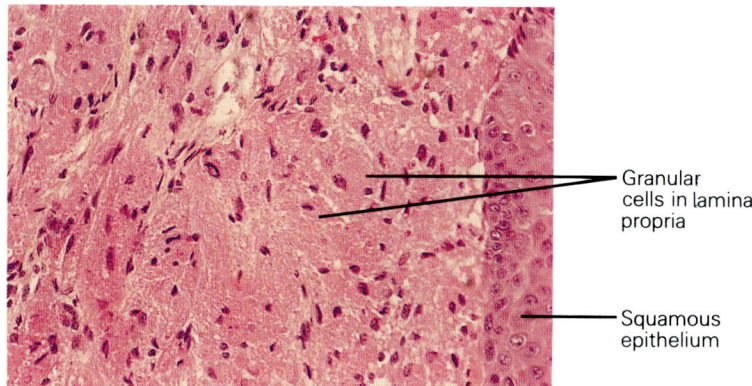

This benign tumor of Schwann cell precursors is commonly found in the tongue and subcutaneous tissues.

Figure 14.28
Kaposi's sarcoma

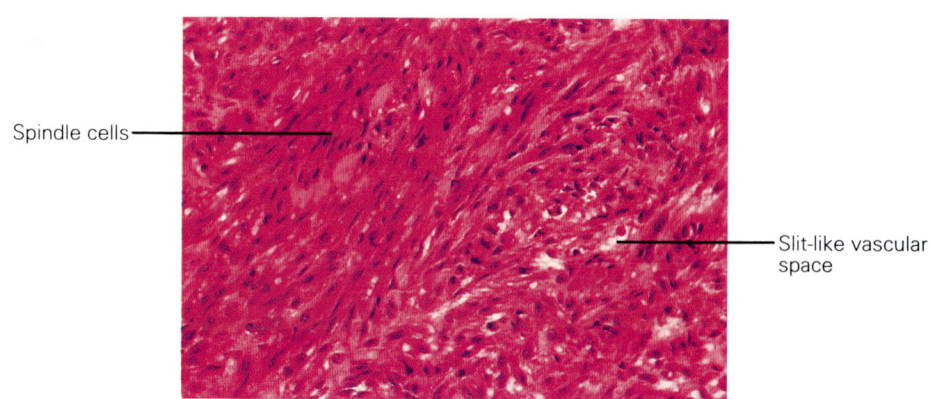

These vascular malignant tumors present as bluish skin nodules in the extremities of elderly males or in multiple sites in individuals with acquired immune deficiency syndrome (AIDS).

Figure 14.29
Hemangiopericytoma (soft palate)

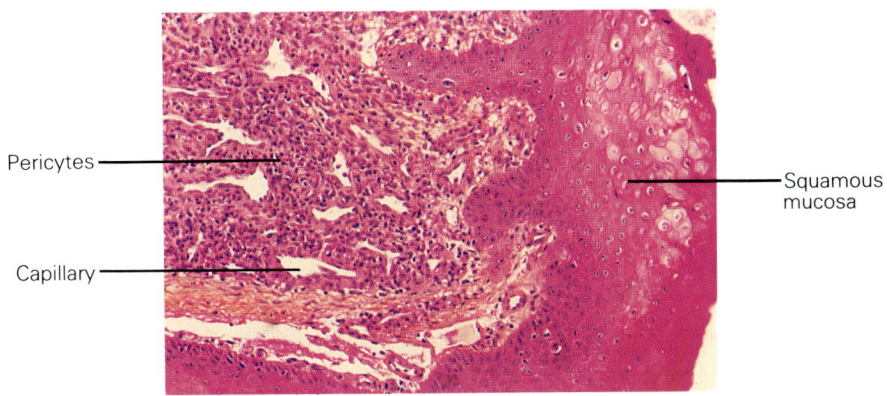

This tumor develops from pericytes, a spindle cell population within the walls of capillaries and surrounding the endothelium. The tumor shows vascular channels enclosed by nests of neoplastic pericytes.

Figure 14.30
Glomus tumor

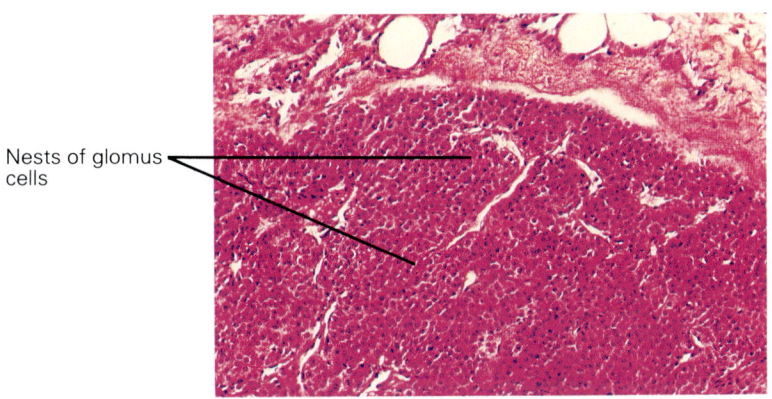

These are painful, small benign tumors of the modified smooth muscle cells comprising glomus bodies (neuromyoarterial receptors).

CHAPTER 15

DERMATOPATHOLOGY

Figure 15.1
Normal skin

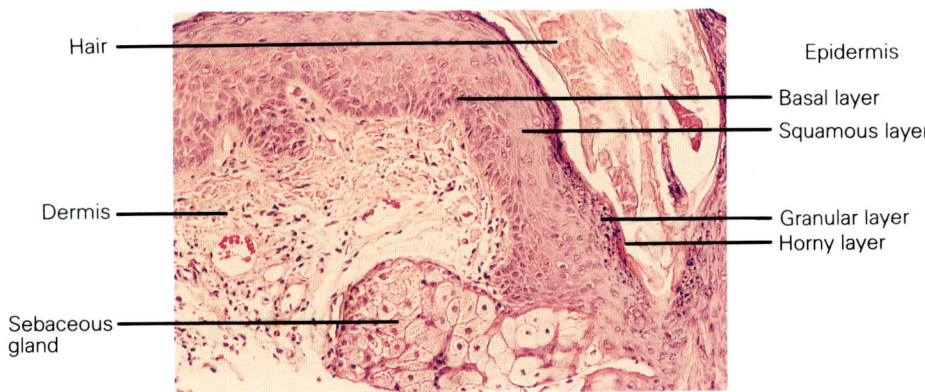

Routine evaluation should include examination of the epidermis, dermis, and adnexal structures for evidence of inflammation or neoplasia.

Figure 15.2
Eczema (dermatitis)

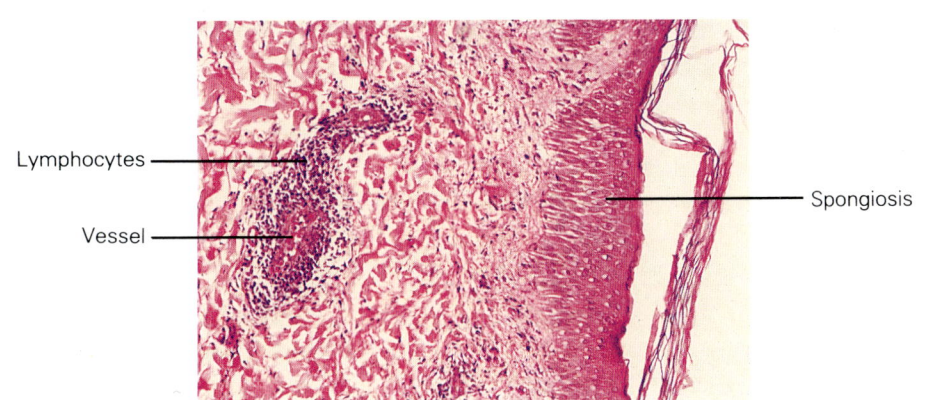

Some of the changes seen in dermatitis include spongiosis (intercellular edema) and perivascular dermal infiltrates of lymphocytes.

Figure 15.3
Pemphigus vulgaris

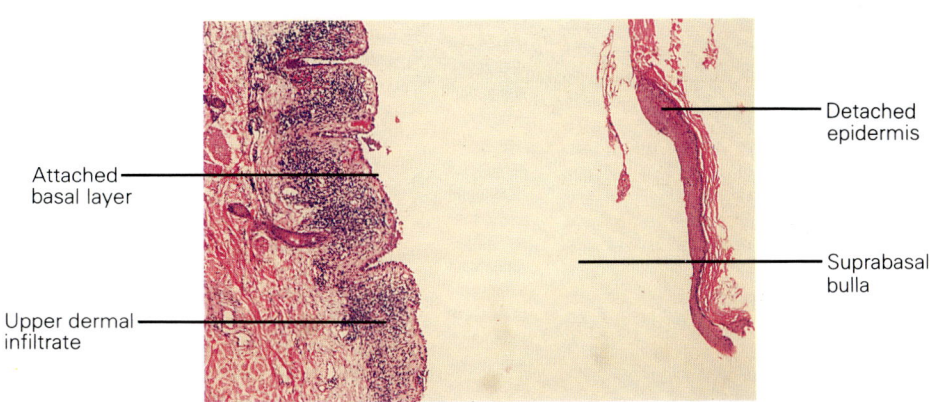

This bullous disease results from loss of coherence of epidermal cells (acantholysis) leading to suprabasal cleft formation and, ultimately, denudation of epidermis.

Dermatopathology 201

Figure 15.4
Dermatopathology: major pathologic lesions

Normal skin

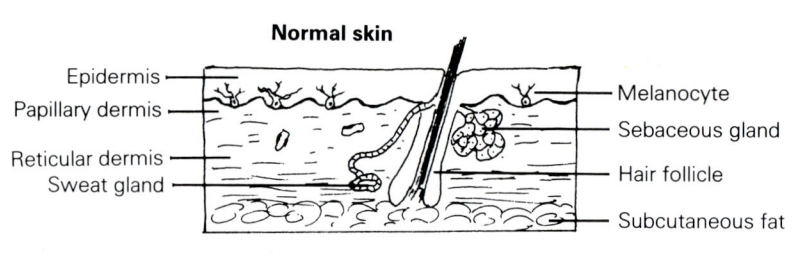

Epidermal tumors

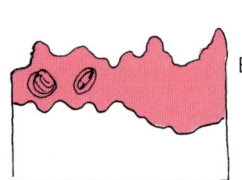 Benign
- Seborrheic keratosis
- Keratoacanthoma

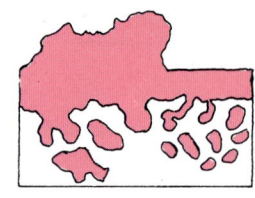 Premalignant
- Actinic keratosis

Malignant
- Squamous cell carcinoma
- Basal cell carcinoma

Melanocytic lesions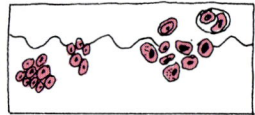
- Nevi
- Malignant melanoma

Adnexal tumors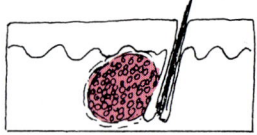
- Nevus sebaceous
- Trichoepithelioma
- Pilomatrixoma
- Cylindroma

Inflammatory dermatoses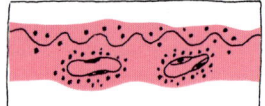
- Eczema
- Erythema multiforme
- Acne vulgaris
- Lichen planus
- Psoriasis

Blistering (bullous) diseases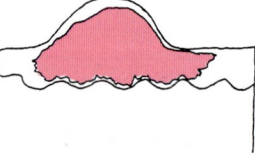
- Pemphigus
- Bullous pemphigoid
- Dermatitis herpetiformis
- Porphyria

Infections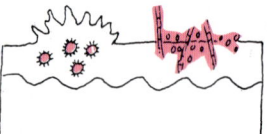
- Verrucae (warts)
- Impetigo
- Fungi and arthropods

Figure 15.5
Erythema multiforme

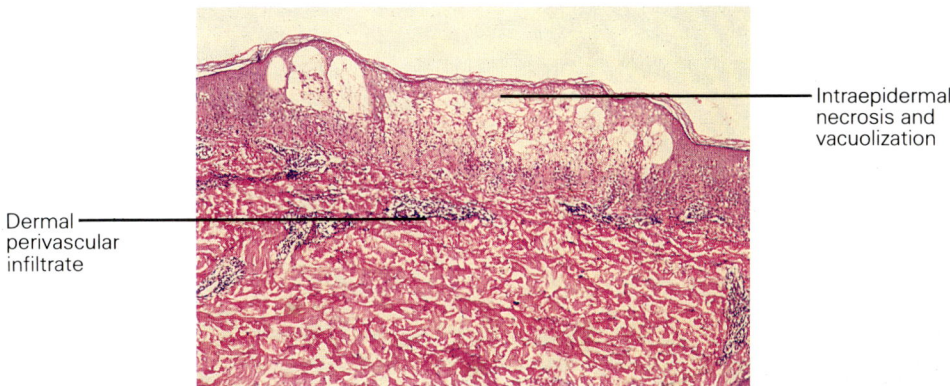

The major changes in the epidermal form of this condition shown include necrosis and lysis of epidermal cells. A mild dermal mononuclear infiltrate is present. The lesion reflects a hypersensitivity reaction to drugs, or is idiopathic.

Figure 15.6
Dermatitis herpetiformis

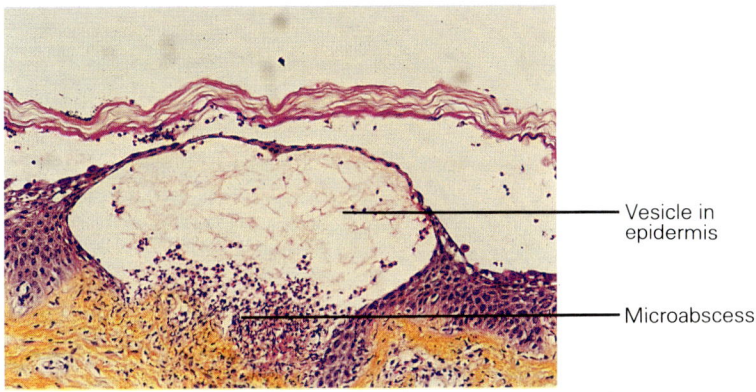

This chronic disease of the extensor surfaces of the extremities, shoulders, and buttock shows epidermal vesicles and microabscesses involving dermal papillae.

Figure 15.7
Psoriasis

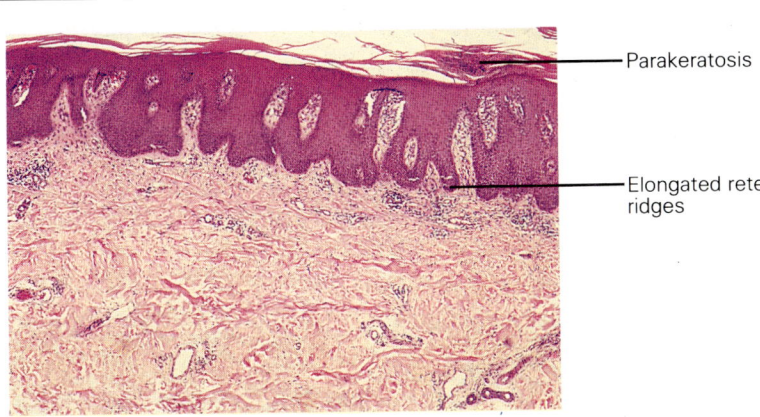

Heightened epidermal cell replication in psoriasis produces elongated rete ridges and parakeratosis (nuclei persisting into horny layer).

Figure 15.8
Lichen planus

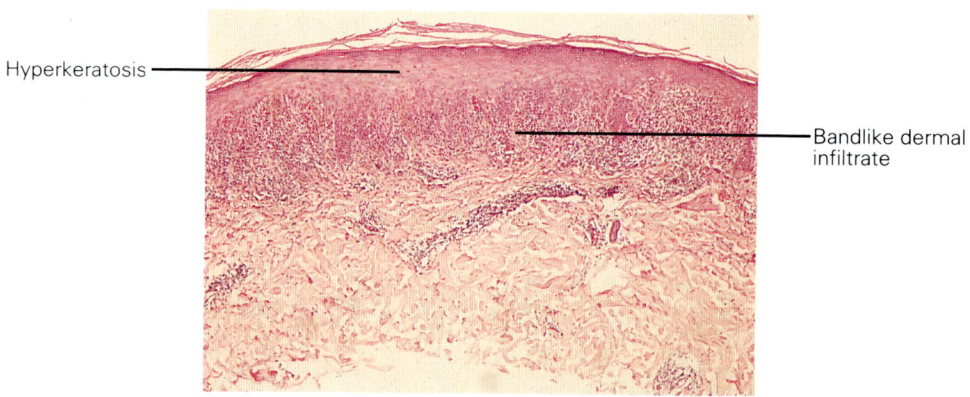

Lesions of lichen planus show hyperkeratosis and hypergranulosis, basal cell layer damage, and a bandlike dermal infiltrate.

Figure 15.9
Lichen sclerosus et atrophicus

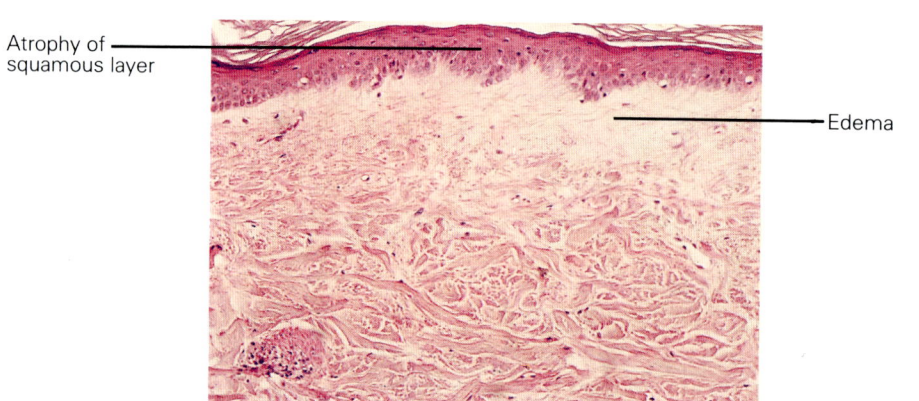

The stratum germinativum (squamous layer) is reduced to a few cells in thickness and there is edema of the upper dermis.

Figure 15.10
Molluscum contagiosum

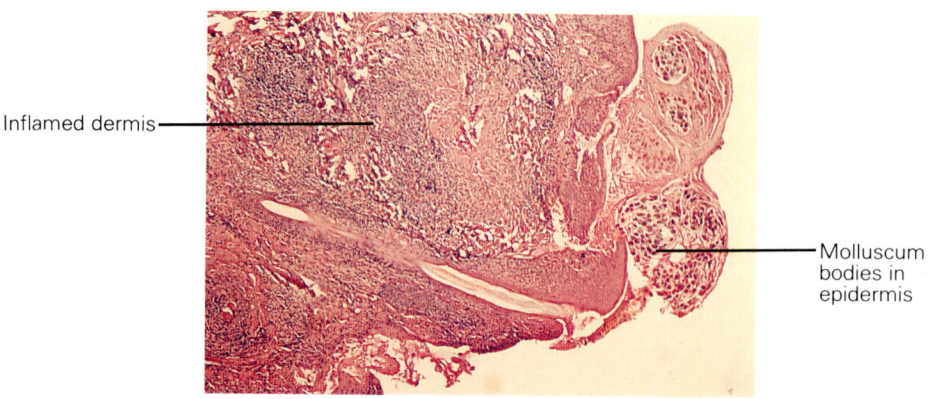

Poxvirus (DNA virus) infection of the skin of the trunk produces umbilicated papules composed of downward-projecting hyperplastic epidermal lobules. The epidermis contains red-purple "molluscum bodies" (intracellular inclusions of poxvirus).

Figure 15.11
Verruca vulgaris (wart)

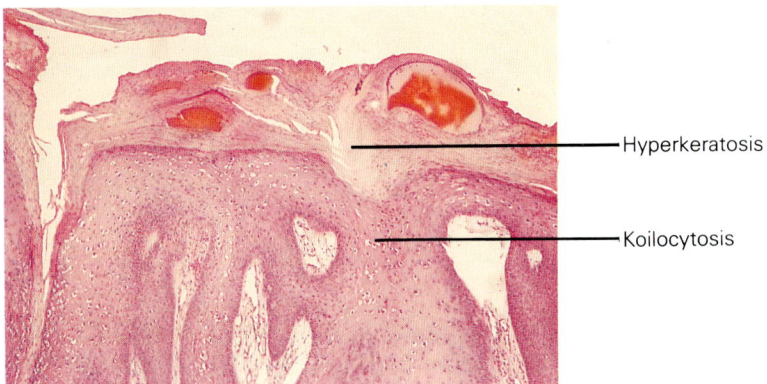

These papillary, epidermal hyperplastic lesions show hyperkeratosis and epithelial cell vacuolization (koilocytosis). The papilloma virus is the causative agent.

Figure 15.12
Sebaceous (epidermal) cyst

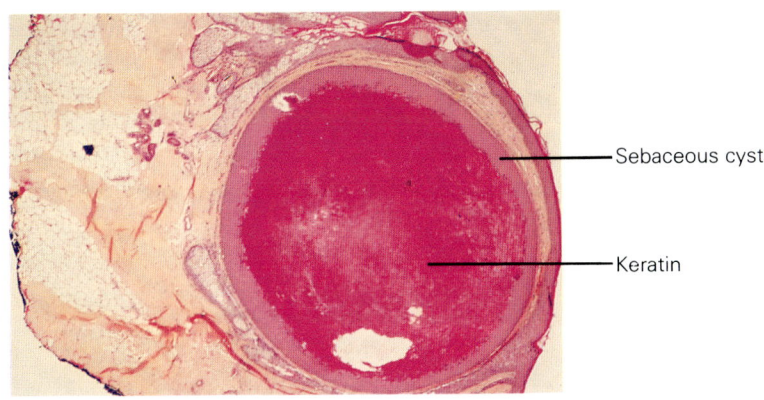

Cystic epidermal structures containing keratin become enclosed in the dermis in this common lesion of the head, neck, and trunk.

Figure 15.13
Keloid

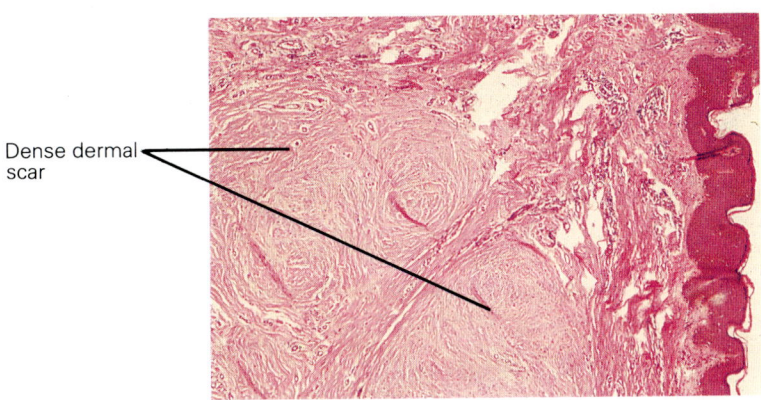

Protuberant scars in areas of wound healing are termed keloids, and consist of dense, dermal collagenous scar tissue.

Dermatopathology 205

Figure 15.14
Seborrheic keratosis

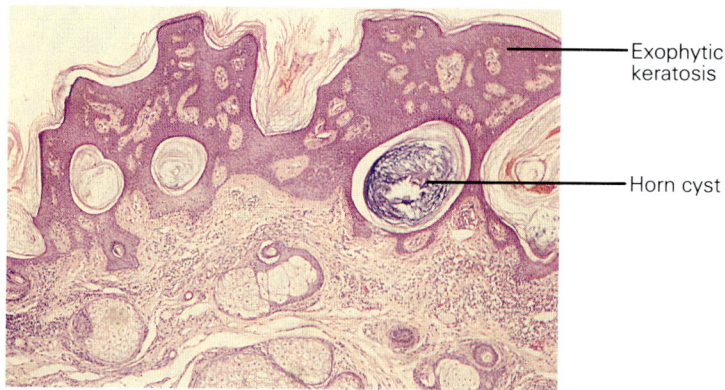

This is a benign tumor of basal cell-like cells which proliferate to form exophytic lesions with regions of keratin-filled "horn cysts."

Figure 15.15
Actinic keratosis

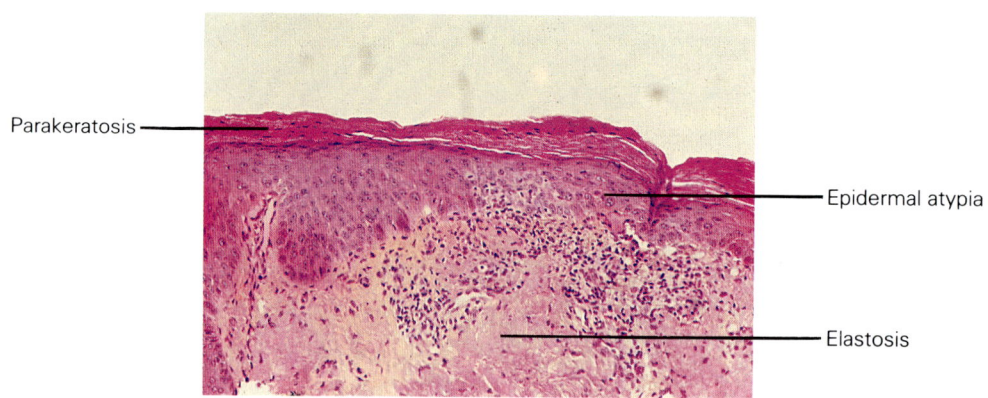

Sun exposed skin may develop this premalignant lesion, characterized by lower epidermal atypia, dermal elastosis, hyper- and parakeratosis.

Figure 15.16
Basal cell carcinoma

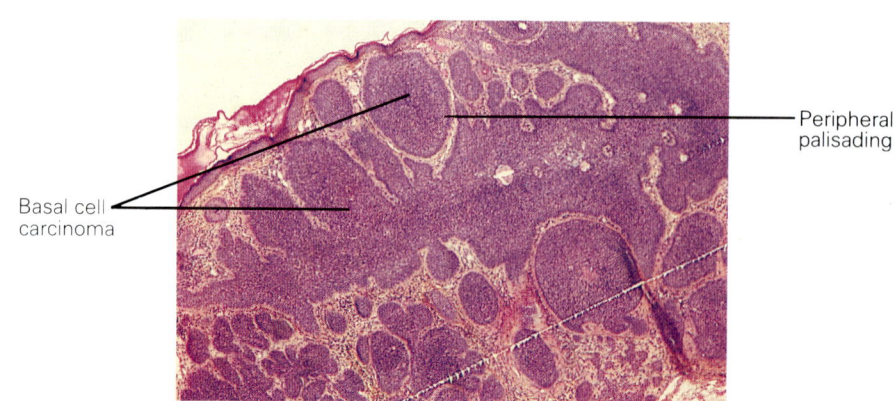

This locally aggressive tumor consists of basal epidermal cells growing in nests and islands into the dermis. Tumor cell palisading at the periphery of nests is common.

Figure 15.17
Squamous cell carcinoma

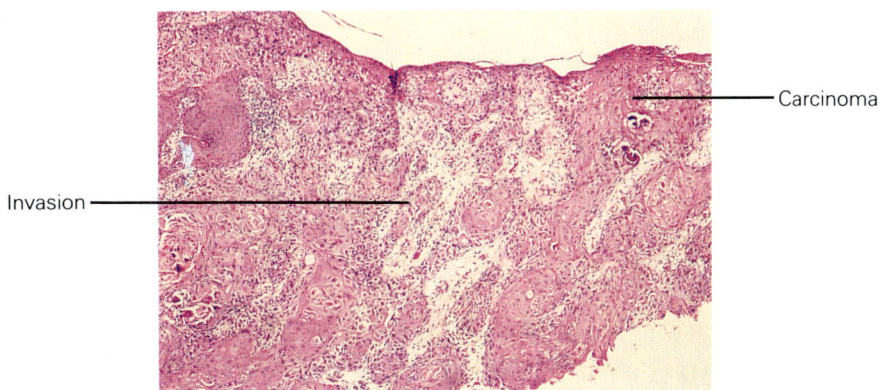

Note the atypia of the squamous cells within the epidermis and the invasive nests of tumor. These tumors are related to chronic sun exposure.

Figure 15.18
Keratoacanthoma

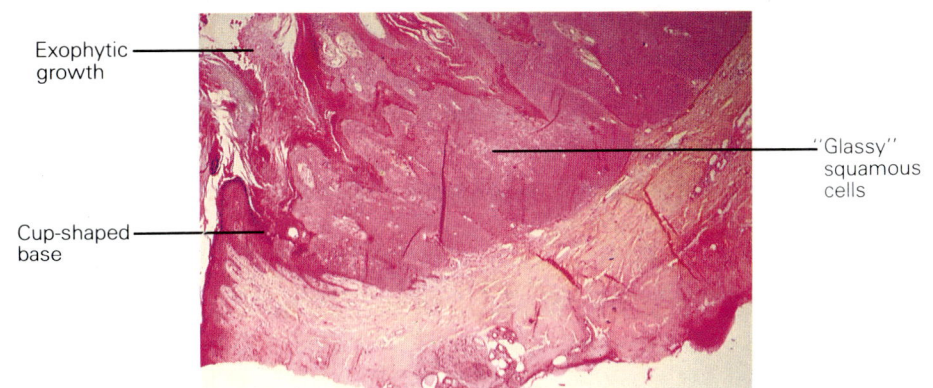

This rapidly growing, benign squamous cell tumor must be differentiated from squamous cell carcinoma. A volcano-like mass of well differentiated squamous cells with little atypia is present.

Figure 15.19
Junctional nevus

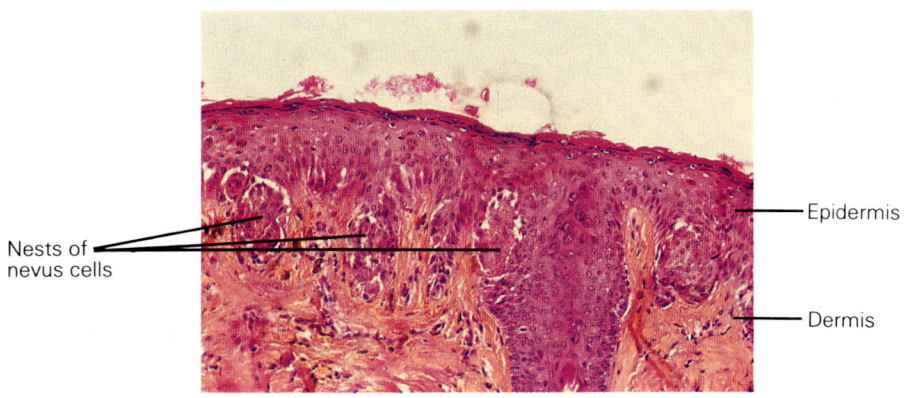

This form of pigmented mole shows nests of nevus cells (melanocytes) at the epidermal-dermal junction.

Figure 15.20
Intradermal nevus

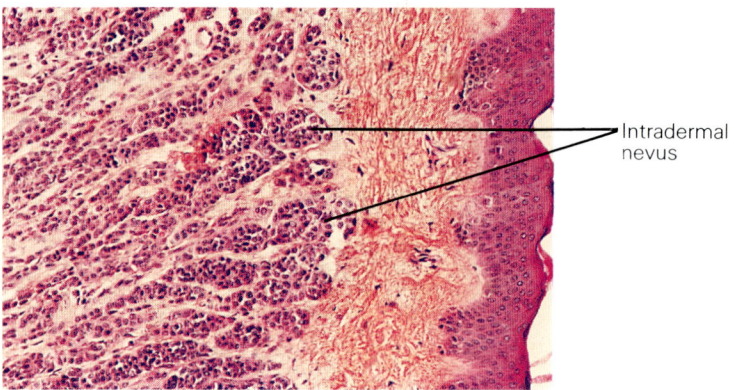

Nests of nevus cells are present within the dermis.

Figure 15.21
Compound nevus

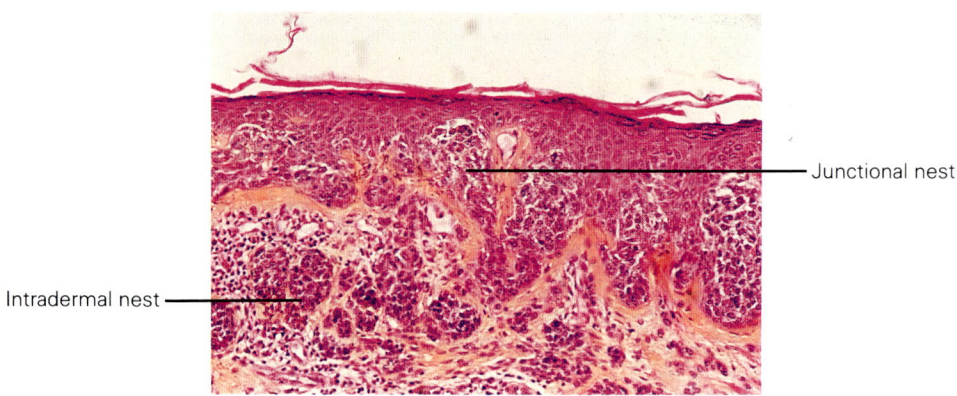

This form of nevus combines nests of nevus cells at the epidermal-dermal junction with intradermal nests.

Figure 15.22
Blue nevus

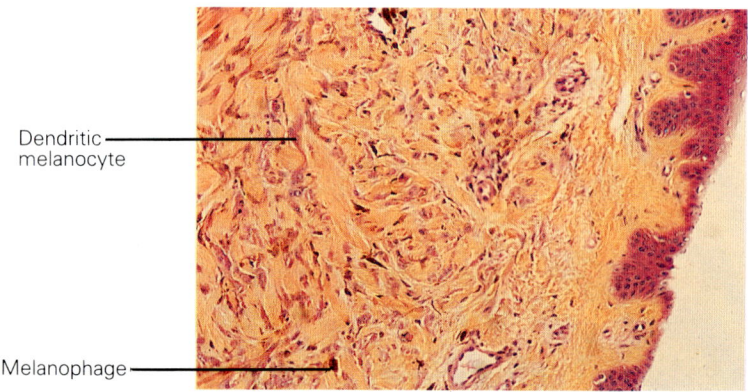

This lesion is characterized by spindle-shaped, dendritic cells in the dermis. Melanophages (melanin-containing macrophages) within the dermis may also be present.

Figure 15.23
Lentigo maligna (in situ melanoma)

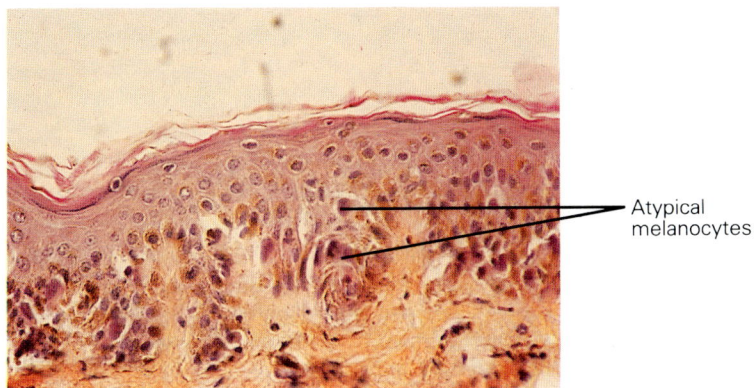

In this in situ melanoma, pleomorphic melanocytes occur at the epidermal-dermal junction, without dermal or epidermal invasion.

Figure 15.24
Superficial spreading malignant melanoma

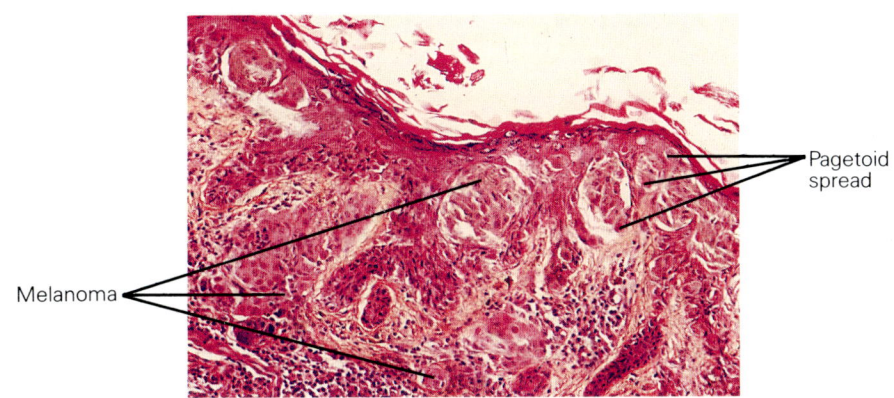

A radial growth phase of single cells and nests of melanoma within the epidermis is seen in this lesion prior to dermal invasion.

Figure 15.25
Nodular melanoma

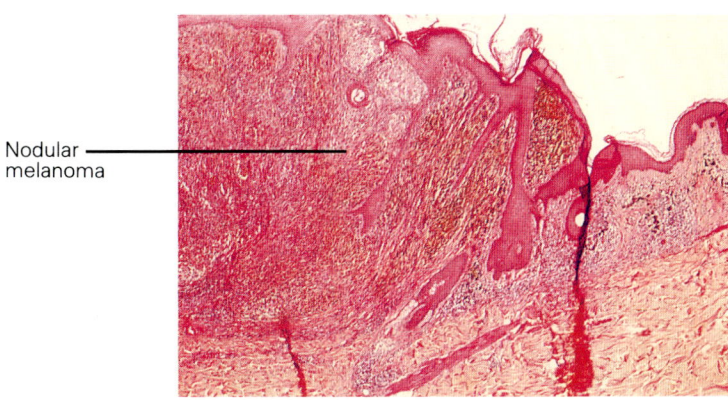

These tumors show no radial growth and often are prognostically poor because of depth of invasion.

CHAPTER 16
NEUROPATHOLOGY

Figure 16.1
Normal brain

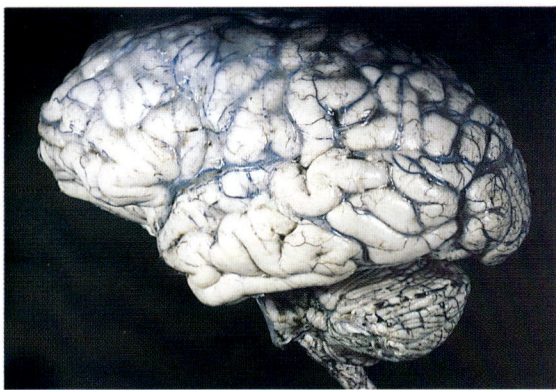

Normal weight: 1396 g (male) and 1234 g (female).

Figure 16.2
Normal anterior horn neurons

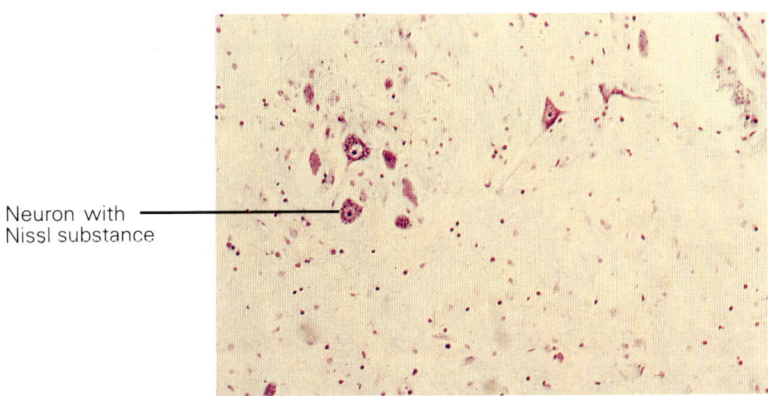

In this cresyl violet stain, the neurons show round pale nuclei, central purple-blue Nissl granules and dendritic processes.

Figure 16.3
Retrograde degeneration of neurons

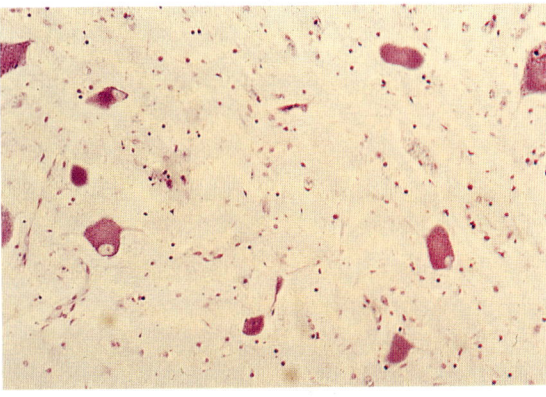

Following nerve root injury, retrograde degeneration (central chromatolysis) develops. The anterior horn cells are larger than those in Figure 16.2 and show eccentric nuclei, and loss of Nissl substance.

Neuropathology

Figure 16.4
Nervous system and muscle: major pathologic lesions

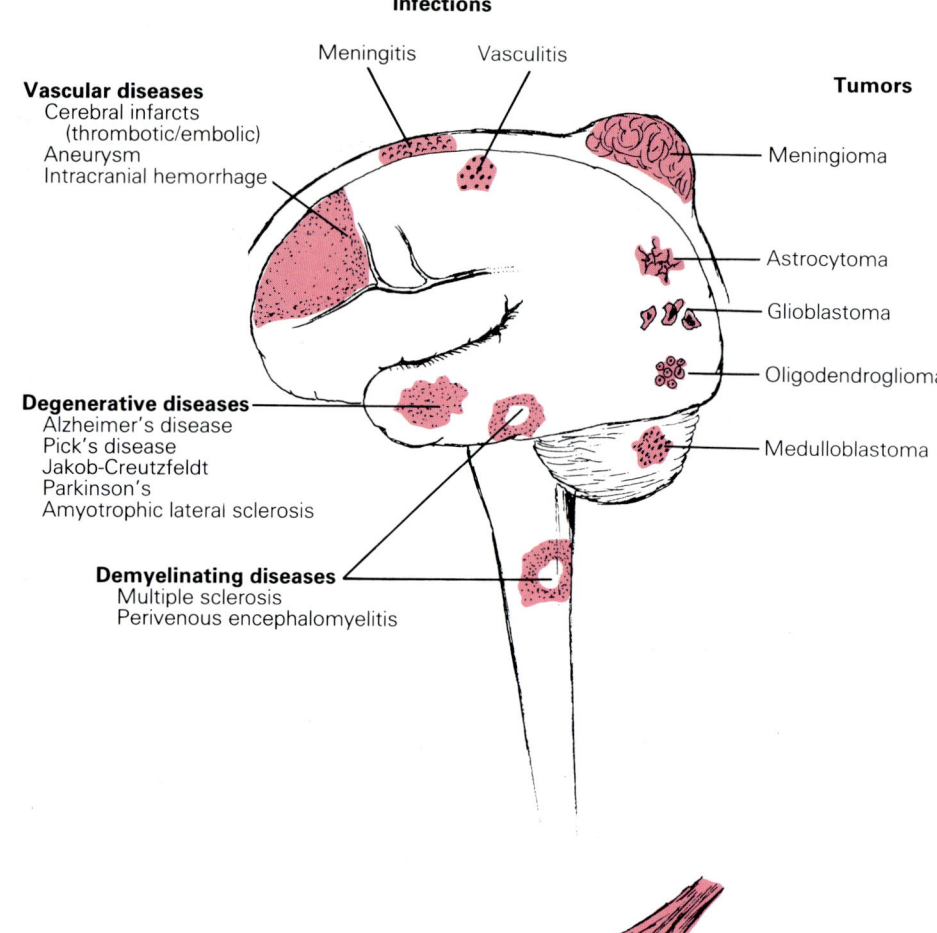

214 *Histopathology of Disease*

Figure 16.5
Encephalomalacia (cerebral infarct)

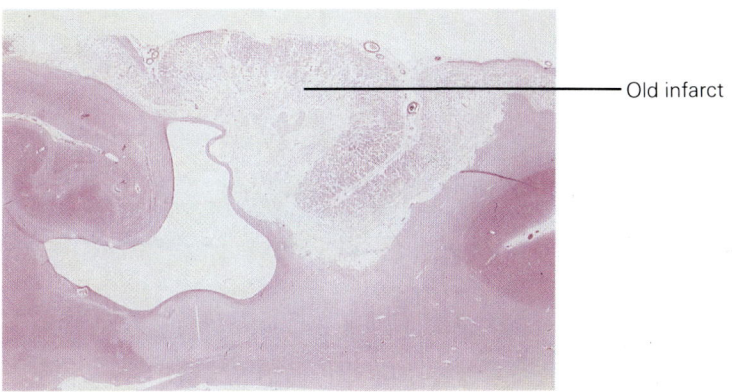

The infarcted area is covered by the meninges and shows degenerated cortical tissue and hypertrophied astrocytes.

Figure 16.6
Recent infarction

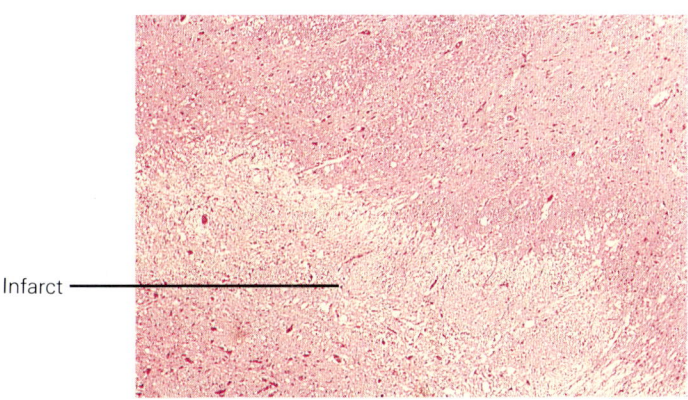

The lower left neural tissue appears pale and edematous with loss of staining of myelin structures. In this zone, neurons show ischemic damage and macrophages begin to accumulate.

Figure 16.7
Recent infarction

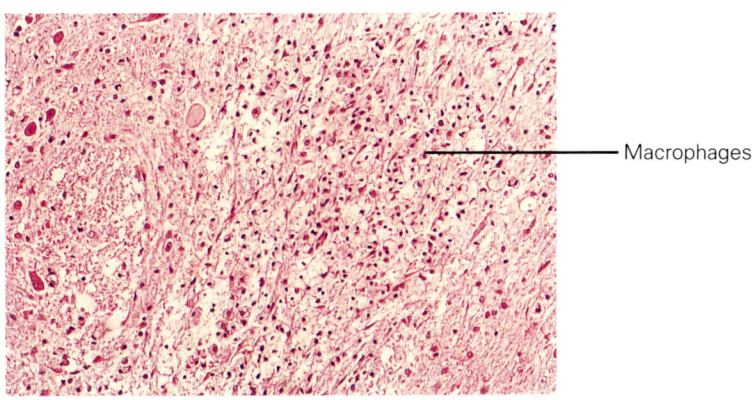

The central part of this field shows edema and degeneration of the neural tissue with infiltration by foamy macrophages containing myelin breakdown products. Peripheral tissue (at left and lower right) appears better preserved.

Figure 16.8
Ischemic necrosis of neurons

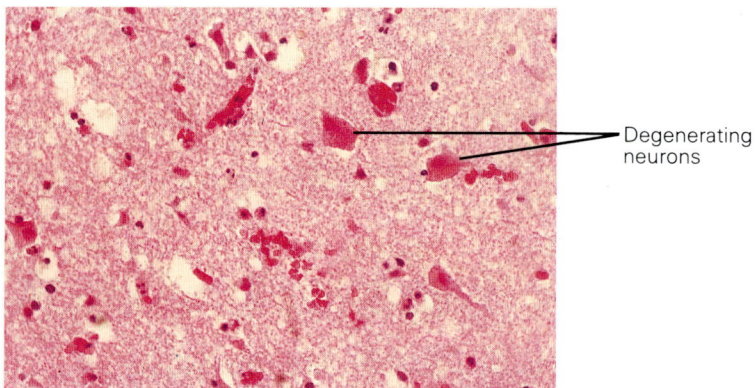

Ischemic damage to neurons results in coagulative necrosis, seen here as dense acidophilic damage of the cytoplasm.

Figure 16.9
Arteriovenous malformation (Trichrome stain)

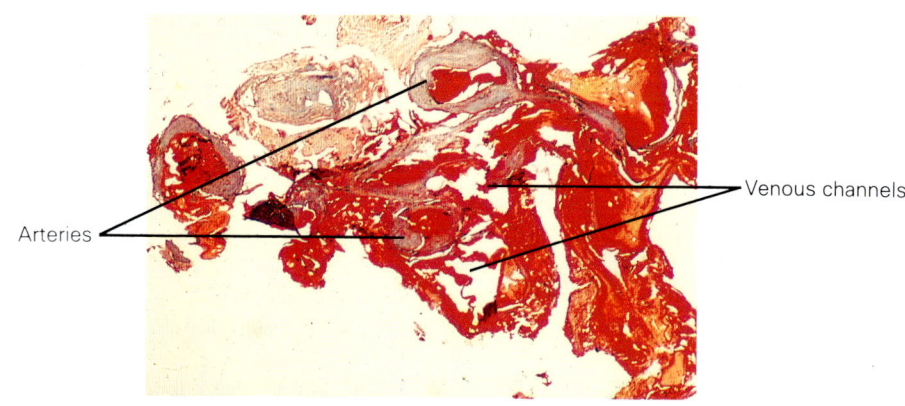

These clusters of abnormal communicating arteries and veins are found predominantly on the surfaces of the cerebral hemispheres. Their major complication is rupture.

Figure 16.10
Meningitis

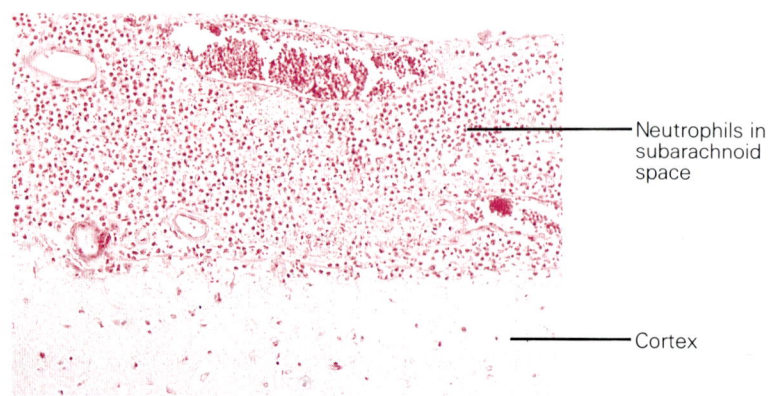

Purulent meningitis is due predominantly to pneumococcal or meningococcal infection.

Figure 16.11
Encephalitis

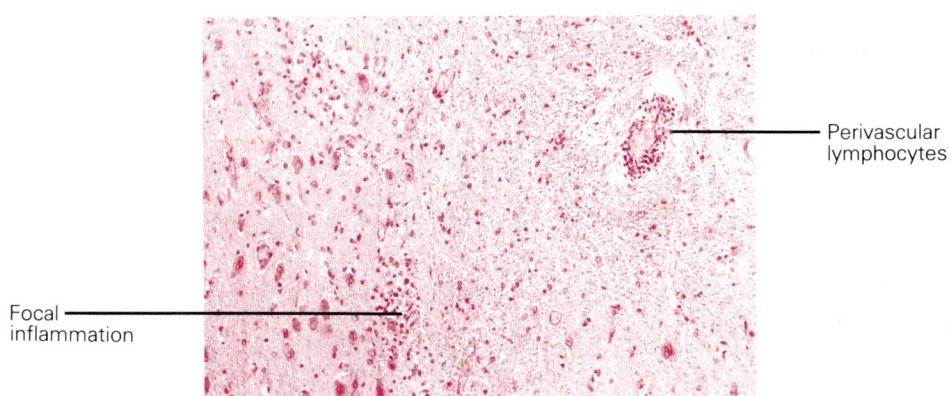

The case illustrated is representative of some of the changes of viral encephalitis, which include destruction of nerve cell bodies, perivascular infiltrates of lymphocytes and plasma cells, and microglial proliferation.

Figure 16.12
Multiple sclerosis

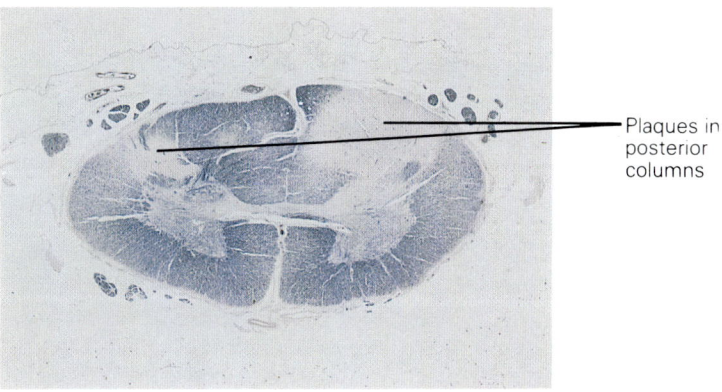

Mahon myelin stain demonstrating plaques (regions of demyelination) within the posterior columns of the spinal cord.

Figure 16.13
Amyotrophic lateral sclerosis

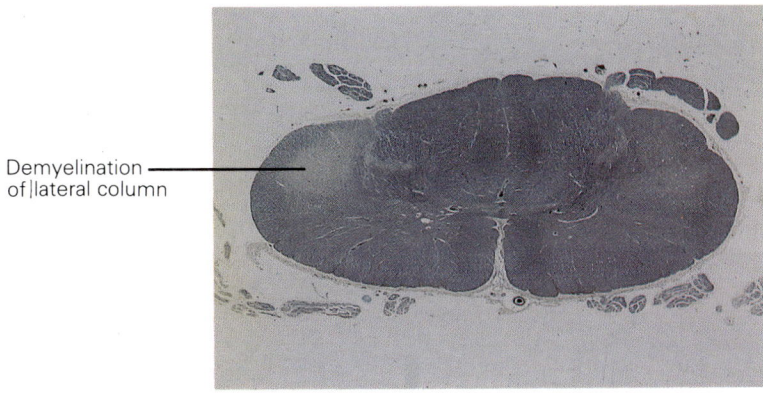

This degenerative disease combines lower motor neuron loss and muscle atrophy with upper motor neuron damage associated with lateral corticospinal tract demyelination.

Neuropathology

Figure 16.14
Tabes dorsalis

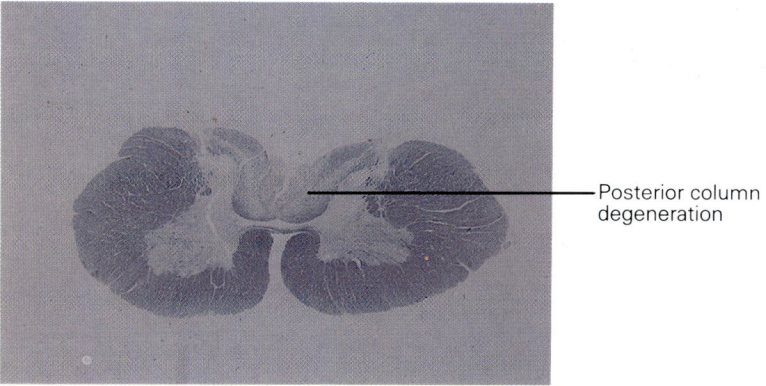

Neurosyphilis (tertiary stage of *Treponema pallidum* infection) is associated with degeneration of the posterior columns and locomotor ataxia.

Figure 16.15
Alzheimer's disease

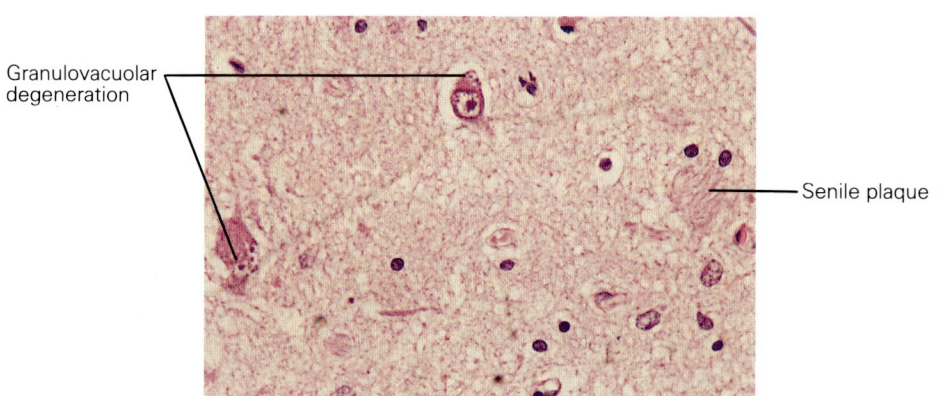

Granulovacuolar degeneration and senile plaques are features of Alzheimer's disease. Granulovacuolar degeneration consists of clear neuronal cytoplasmic vacuoles containing argyrophilic granules. Senile plaques show amyloid cores surrounded by cellular processes.

Figure 16.16
Alzheimer's disease

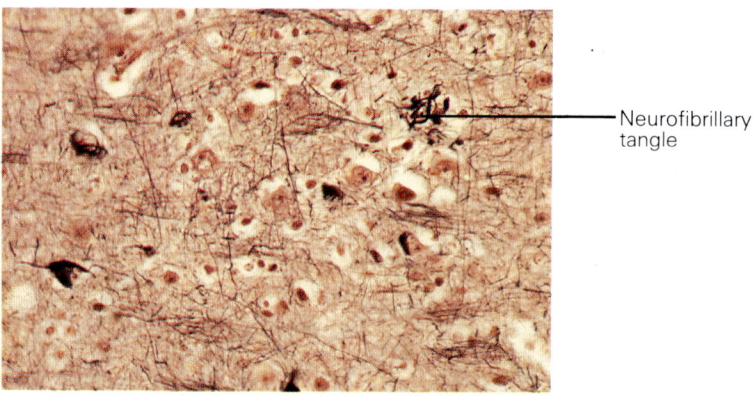

Bielshowsky stain demonstrating neurofibrillary tangles in Alzheimer's disease.

Figure 16.17
Meningioma

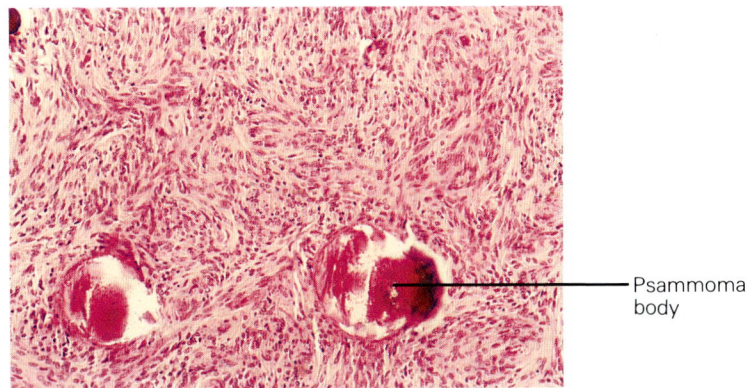

Syncytial, fibroblastic, angioblastic, and transitional (shown) histologic forms exist. The transitional type shows whorled cells and laminated calcium concretions (psammoma bodies).

Figure 16.18
Craniopharyngioma

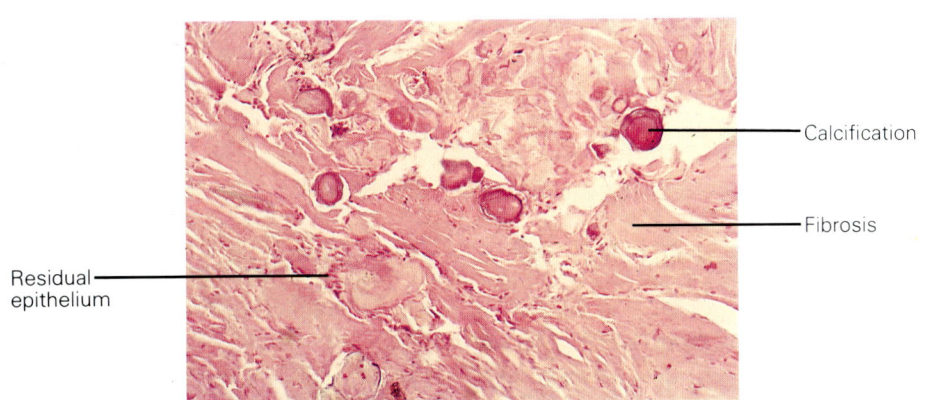

These tumors consist of cords and sheets of epithelial cells with foci of keratinized "horny pearls." The example shown above is largely degenerated and fibrotic, with little flattened residual epithelium and scattered calcifications.

Figure 16.19
Chromophobe adenoma of pituitary

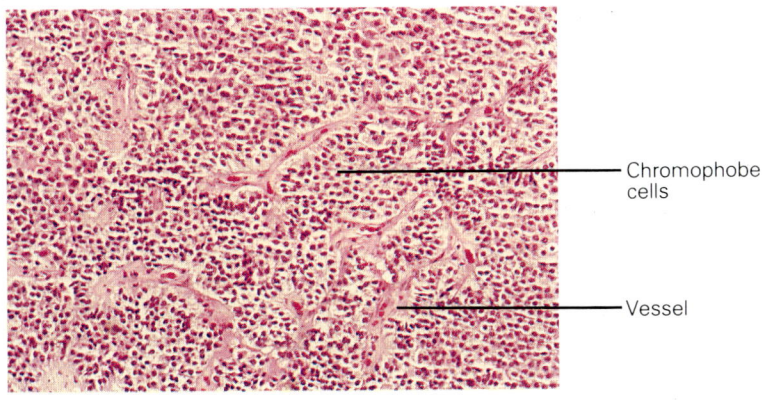

These benign tumors grow in sheets, cords, and nests and may be inactive (chromophobe adenoma) or secretory (acidophilic and basophilic adenomas).

Figure 16.20
Astrocytoma

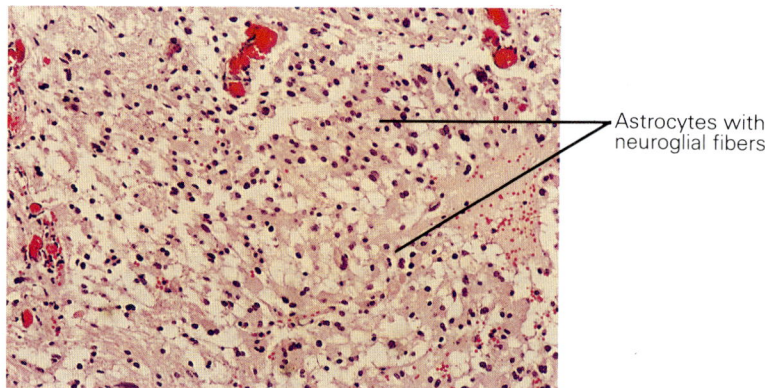

The example shown consists of astrocytes with abundant cytoplasm and cellular processes. These tumors range from well differentiated lesions to anaplastic glioblastomas.

Figure 16.21
Glioblastoma multiforme

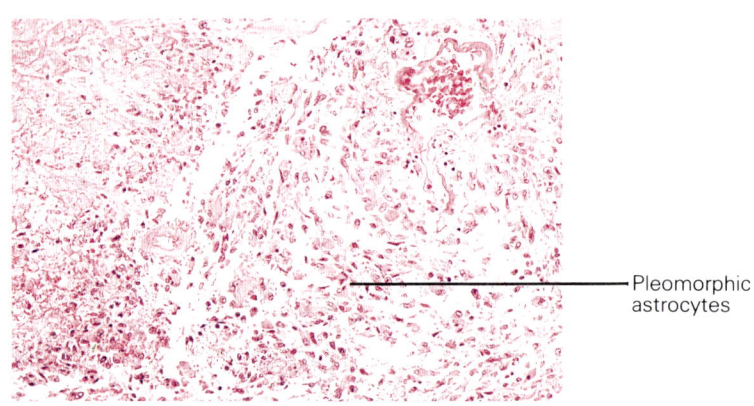

Poorly differentiated, anaplastic astrocytomas (glioblastomas) show high cellularity, pleomorphism, mitoses, and necrosis. The prognosis is poor.

Figure 16.22
Oligodendroglioma

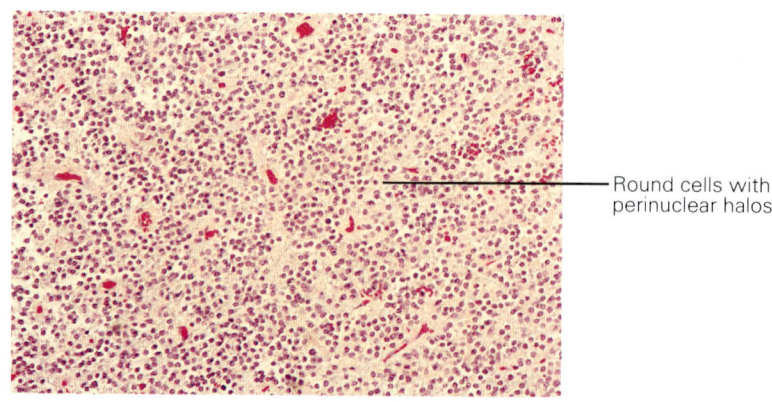

These uncommon glial tumors develop in the cerebral hemispheres and consist of sheets of cells with round nuclei and clear cytoplasm (appearing as a perinuclear halo).

Figure 16.23
Medulloblastoma

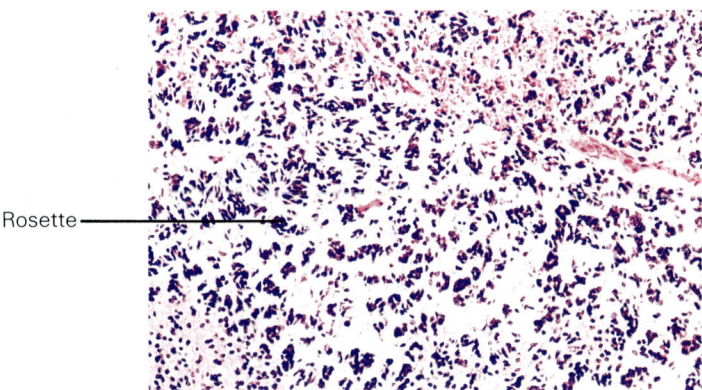

These malignant tumors of the cerebellar vermis in children show highly cellular sheets of cells with round or oval nuclei, arranged in parallel or rosettes.

Figure 16.24
Neuroblastoma

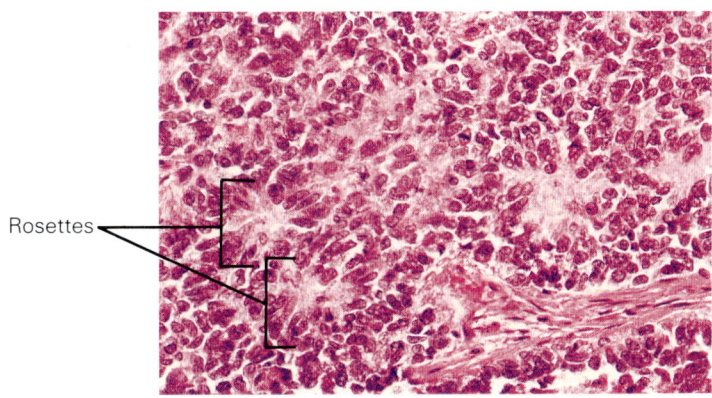

The cells of this highly malignant tumor (usually of the adrenal medulla) form rosettes with young nerve fibrils growing into the rosette center.

Figure 16.25
Normal skeletal muscle

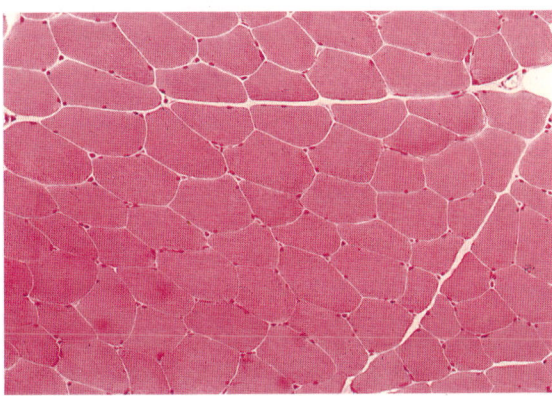

Note the uniformity of cross-sectional fiber size, peripheral nuclei, and absence of interstitial inflammation or fibrosis.

Figure 16.26
Denervation atrophy of muscle

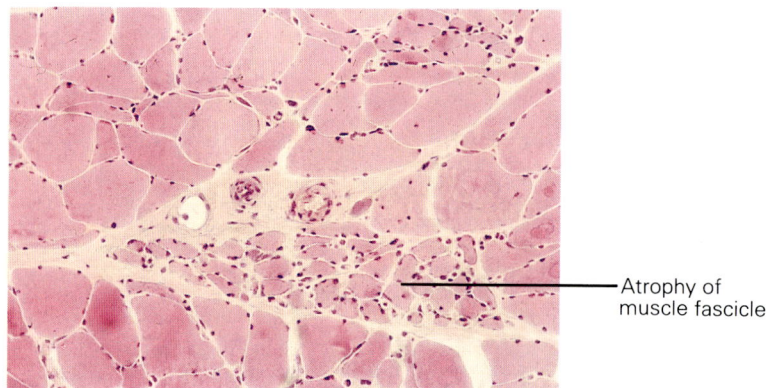

Spinal cord or peripheral nerve injury over time results in diminished fiber size in a fascicular distribution.

Figure 16.27
Muscular dystrophy

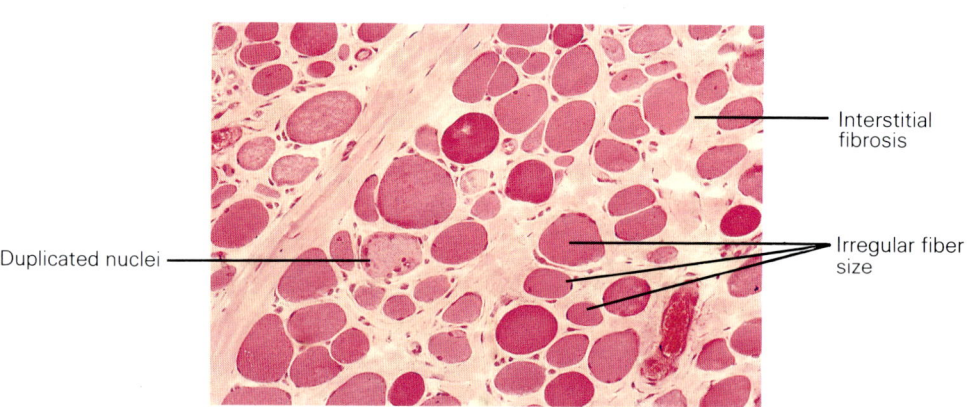

The muscular dystrophies have in common fiber degeneration and regeneration, manifested as variations in fiber size, multinucleation, and interstitial fibrosis.

Figure 16.28
Polymyositis

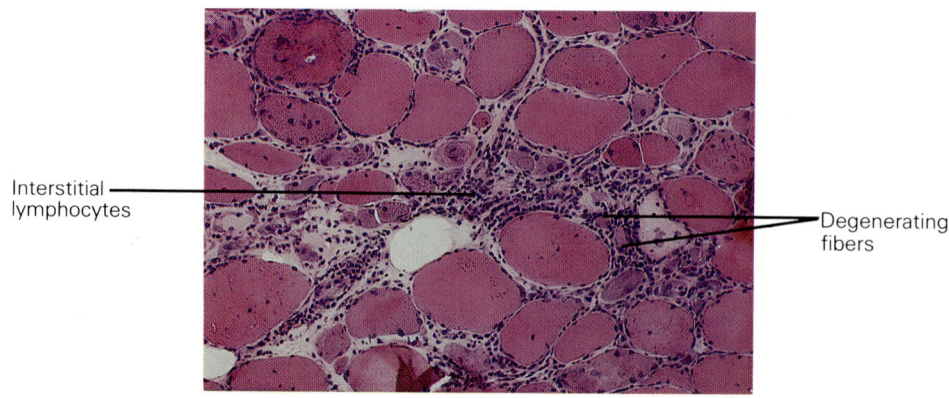

This haphazard, degenerative, and inflammatory muscle disease may be idiopathic or associated with visceral malignancy.

INDEX

Numbers printed in boldface indicate figures.

A

Abscess, 7, **13**
  crypt, 113, **114**
Acantholysis, 201
Acetaminophen hepatitis, **129**
Acinic cell carcinoma, 107, **120**
Acne vulgaris, 202
Acquired immune deficiency syndrome (AIDS), 36, 37, 196
  brain in, **37**
  liver in, **138**
  lung in, **58**
  lymph node in, **76**
Actinic keratotis, 202, **206**
Acute tubular necrosis, 90, **96**
Actinomyces, **85**
Acute tubular necrosis, 90
Addison's disease, 177
Adenocarcinoma, **17, 18, 20**
  lung, **26**, 60
  mucinous, **20**
  papillary, **20**, 148, 176, **181**
  vacuoles in, **26**
Adenoid cystic carcinoma, 107, **120**
Adenolymphoma (*see* Warthin's tumor)
Adenoma, **17, 18, 116**
  adrenocortical, **18, 178**
  liver cell, 124, **141**
  parathyroid, 176, **183**
  pituitary, 176, **219**
  renal, 90
  thyroid, 176, **181**
  villous, **115**
Adnexal tumors, 202
Adrenal gland
  adenoma, 176
  atrophy, 176, **177**
  carcinoma, **178**
  hyperplasia, 176, **178**
  metastasis to, 176, **179**
  normal, **175**
  tuberculosis, 176
  Waterhouse-Friderichsen syndrome, 176
Adult respiratory distress syndrome (ARDS), 52, **56**
Aging, bone marrow, **70**
Alcoholic hepatitis, 124, **130**, 140
Alpha-1-antitrypsin, 163
Alpha-1-antitrypsin deficiency, 55, 124, **131**
Alphafetoprotein (AFP), 22, 163, 170
Alzheimer's disease, 214, **218**
Amebiasis, 35
  Entamoeba histolytica, **35**
Ameloblastoma, **118**

Amine precursor uptake and decarboxylation (APUD) tumors, 111
Amyloidosis, **90**
  congo red stain, **99**
  liver, 124, **132**
  renal, **98**
  thyroid carcinoma, **182**
Amyotrophic lateral sclerosis, 214, **217**
Anaplasia, **16**
Anemia, 68
  aplastic, 68, **69**
  iron deficiency, 68, **69**
  megaloblastic, 68, **69**
  sickle cell, 68, **69**
Aneurysm, 3, 42
  cerebral, 214
Angioimmunoblastic lymphadenopathy, **76**
Angiomyolipoma (*see* Mesenchymoma)
Angiosarcoma, 124, **143**, 188
Angiotensin converting enzyme (ACE), 59
Anitschkow cells, 43
Anthracosis, **53**, 60
Anthrax, 5
Antibiotics, 47
  toxicity, **47**, 96
Antibodies, **15**
  basement membrane, 58, 93
  mitochondrial, 135
  monoclonal, 5
Antigen, 22
  carcinoembryonic, **22**
  oncofetal, 22
  tumor cell, 22
Antoni regions, in Schwannoma, **195**
Aplastic anemia, 68, **69**
Appendicitis, 107, **112**
Appendix
  appendicitis, **112**
  carcinoid tumor, **112**
Arteriosclerosis, 42
  arteriolosclerosis, 42
  atherosclerosis, 42
  Mönckeberg's calcific sclerosis, 42
  nephroarteriolosclerosis, 90, **97**
Arteriovenous malformation, **216**
Arteritis, 42, **48**
  giant cell, 42, **48**
  temporal, 42, **48**
Artery, **48**
Arthropods, 202
Asbestosis, 52, **61**
  asbestos body, **61**
  ferruginous body, 61
Aschoff body, 43

Aschoff cells, 43
Asthma, 52
Astrocytoma, 214, **220**
Atelectasis, **54**
Atherosclerosis, **41**, **43**, **44**
    pathogenesis, 42
    plaques, **43**, **44**
Atrial septal defect, 42
Atrophy, **16**, **111**, **160**
Auer rod, 71
Autopsy, 4

B

Bacteria, 3, **31**
    cocci, **31**
    gram-negative, **31**
    gram-positive, **31**
Barrett's esophagus, 107, **108**
Basal cell carcinoma, 202, **206**
Basement membrane, **17**, 58
    kidney, **91**, **92**
    "spikes" in renal disease, **95**
    "tram-track," **95**
Benign cystic teratoma, **162**
Benign mixed tumor, **119**
Benign nephroarteriolosclerosis, **89**, **90**, **97**
Benign prostatic hypertrophy,
Benivenii, Antonio, 3
Bernard, Claude, **5**
Berylliosis, 52
Bichat, Marie-François Xavier, **4**
Bile, **133**
Bile duct
    carcinoma, 124, **142**
    malformation, **135**
    obstruction, **133**, **134**
Biliary atresia, 124
Bladder (*see* Urinary bladder)
Bone, **185**–**191**
    metastasis, 19
    tumors, **189**–**191**
Bone marrow
    aging, **70**
    erythroid hyperplasia, 68
    granulocytosis, **67**
    granuloma, **70**
    hemosiderosis, **70**
    leukemia, **71**
    lymphoma, 79
    myeloid hyperplasia, 68
    normal, **67**
Bowman's space, **91**, **93**
Bowen's disease, 156, **158**
"Boxcar" nucleus, 46
Brain, 37
    cysts, 37
    normal, **213**
Breast, 155, **165**–**169**
    atrophy, **166**
    carcinoma, 155, **167**
    cystic disease, 155, **165**
    cystosarcoma phyllodes, 155, **169**
    fibroadenoma, 155, **165**
    gynecomastia, 155, **166**
    intraductal papilloma, 155, 166
    lobular carcinoma, 155, **168**
Brenner tumor, **161**
Bridging hepatic necrosis, **125**
Bronchiectasis, 42, 52
Bronchiolitis obliterans, **57**
Bronchioloalveolar carcinoma, **61**
Bronchitis, 52, **55**
Bronchogenic carcinoma, **60**
Bronchopneumonia, 52, **57**
    gray hepatization, 57
    organizing, **57**
    red hepatization, 57
Budd-Chiari syndrome, 124, **137**
Buerger's disease, 42
Bullous pemphigoid, 202
Burkitt's lymphoma, **80**
    African, 80
    American, 80

C

Calcification, 43
Calcium, 44
Call-Exner bodies, **164**
Calor, 15
Candida, **28**
Capillary, **11**, **12**
Capsule, **18**
Carcinoembryonic antigen (CEA), **22**
Carcinoid tumor, 52, **112**
    appendix, 107, **112**
    bronchial, 52
    small intestine, **111**
Carcinoma,
    acinic cell, 107, **120**
    adenoid cystic, 107, **120**
    bile duct, 19, 124, **142**, **143**
    breast, 19, 155, **167**, **168**
    bronchioloalveolar, 52, **61**
    bronchogenic, 52, 60
    cervix, **160**
    clear cell, **100**
    colon, 107, **116**
    endometrium, 155, **157**
    esophagus, 107, **109**
    gallbladder, 148, **148**
    hepatocellular (liver cell), 124, **140**, 143
    invasive, **17**, **19**
    kidney, 90, **100**
    large cell, 52
    larynx, **63**
    lung, 52
    medullary, **168**
    mucoepidermoid, 107, **120**
    nasopharyngeal, 63
    oat cell, **27**, **61**
    pancreas, **149**
    papillary, **20**, **101**
    poorly differentiated, **21**
    prostate, 19, 156, **172**

renal cell, 100
salivary gland, **120**
skin, **207**
small cell, 52, **61**, **168**
stomach, 107, **110**
squamous cell, **17**, **21**, 52, **60**, 63, 107, **109**, 202, **207**
thyroid, **181–182**
transitional cell, 90, **101**
Carcinoma in situ, **17**, 156, **158**
Carcinosarcoma, **22**
Cardiac muscle, **41**
Cardiomyopathy, 42, **47**
Cardiovascular system, 39–48
Caroli's disease, **136**
Cartilage, 60
    in hamartoma, 60
    tumors of, 188
Cascara cathartics, 117
Caseation necrosis, **13**, **59**
Celiac disease (*see* Sprue)
Cell membrane, **25**
Cell theory, 4
Cellular pathology (cellularpathologie), 1, 5
Central nervous system
    tumors of, 214, **219–221**
Cerebral infarct, 214, **215**
Cervical intraepithelial neoplasia (CIN), 155, **159**
Cervix, 155
    carcinoma, 155, **160**
    squamocolumnar junction, **159**
    transformation zone, **159**
Chemotherapy, 5, 27
Cholangiocarcinoma, **142**, 143
Cholangitis, **134**, 136, **139**
Cholecystitis, **147**, 148
Cholelithiasis, 148
Cholera, 5
Cholestasis, **133**, 134
Cholesterol, 44, 147
    cleft, 44
Cholesterolosis, **147**, 148
Chondroma, 188, **190**
Chondrosarcoma, 188, **190**
Choriocarcinoma, **163**
Chromatolysis of neurons, 213
Chromophobe adenoma of pituitary, **219**
Chronic obstructive pulmonary disease, 42, 52
Cigarette smoking, 55, 60, 61, 62
    bronchitis and, 55
Cirrhosis, 124, 126, **127**, 133, **139**
    alcoholic, 108, **130**
    biliary, **134**
    macronodular, 124, **127**, **140**
    micronodular, 124, **140**
    varices in, **108**
Clear cell carcinoma
    kidney, **100**
    vagina, 155, **158**
Coagulation, 14, 15
    intrinsic pathway, 14
Coagulative necrosis, **45**
    myocytes, **45**
Coal workers' lung, 52

Coarctation of aorta, 42
Colon
    carcinoma, 107, **116**
    normal, **106**, **116**
Common ALL antigen (CALLA), 71
Complement, **15**, 92, 95
Condyloma accuminatum, 155, 156, **159**
    penis, **172**
    vulva, **159**
Congenital heart disease, 42
Congenital hepatic fibrosis, **136**
Congestion, 53
    hepatic, **136**
    pulmonary, **53**
Constrictive pericarditis, 42
Copper, 124, **133**
Cor pulmonale, 42
Coronary artery, **41**
    atherosclerosis, **41**
    thrombosis, **44**
Corticosteroids, and fatty liver, **129**
Cowdry type A inclusion, **34**
Craniopharyngioma, **219**
Crescents, in renal disease, **93**
Crohn's disease (*see* Regional enteritis)
Crypt abscess, **114**
Cryptosporidia, **37**
Cushing's syndrome, 178
Cutaneous T-cell lymphoma, **81**
Cylindroma, 202
Cylindromatous carcinoma (*see* Adenoid cystic carcinoma)
Cyst
    ovary, 155
    pancreatic, 148
    pneumocystis, **36**
Cystadenoma, **161**
Cystadenocarcinoma, **161**
Cystic disease, 155, **165**
Cystitis, cystica et glandularis, **100**
Cystosarcoma phyllodes, 155, **169**
Cytomegalovirus (CMV), **34**, **58**, **139**
    pneumonia, **58**
Cytopathology, 23–28
    "molding" of cells, **27**
    vacuoles, **26**
Cytotrophoblast, **163**

D

da Vinci, Leonardo, 3
Dane particle, **128**
Demyelinating diseases, 214, **217**
Dermatitis (*see* Eczema)
Dermatitis herpetiformis, 202, **203**
Dermatopathology, 199–209
Dermis, **201**, 202
Dermoid cyst (*see* Benign cystic teratoma)
Desmoid tumor, 193
Desmoplasia, **167**
Desquamative interstitial pneumonia, 52, **56**
Di Guglielmo's syndrome, 73

Diabetes,
    islets in, 176, **183**
    kidneys in, 90, **91**, **98**
    liver in, 124, 129
Diabetic glomerulosclerosis, 90, **91**
Diarrhea, 35, 37
Diethylstilbesterol (DES), 158
Diffuse alveolar damage (DAD), **56**
Diffuse proliferative glomerulonephritis, **96**
Disseminated intravascular coagulation, **14**
Diverticulum
    colon, 107, **117**
    urinary bladder, 90
Dolor, 15
Drug hepatitis, 124, **129**, 130
Dukes, staging for carcinoma of colon, **116**
Duodenum, normal, **106**
Dysgerminoma, **162**
Dysplasia, **16**, **159**
    liver cell, **140**

E

Echinococcus, **35**
Eczema, **201**, 202
Edema, **15**
    pulmonary, 53, **56**
Egg, parasitic, 35
Ehrlich, Paul, **5**
Elastosis, **206**
Electron microscope, 5
    and microscopy, 23
Embryonal carcinoma, 156, **170**
Emphysema, **55**
    centrilobular, 55
    panacinar, 55
Encephalitis, **217**
Encephalomalacia, **215**
Encephalomyelitis, 214
Enchondroma (see Chondroma),
Endocarditis, 3, 42, **43**
Endocrine glands, 173–183
Endodermal sinus tumor, **163**
Endometriosis, 155, **157**
Endometrium, 155
    carcinoma, 155, **157**
    hyperplasia, 155, **157**
    menstrual, **154**
    proliferative, **153**
    secretory, **153**, 154
Endoplasmic reticulum, 23, **25**
    rough, 23, **25**
    smooth, 23
Endstage kidney, **99**
Enterochromaffin cells, 111
Eosinophil, **9**
    drug hypersensitivity, 47
    in vasculitis, 47
Epidermis, **201**
    tumors of, 202
Epithelium, **16**
    glandular, **16**
    squamous, 25, **26**

Epstein-Barr virus, 63, 80
Erythema multiforme, 202, **203**
Erythroleukemia, **73**
Escherichia coli, 133, 134
Esophagitis, 107, **108**
Esophagus
    Barrett's, 107, **108**
    carcinoma, **109**
    esophagitis, 107, **108**
    Mallory-Weiss tear, 107
    normal, **105**
    varices, 107, **108**
Ewing's sarcoma, 188, **190**
Experimental pathology, 5
Extramedullary hematopoiesis, 68, 73
    spleen, 68, **84**
Extravascular space, 11
Exudate, 36
    in Pneumocystis pneumonia, **58**

F

Fasciitis, 188, **193**
Fat, **129**
    in liver, 129, **130**
    microvesicular, **130**
Fat necrosis, 148, **149**
Ferruginous body
Fibrin, 14, 43, **47**
Fibrinoid necrosis, 43, **48**, **97**
Fibrinolysis, **15**
Fibroadenoma, 155, **165**
Fibroblast, 17
Fibroma, 17
    ovary, **164**
    palate, **118**
Fibromatosis, 188, **193**
Fibrosarcoma, 17, 188
Fibrosis
    interstitial, 42
    perivascular, 46
Fibrothecoma, 164
Fibrous dysplasia, 188, **189**
Fibrous histiocytoma, 188
    benign, **193**
Foam cells, 43
    in atherosclerosis, 43
    in storage disorders, **131**
Focal nodular hyperplasia, **141**
Focal segmental glomerulosclerosis, 90, **94**
Folate deficiency, 69
Follicular hyperplasia, **75**
Functio laesa, 15
Fungi, 32–34, 202
    Aspergillus, **33**
    Candida, 28, **32**
    coccidioidomycosis, **34**
    Cryptococcus, **32**
    histoplasmosis, **33**
    hyphae, 33
    mucormycosis, **33**
    mycelia (see Hyphae)
    yeast, 32, 33

G

Galen, 3
Gallbladder, 145–148
Gallstones, 124, 142
Ganglion, **192**
Gastritis, 107
  chronic atrophic, **109**
Gastrointestinal tract, 103–120
Gaucher's disease, **70**
General pathology, 9–22
Germ cell tumors, 162, **163**
  ovary, 155, **162–163**
  testis, 156
Ghon complex, 52
Ghon focus, 52
Giant cell, **11**
  foreign body type, 11
  Langhans' type, **11**, 13, **59**
  urate nephropathy, **96**
Giant cell arteritis (*see* Arteritis)
Giant cell tumor, 188, **191**
Giardiasis, **37**
Gliadin, 111
Glioblastoma, 214, **220**
Glisson's capsule, **123**
Glomerulonephritis, 90, 91
  acute post-streptococcal, 90, 91, 92
  diffuse proliferative, **96**
  Goodpasture's syndrome, **58**
  lupus, **90**
  membranoproliferative, 90, **91**
  membranous, 90, 91, **94**, **95**
  rapidly progressive, 58, 90, 91, **93**
Glomerulus, 91
Glomus tumor, **197**
Glucocerebroside, 70
Gluten, 111
Gluten-sensitive enteropathy (*see* Sprue)
Glycogen, 5, **25**, 100, 158
  storage disease, **131**
Gohn complex, 52
Gohn focus, 52
Gold therapy, 94
Golgi apparatus, 10
Goodpasture's disease, 52, **58**
  glomerulonephritis in, 58, **93**
Gout, 188
Graft vs. host disease, 124
Granular cell tumor, **196**
Granulation tissue, 7, **12**
  in myocardial infarction, **45**
Granules, 9
Granulocytosis, **67**
Granuloma, 7, **12**, **13**, 52, 96, 113, 124
  in arteritis, **48**
  bone marrow, **70**
  caseating, **13**, 52
  liver, **138**
  noncaseating, **12**
Granuloma-theca cell tumor, **164**
Granulovacuolar degeneration, **218**
Graves' disease, 176, **180**

Ground-glass hepatocytes, **128**
  orcein stain, **128**
Ground-glass nuclei
  in thyroid carcinoma, **181**
Ground substance, **12**, 44, **45**
Gynecomastia, 155, **166**

H

Hamartoma, 60
  lung, 60
Hairy cell leukemia, **73**
Hashimoto's thyroiditis, **180**
Hassall corpuscle, **85**
Heart, 41
  normal, **41**
  tumors, **42**
  valves, 41, **42**
  weight, 41
Heart failure, 53
  spleen in, 83
"Heart failure" cells, **53**
Heavy metals, 96
Hemangioma, 188
  buccal, **118**
  liver, 124, **141**
Hemangiopericytoma, 188, **197**
Hematopoietic system, 65–85
Hemochromatosis, 124, **132**, 140
Hemoptysis, 54
Hemorrhage, 52
  in adult respiratory distress syndrome, 52, **56**
  cerebral, 214
  in Goodpasture's syndrome, **58**
Hemorrhoids, 107
Hemosiderin, **53**, **132**
  "heart failure" cells, **53**
Hepatitis,
  acute, **125**
  alcoholic, 124, **130**
  autoimmune, 124, 140
  chronic active, **126**, **127**, 133, 140
  chronic lobular, **126**
  chronic persistent, **126**
  cytomegalovirus, **139**
  drug, 124, **129**, 130
  giant cell, 124, **129**
  lupoid, 124, 140
  neonatal, 124
  viral, 48, 124, 140
Hepatitis B virus, 48, 125, 127, 140
  ground-glass cells, **128**
  membranous glomerulonephritis, 90, **94**, **95**
  polyarteritis nodosa, **48**
  surface antigen, **128**
Hepatitis viruses
  A, 125
  B, 48, 94, 125, 127, **128**, 140
  Delta, 125
  Non-A, non-B, 69, 125
Hepatocellular carcinoma, 124, **140**
Hepatocyte, **25**

Hernia sac, **117**
Hippocrates, **3**
Histamine, **15**
Histocompatibility antigens, 143
Histiocyte (*see* Macrophage)
Hodgkin's lymphoma, **82–83**
    lymphocyte-depleted, 77, **82**
    lymphocyte-predominant, 77, **82**
    mixed cellularity, 77, **82**
    nodular sclerosing, 77, **82**
    Reed-Sternberg cell, 77, **82**
Human chorionic gonadotrophin (HCG), 170
Humoral pathology, 1
Hunter, John, 4
Hürthle cells, **180**
Hyaline membranes, 52, **56**
    adult respiratory distress syndrome, 52
Hyalinosis, pancreatic islet, 176
Hybridomas, 5
Hydatid disease (*see* Echinococcus)
Hyperlipidemia, 42
Hyperplasia, **16**
Hypertension, 42
    heart disease in, 42, 46
    malignant, **90**
    pulmonary, 42
Hypertrophy, **16**
    left ventricular, 42, **46**
Hyphae, **33**
    pseudohyphae, **28**, **32**

I

Immune complexes, renal disease and, **91**, **92**, 95
Immunoglobulin
    in multiple myeloma, 74
    IgG, 92, **93**, 95
    IgM, 74
Immunoperoxidase, **22**
Impetigo, 202
Inclusions, **34**
Infarction, 14
    brain, 43, 214, **215**
    kidney, 43, **90**
    myocardial, 42, **44**, **45**
    pituitary, 176
    pulmonary, **54**
    spleen, 43, 68
Infectious disease, 5, 29–37
Inflammation, 7
    acute, 7
    cellular phase, **15**
    chronic, 7
    vascular phase, **15**
Insulitis, pancreatic islets, 176
Interleukin, **15**
    type 1, **15**
    type 2, **15**
Intima, **43**
    in atherosclerosis, 43
Invasion, 18, 19
    lymphatic, **19**
    perineural, **19**
    stroma, **18**
    vascular, **19**
    veins, 19
Iron, 124, **132**
Iron deficiency anemia, 68, 69
Islets of Langerhans, in diabetes, **183**

J

Jakob-Creutzfeldt disease, 214
Jejunum, normal, **106**
Jenner, Edward, 4

K

Kaposi's sarcoma, 188, **196**
Karyolysis, 12
Karyorrhexis, **12**
Keloid, **205**
Keratin, **21**
    pearl, 21
Keratoacanthoma, 202, **207**
Kidney, **87–100**
    adenoma, 90
    benign nephroarteriolosclerosis, **89**, **90**, **97**
    electron microscopy, 89, **92**, **94**, **95**
    endstage, **99**
    foot process, **89**
    normal, **89**
    sickle cell disease, 90
    tumors, 90
    ultrastructure, **89**
    vascular disease, 90
Kimmelstiel-Wilson disease, **98**
Kinins, **15**
Kohn, 57
    pores of, **57**
Koilocytosis, **159**, **172**, **205**
Kulchitsky cells, 111
Kupffer cell, **25**, **132**
Kveim test, 59

L

Lacunar cell, 82
Lamina densa, **91**
Langhans' giant cell, **11**, **13**, **59**
Larynx, 62
    squamous cell carcinoma, **63**
Leeuwenhoek, Anton Von, 3
Leiomyoma, 17, 188
    stomach, 107, **110**
    uterus, **153**, **155**, **158**
Leiomyosarcoma, 17, 188, **195**
    stomach, 107
    uterus, 155
Lentigo maligna, **209**
Leukemia, 22, 68, **71–73**
    acute lymphocytic, **71**
    acute myelogenous, **71**

chronic lymphocytic, **72**
chronic myelogenous, **72**
erythroid, **73**
hairy cell, **73**
Leukemoid reaction, 68
Leukocytosis, 67, 68
Leukopenia, 68
Leukotrienes, **15**
Leydig cells, 164, **169**
Lichen planus, 202, **204**
Lichen sclerosus et atrophicus, **204**
Limiting plate, hepatic, **123**, **126**
Lipocyte, 17
Lipoid nephrosis, 90, 91, 93, **94**
Lipoma, **17**, 188, **194**
Liposarcoma, **17**, 188, **194**
Liver, 121–143
  biliary tract disease, 124, **133**, 140
  cirrhosis, 124, 130
  electron microscopy, **25**
  fatty change, **129**, **130**
  hepatitis, 124
  metabolic disease, 124, 131
  metastasis, 19, 124
  normal, **123**
  shock, **137**
  systemic disease, 124
  tumors, 124
  vascular diseases, 124
Liver cell dysplasia, 140
Lobular carcinoma (*see* Lobular neoplasia)
Lobular neoplasia, 155, **168**
Lung, 49–63
  adenocarcinoma, **26**
  interstitial fibrosis, 42
  metastasis, 19
  normal, **51**
  tumors (*see specific type.*)
Lupoid hepatitis, 124
Lymph node
  in acquired immune deficiency syndrome, **76**
  hyperplasia, 68, **75**
  metastasis, 17, 19
  normal, **75**
  sinus
    medullary, 19, **75**
    subcapsular, 19, **75**
Lymphatic, 19
Lymphocyte, 10, 12, **13**
  T-, 143
Lymphocyte-depleted Hodgkin's lymphoma, 77, **82**
Lymphocyte-predominant Hodgkin's lymphoma, 77, **82**
Lymphokines, **15**
Lymphoma, 22, 68, 76–84
  Burkitt's, **80**
  classification, 77
  cleavage, **80**
  diffuse, **77**, **78**
  follicular, **77**, **78**
  gastric, **79**, 107
  histiocytic, **27**
  Hodgkin's, **77**
  immunoblastic, 77, **81**
  large cell, 77, **79**
  lymphocytic, **27**
  mixed, **80**
  nodular, **77**
  noncleaved, 77
  non-Hodgkin's, 77, **79**
  small cell, 77, **79**
  T-cell, **81**
  working formulation for clinical usage, 77
Lysosomes, 9

M

Macrophage, **10**, **12**, **15**
  hemosiderin-laden, 45, **53**
  in myocardial infarction, **45**
  pigmented, **45**
Malignant hypertension (*see* Hypertension)
Malignant melanoma, 202
  nodular, **209**
  superficial spreading, **209**
Mallory bodies, **130**
Mallory-Weiss tear, 107
Marantic endocarditis, 42, **43**
Massive hepatic necrosis, **125**
Mast cell, 9, **15**
Media, **43**
  in atherosclerosis, **43**
Medullary carcinoma,
  breast, **168**
  thyroid, **182**
Medulloblastoma, 214, **221**
Megakaryocyte, 67
Megaloblastic anemia, 68, **69**
Meig's syndrome, 164
Melanocyte, tumors of, 202, **207–209**
Melanophage, **208**
Melanosis coli, **117**
Membranoproliferative glomerulonephritis, 90, **95**
Membranous glomerulonephritis, 90, 94, **95**
Meningioma, 214, **219**
Meningitis, 214, **216**
Mesangial matrix, 91, **94**
Mesenchyme, 17
Mesenchymoma, 194
Mesothelioma, **62**
Mesothelium, **41**
  in hernia sac, **117**
Metaplasia, **16**
  columnar, **108**
  goblet cell, **55**
Metastasis, **17**, **19**, 124
Microangiopathic disorders, and renal disease, 90
Microhamartoma,
Microvillus, **25**
Milstein, Cesar, **5**
Mitochondria, **25**, 119, 135
Mixed cellularity Hodgkin's lymphoma, 77, **82**
Molluscum contagiosum, **204**
Mönckeberg's calcific sclerosis, 42
Monoclonal protein, 74
Morgagni, Giovanni Battista, **3**
Mucin, 20

Index 229

Mucoepidermoid carcinoma, 107, **120**
Multiple myeloma, **74**
Multiple sclerosis, 214, **217**
Mummy, Egyptian, 3
Muscle, 214, **221–222**
    denervation atrophy, 214, **222**
    dystrophy, 214, **222**
    polymyositis, 214, **222**
Muscular dystrophy, 214
Myasthenia gravis, and thymoma, 85
Mycobacteria, **31**
    avium-intracellulare, **138**
    tuberculosis, **31**
Mycosis fungoides, **81**
Myelofibrosis, 68
Myeloid metaplasia, **73**
Myeloma kidney, **90**
Myelophthisis, 68, **74**
Myocardial infarction, 42
    acute, **44, 45**
    healed, **46**
    histologic changes, **44–46**
Myocarditis, 42, **46**
Myocyte, **13**
    cardiac, 13
Myxoma, 42
    atrial, 42

N

Necrosis, **11**, 124
    caseation, **13**, 59
    coagulative, **45**
    fibrinoid, **43, 48**
Neoplasia, 7, **16, 17**
Nephritis, **90**
Nephroblastoma (*see* Wilm's tumor)
Nephrotic syndrome, 93
Nerve, 188
Neurilemmoma (*see* Schwannoma)
Neuroblastoma, **221**
Neurofibrillary tangle, **218**
Neurofibroma, 188, **196**
Neuromyoarterial receptor, 197
Neurons
    normal, **213**
    retrograde degeneration, **213**
Neuropathology, 211–222
Neurosyphilis, 218
Neutrophilic leukocytes, 9, **12, 15**, 67
    emigration, 11
    hypersegmentation, **69**
    pavementing, 11
Nevus, 202
    blue, **208**
    compound, **208**
    intradermal, **208**
    junctional, **207**
    sebaceous, 202
Niemann-Pick disease, **131**
Nil disease (*see* Lipoid nephrosis)
Nissl substance, **213**
Nobel Prize, 5

Nodular regenerative hyperplasia, **142**
Nodular sclerosing Hodgkin's lymphoma, 77, **82**
Non-A, non-B hepatitis, 69
    aplastic anemia in, **69**
Nonbacterial, thrombotic endocarditis (*see* Marantic endocarditis)
Nontoxic nodular goiter, 176
Nucleolus, **17, 18**
Nucleus, 12, **25**
    hyperchromatism, **17, 18**
    inclusions, **34**
"Nutmeg" liver, **136**

O

Oat cell carcinoma, **27, 61**
Obesity, liver in, 124, 129
Oligodendroglioma, 214, **220**
Oncocytes, in Warthin's tumor, 119
Oral contraceptives, 141
Organic solvents, 96
Organization, 44
    of pneumonia, **57**
    of thrombi, **44**
Osteitis deformans (*see* Paget's disease)
Osteoarthritis, 188
Osteogenic sarcoma, 188, **189**
Osteoid, **189**
Osteoid osteoma, 188, **189**
Osteomyelitis, **187**
Osteoporosis, **187**, 188
Ovary, 153
    atrophy, **160**
    tumors of, 155, **161–164**

P

Paget's disease
    bone, **187**, 188
    breast, **167**
Paleopathology, 3
Pancreas, 148–149
    carcinoma, 124, 148
    cyst, 148
    islets, 176
    pancreatitis, 124, 148, **149**
    pseudocyst, 148
Pancreatitis, 124
    acute, 148, **149**
    chronic, 148, **149**
Pannus, **191**
Papanicolaou (PAP) smear, **25, 28**
Papilloma, **17, 62**
    intraductal, 155, **166**
    laryngeal, **62**
    squamous, **62**
Parakeratosis, **203, 206**
Parasites, **35–37**
Parathyroid gland, 175
    adenoma, 176
    hyperplasia, 176, **182**
    normal, **175**

Parkinson's disease, 214
Pasteur, Louis, **5**
Pautrier microabscess, **81**
Peliosis hepatis, 124, **137**
Pelvic inflammatory disease (PID), 155, **165**
Pemphigus vulgaris, **201**, 202
Penis, condyloma acuminatum, 156, **172**
Peptic ulcer disease, 107, **109**
Pericarditis, 42
    constrictive, 42
    fibrinous, **47**
Pericardium, 42, **47**
Pericytes, tumor of, **197**
Pernicious anemia, 69
Peroxisome, **25**
Pheochromocytoma, 176, **179**
Pick's disease, 214
Piecemeal necrosis, **126**, **127**
Pigmented villonodular synovitis, **192**
Pilomatrixoma, 202
Pineal gland, 175
Pituitary gland, 175
    adenoma, 176, **219**
    Sheehan's postpartum necrosis, 176
Plaque
    in Alzheimer's disease, **218**
    in multiple sclerosis, **217**
Plasma cell, **10**, **15**, **25**, 74
Platelets, **14**, 43, 68
Pleomorphic adenoma (see Benign mixed tumor)
Pleural fluid, **25**, **27**
Pneumoconiosis, 52
    asbestosis, 52, **61**
    berylliosis, 52
    coal workers' lung, 52
    silicosis, 52
Pneumocystis carinii, **36**, 58
    cysts, **36**
    pneumonia, **58**
    trophozoites, **36**
Pneumonia, 3, **57**
    bronchopneumonia, 52, **57**
    desquamative interstitial, 52, **56**
    lobar, 3
    organizing, **57**
    usual interstitial, 52, **56**
Polyarteritis nodosa, 42, **48**
    hepatitis B virus and, **48**
    kidney in, **97**
    liver in, **48**, 124
Polycythemia vera, 73
Polymyositis, 214
Polyp, 107
    adenomatous, **115**
    endocervical, 155
    endometrial, 155
    hyperplastic, **115**
    vocal cord, **62**
Porphyrias, 124, 202
Portal hypertension, 83, 136, 142
Premalignant change, 16
Pregnancy, fatty liver of, 130
Primary biliary cirrhosis, 124, **135**
Primary sclerosing cholangitis, 124, **135**, 142

Prostate, 153
    carcinoma, 156, **172**
    hyperplasia, 156, **172**
    normal, **171**
    prostatitis, 156, **171**
Prostatitis, 156, **171**
Protozoans, 35, **36–37**
    Amebiasis, 35
    Cryptosporidia, **37**
    Giardiasis, **37**
    Toxoplasmosis, **37**
    Trichomonas, **28**
Psammoma bodies, **161**, **181**, **219**
Pseudohyphae, **28**, **32**
Pseudopolyps, in ulcerative colitis, **114**
Pseudosarcomatous fasciitis (see Fasciitis)
Psoriasis, 202, **203**
Pulmonary embolism, 42, 52, **54**
Pulmonary hypertension, 42, 52
Pulmonary infarct, 52, **54**
Pyelonephritis, **90**, **97**
Pyknosis, **12**

R

Rabies, 5
Radiation, 56
    diffuse alveolar damage, 56
    adult respiratory distress syndrome, 56
Rapidly progressive glomerulonephritis, 58, **93**
Red blood cells, **14**, 43
Reed-Sternberg cell, **77**, **82**
Regional enteritis, 107, **113**
Renaissance, 3
Renal artery stenosis, **90**
Renal cell carcinoma,
Repair, 7
Reproductive organs, 151–172
Reye's syndrome, 130
Rhabdomyosarcoma, **21**, 188, **195**
Rheumatic heart disease, 43
Rheumatoid arthritis, 75, 188, **191**
Riedel's struma, **180**
Rokitansky, Carl, 4
Rokitansky-Aschoff sinus, **147**
Rosette
    cholestatic, **133**
    neuroblastoma, **221**
Rubor, 15
Ruska, Ernst, **5**
Russell bodies, 74
Rye classification of Hodgkin's disease, 77

S

Salivary glands, **107**
    atrophy, 107
    tumors, 107, **119–120**
Salvarsan, 5
Sarcoidosis, 12, 42, 52, 59
    liver, **12**, **138**
    lung, 52, **59**

Sarcoma, 19, **21**
Scar, 7, **13**
   myocardial, **13**, **46**
Schistosomiasis, **35**
   hematobium, 35
   japonicum, 35
   mansoni, **35**
Schleiden, Mathias Jakob, **4**
Schiller-Duval body, **163**
Schwann, Theodor, **4**
Schwannoma, 188, **195**
Scolices, 35
   Echinococcus, **35**
Sebaceous cyst, **205**
Seborrheic keratotis, 202, **206**
Seminoma, 156, 162, **170**
Senile plaque, **218**
Sepsis, 133, 177
   spleen in, **84**
Sertoli cells, 164, **169**
Sertoli-Leydig cell tumor, **164**
Sheehan's postpartum pituitary necrosis, 176
Sickle cell disease, 68, **69**, 90
   osteomyelitis in, 187
Signet ring cells, in gastric cancer, **110**
Silicosis, 52
Silo filler's disease, 57
Singer's node, 62
Sinus histiocytosis, **75**
Sinusoid, **123**
Sjögren's disease, 107, **119**
Skeletal muscle, 21
   normal, **221**
Skin, 199–209
   basal cell carcinoma, 202
   normal, **201**
   squamous cell carcinoma, 202
Small cell carcinoma
   breast, **168**
   lung, **27**, **61**
Small intestine
   normal, **106**
   regional enteritis, 107
   sprue, 107
Smallpox, 4
Smith, Edwin, 3
   papyrus, 3
Smooth muscle, 17
Soft tissues, 188, **191–197**
Spermatozoa, 3
Sphingomyelin, 131
Spindle cell, 21
Spirochetes, **32**
   Treponema pallidum, 32
Spleen, 68
   congestive, 68, **83**
   extramedullary hematopoiesis, 68, **84**
   lymphoma, 68, **84**
   normal, **83**
   septic, 68, **84**
Splenitis, 84
Spongiosis, **201**
Sprue, 107, **111**
Sputum, 27

Squamous cell, 17, 18, **25**
   basal, **201**
   cervix, **26**
   intermediate, **26**
   parabasal, **26**
   superficial, **25**
Squamous cell carcinoma, 60, 109
   cervix, 26
   larynx, 63
   lung, 60
   skin, 202, **207**
Stains
   Bielschowsky, **218**
   Brown-Brenn, **31**
   Congo red, **99**
   Cresyl violet, **213**
   Giemsa, **36**
   Gomori methenamine silver, **32, 33, 34, 36**
   Grimelius, **112**
   Immunoperoxidase, **22**
   Mahon, **217**
   Mucicarmine, **110**
   Orcein, **128**
   Periodic acid-Schiff (PAS), **70, 94, 95**
   Periodic acid-Schiff (PAS) with diastase, **33**
   Prussian blue iron, **132**
   Rhodanine, **133**
   Reticulin, **73**
   Silver, **112**
   Trichrome, **216**
   Warthin-Starry, **32**
   Ziehl-Neelsen, **31, 138**
"Starry Sky" pattern, **80**
   in Burkitt's lymphoma, **80**
Stomach
   adenocarcinoma, 107
   gastritis, 107, **109**
   leiomyoma, 107
   leiomyosarcoma, 107
   lymphoma, **79**
   normal, **105**
   ulcer, 107
Storiform pattern, **193**
Stricture, biliary, 124
Sulfur granules, 85
Surfactant, 54
Syncytiotrophoblast, **163**
Synovial sarcoma, **192**
Synovitis, **191**
Syphilis, 5, 75, 218
   congenital, **32**
Systemic lupus erythematosus, 94, 95

T

Tabes dorsalis, **218**
Takayasu's pulseless aortitis, 42
Tartrate-resistant acid phosphatase, 73
Temporal arteritis (*see* Arteritis)
Teratocarcinoma, **171**
Teratoma, 156, **162**
Testis, 153
   atrophy, **169**

normal, **169**
tumors, 156, **170–171**
Tetracycline hepatotoxicity, 130
Tetralogy of Fallot, 42
Thorotrast, **142**, **143**
Thromboangiitis obliterans, 42
Thrombocythemia, idiopathic, 73
Thrombocytopenia, 68
Thrombocytosis, 68
Thromboembolism, 14
Thrombophlebitis, 42
Thrombosis, 7, **14**
organization of, **44**
Thrombus, 14
Thymoma, **85**
Thymus, normal, **85**
Thyroid gland, 175, **179–182**
adenoma, **181**
carcinoma, 176, **181**, **182**
Graves' disease, 176, 180
nontoxic nodular goiter, 176, **179**
normal, **175**
Thyroiditis, 176, **180**
Thyrotoxicosis (see Graves' disease)
Tissues, 4
Tonsillitis, **85**
Toxoplasmosis, **37**
Transplant
liver, 124, **143**
renal, 99
Transposition of great vessels, 42
Treponema pallidium, **32**, **218**
Trichoepithelioma, 202
Trichomonas, **28**
Tuberculosis, 4, 52, **59**
late progressive, 52
primary, 52
secondary, 52
Tubulointerstitial disease, 90, 99
Tumor, 3, 15
benign, **17**
malignant, **17**

U

Ulcerative colitis, 107, **113**, **114**, 135
Ultrastructure, of cell, 23, **25**
Uric acid, and renal disease, 90, 96
Urinary bladder, 89, 90, 101
calculus, 90
cystitis, 90, **100**
diverticulum, 90
transitional cell carcinoma, 90
Usual interstitial pneumonia (UIP), 52, **56**
Uterus
leiomyoma, **153**, 155, **158**
leiomyosarcoma, 155, **158**

V

Vacuoles, **26**
Vagina, adenocarcinoma, 155, **158**

Valproic acid hepatotoxicity, 130
Valves, **41**
calcification, **43**
cardiac, **41**, 42
vegetations, **43**
Valvular heart disease, 42
aortic stenosis, 42
endocarditis, 42
mitral prolapse, 42
rheumatic, 42
Varices, 107, **108**
Varicose veins, 42
Vascular disease, 42
Vasculitis
central nervous system, 214
hypersensitivity, **47**
Vasoconstriction, 15
Vasodilatation, 15
Vegetations, **43**
Veno-occlusive disease, 124
Ventricular septal defect, 42
Verrucae, 202, **205**
Vesalius, Andreas, 3
Villous atrophy, **111**
Virchow, Rudolph, 1, **5**
Virus, 34
adenovirus, 57
cytomegalovirus, **34**, **139**
Epstein-Barr, 63, 80
hepatitis, 124, 125
herpes, **34**, 158
human papilloma, 62, 159, 172
pox, 204
respiratory syncytial, 57
Vocal polyp, **62**
von Recklinghausen's disease (see Neurofibroma)
Vulva, intraepithelial neoplasia, 155, **158**
Vulvar intraepithelial neoplasia, **158**

W

Waldenstrom's macroglobulinemia, **74**
Wart (see Verrucae)
Warthin's tumor, 107, **119**
Waterhouse-Friderichsen syndrome, 176, **177**
Wegener's granulomatosis, 52, **59**
Wilms' tumor, 90, **100**
Wilson's disease, 124, **133**
"Wire-loop" lesion, in glomerulonephritis, 96
Wound, 12

Y

Yeast (see Fungi)
Yolk sac tumor, 156, **163**

Z

Zahn, lines of, **14**

25 430BR2 181 BR 6060
89   4   1